■ ■ ■

"What an outstanding text you have produced to guide health care practitioners through the maze of disease! When a patient, for whom poly-pharmacy has been ineffective, walks through your door, and the next step is life-altering surgery, what are you going to do? *Case Studies in Integrative and Functional Medicine* is a superb step-by-step guidebook for approaching severe degenerative disease without dogma or fanaticism. Evidenced-based and rational, the text shows how every case is different and no two treatments are the same. What questions to ask, what tests to run, where do you start? Here you'll see case after case, with different protocols but similar outcomes, which equal higher levels of health and fewer indicators of disease. Great job."

*Tom O'Bryan, DC, CCN, DACBN*

■ ■ ■

"The findings of the historical Human Genome Project elucidate why broad-based therapies and cookie-cutter interventions for individual health problems are often unscientific and unsuccessful. Unique genomes with individual biochemistry necessitate assessment of individual biochemistry in order to determine the underlying molecular factors involved in the etiology of illness in each specific case. We are now at a time of metamorphosis in the provision of health services where it is possible to explore the underlying molecular fingerprint and the mechanisms associated with ill health. By zeroing in on the source cause, the practitioner is able to intervene and to correct the abnormalities at a microscopic level that are causing suffering and disease at a macroscopic level. By use of various patient cases, *Case Studies in Integrative and Functional Medicine* provides examples of how biochemical and molecular testing can offer invaluable assistance in directing the practitioner to the source of the problem and the means to the solution of that problem."

*Stephen Genuis, MD, FRCSC, DABOG, DABEM, FAAEM*
*Clinical Professor, Faculty of Medicine, University of Alberta*

■ ■ ■

"Managing the intractable symptoms of chronic illness is a challenge. Often, however, clues to illness and symptoms can be found by taking a practical and integrative approach to health. Such an approach, if done scientifically, is supported by allopathic medicine, but because of the complexities of the health care delivery system, and lack of time and funding, we often fail to look into such options. These cases illustrate a clinician taking the time to ask some very important questions and getting supportive lab data along the way. The anecdotes reported here show the amazing changes that such inquiry can have on the health and well-being of a few patients. The outcomes here certainly should inspire all health care providers to learn more about integrative care and should stimulate further research."

*Lloyd R. Saberski, MD*
*Advanced Diagnostic Pain Treatment Centers*
*Faculty: Department of Medicine, Yale School of Medicine*

■ ■ ■

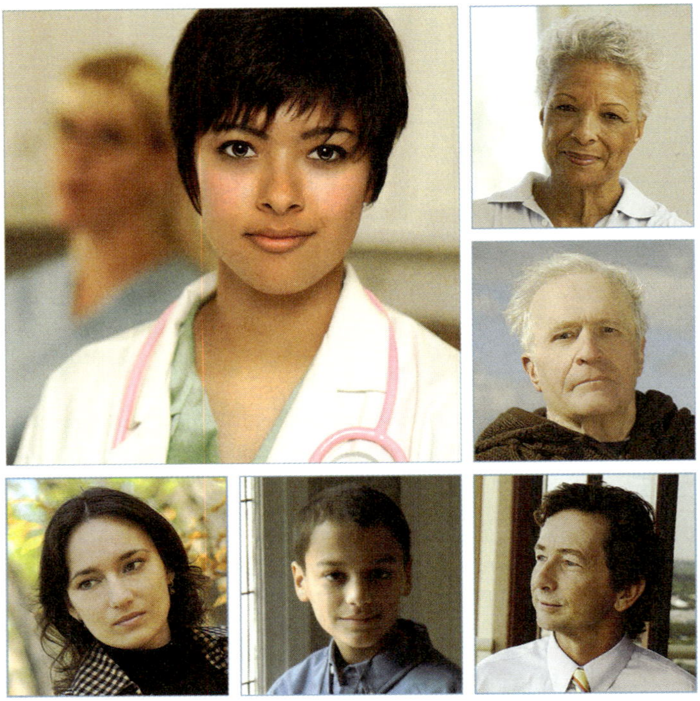

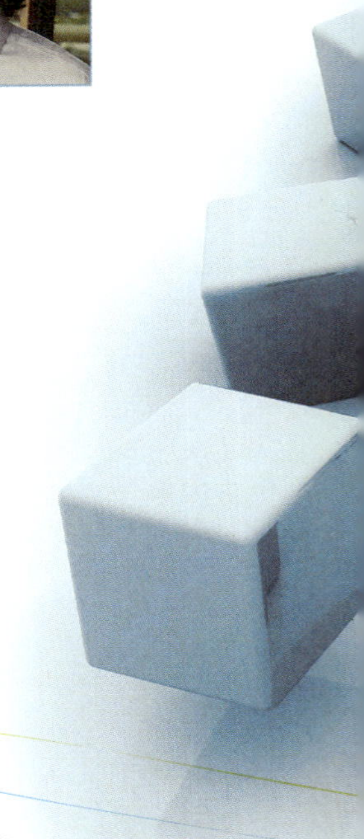

# CASE STUDIES

## in Integrative and Functional Medicine

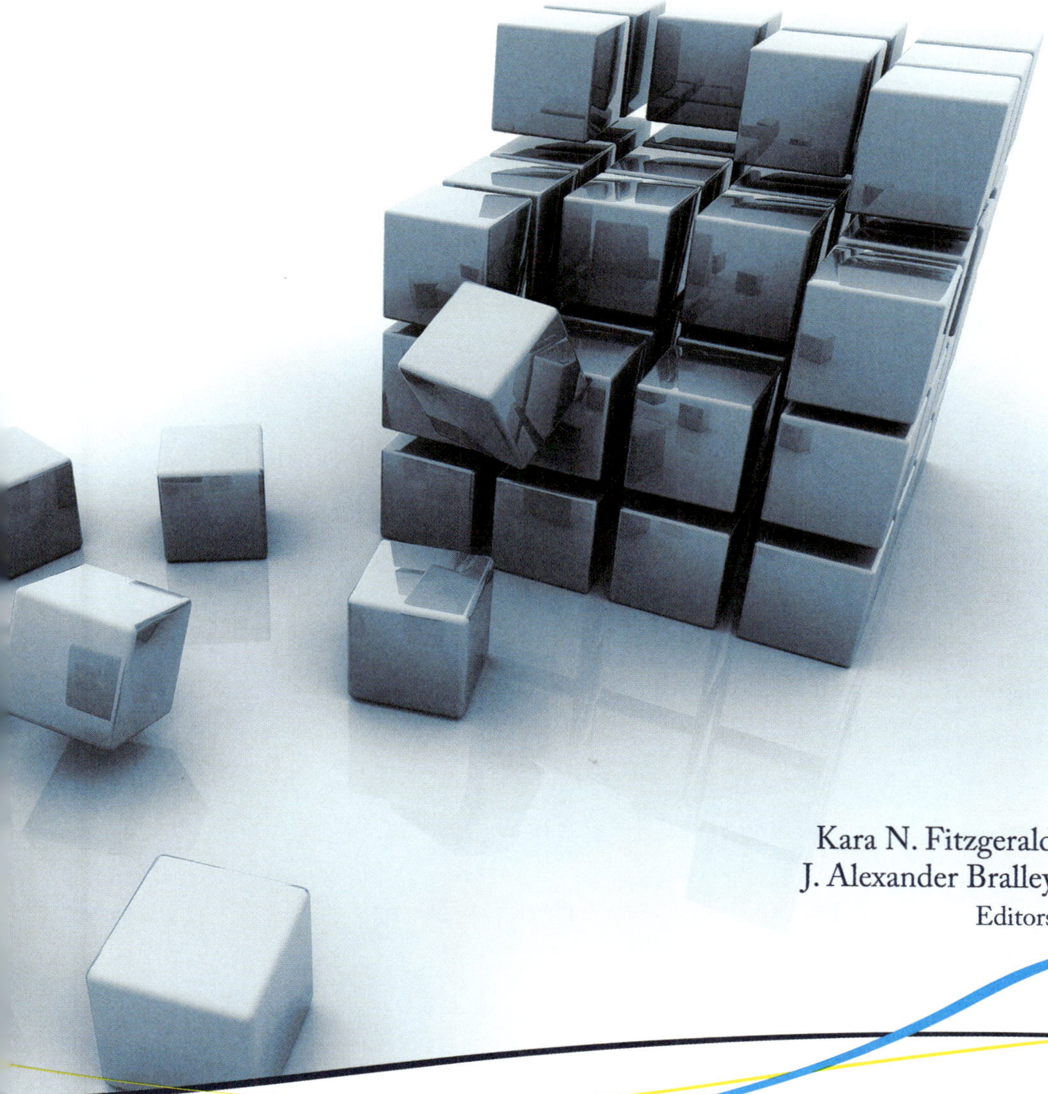

Kara N. Fitzgerald
J. Alexander Bralley
Editors

METAMETRIX INSTITUTE • DULUTH, GEORGIA

**Case Studies in Integrative and Functional Medicine**



**Disclaimer:** Clinical laboratory science and application is a complex and evolving field. No publication can be assumed to encompass the full scope of information that an individual practitioner brings to his or her practice and, therefore, this book is not intended to be used as a clinical manual recommending specific tests and/or treatments for individual patients. It is intended for use as an educational tool, to broaden the knowledge and perspective of the practitioner. It is the responsibility of the healthcare practitioner to make his or her own determination of the usefulness and applicability of any information contained therein. If medical advice is required, the services of a competent professional should be sought. The final decision to engage in any medical treatment should be made jointly by the patient and his or her healthcare practitioner. Neither the publisher, the editors, authors, nor reviewers assume any liability for any errors or omissions or for any injury and/or damage to persons or property arising from the use of information to be found in this publication.

**Library of Congress Cataloging-in-Publication Data**

Case Studies for Integrative and Functional Medicine/Kara N. Fitzgerald and J. Alexander Bralley

Includes bibliographic references

ISBN 978-0-9673949-5-4

I. Kara N. Fitzgerald 1967--. II. J. Alexander Bralley, 1952--.



International Standard Book Number 978-0-9673949-5-4

Printed in USA 10 9 8 7 6 5 4 3 2 1

**Production Team**
Editorial and Project Assistance: Carolyn Bralley, Cathy Morris
Layout and Design: Philip Gómez
Technical and Medical Editor: Sheila Quinn
Printing: ProGraphics Communications • pgc-atl.com

FSC®
www.fsc.org
MIX
From responsible sources
FSC® C010617

# Contents


Foreword . . . . . . . . . . VII

Preface . . . . . . . . . . IX

The Editors . . . . . . . . . . X

Acknowledgments. . . . . . . . . . XI

Introduction . . . . . . . . . . XII

1 **Atopic Disease** **1**

8-Year-Old Male with Atopic Dermatitis . . . . . . . . . . 1

2 **Autoimmune Conditions** **13**

56-Year-Old Male with Psoriatic Arthritis . . . . . . . . . . 13

53-Year-Old Female with Rheumatoid Arthritis and Osteoporosis. . . . . . . . . . 26

3 **Behavioral and Neurodevelopmental Conditions** **47**

2.5-Year-Old Male with Pervasive Developmental Disorder. . . . . . . . . . 47

12-Year-Old Male with Attention Deficit Hyperactivity Disorder . . . . . . . . . . 70

4 **Cardiovascular and Related Conditions** **85**

48-Year-Old Male with Resistant Hypertension on Triple Therapy . . . . . . . . . . 85

57-Year-Old Male with Statin-Induced Myopathy . . . . . . . . . . 95

56-Year-Old Female with Paroxysmal Supraventricular Tachycardia . . . . . . . . . . 101

5 **Endocrine and Metabolic Disorders** **107**

29-Year-Old Female with Adrenal Fatigue . . . . . . . . . . 107

56-Year-Old Female with Type 2 Diabetes Mellitus . . . . . . . . . . 117

6 **Gastrointestinal Disorders** **135**

29-Year-Old Female with Ulcerative Colitis/Pancolitis . . . . . . . . . . 135

38-Year-Old Male with Idiopathic Gastrointestinal Pain . . . . . . . . . . 146

7 **Genetic Diseases** **157**

58-Year-Old Female with Hemochromatosis . . . . . . . . . . 157

2-Year-Old Male with Mitochondrial Disease . . . . . . . . . . 163

8 **Neurodegenerative Diseases** 173

50-Year-Old Male with Amyotrophic Lateral Sclerosis . . . . . 173

9 **Neuropsychiatric and Neuroinflammatory Conditions** 181

40-Year-Old Female with Migraine Headaches and Depression . . . . . 181

66-Year-Old Male with Depression and Sarcoidosis . . . . . 194

10 **Respiratory Disorders** 203

54-Year-Old Female with Chronic Asthma . . . . . 203

11 **Toxic Exposures** 211

16-Year-Old Female with Neurologic Effects of Lead Toxicity . . . . . 211

43-Year-Old Male with Volatile Solvent-Induced Neurotoxicity . . . . . 217

**Appendix A** 231

Introduction to the Functional Medicine Matrix . . . . . 231

Case at a Glance: Migraine and Depression . . . . . 232

Case at a Glance: ADHD . . . . . 234

Case at a Glance: Psoriatic Arthritis . . . . . 236

Case at a Glance: Volatile Solvent-Induced Neurotoxicity . . . . . 238

**Appendix B** 241

Table B1. Select Laboratory Imbalances and Clinical Conditions . . . . . 241

**Appendix C** 243

Web-based Medical and Scientific Resources . . . . . 243

**Appendix D** 245

Select Supplement Companies . . . . . 245

Select Compounding Pharmacies . . . . . 248

Select Distribution Companies . . . . . 248

Quality Assurance Analysis of Nutritional Products . . . . . 248

**Appendix E** 249

Common Abbreviations . . . . . 249

# Foreword

*Case Studies in Integrative and Functional Medicine* may prove to be one of the most important publications about functional medicine currently available. During the last decade, significant textbooks about functional medicine have been published. Initially, functional medicine practitioners celebrated the arrival of *Clinical Nutrition: A Functional Approach* published by the Institute for Functional Medicine (IFM). This important textbook was followed by the first edition of *Laboratory Evaluations for Integrative and Functional Medicine,* published by the Metametrix Institute. In 2005, the comprehensive *Textbook of Functional Medicine* (IFM) provided the evidence and concepts behind the robust architecture and disciplined methodology of functional medicine—a systems approach that addresses what must become the primary challenge of 21st-century medicine: improving prevention and treatment outcomes for complex chronic illness. Together, these textbooks define an effective, systems-based and clinically-relevant approach to achieving this urgent goal.

Health care in the industrialized world relies primarily on the 20th-century, acute-care medical model, which is characterized by rapid differential diagnosis aimed at prescribing a drug (or procedure) that will ameliorate the patient's presenting symptoms and avert the immediate threat.[1] This model evolved in response to the primary causes of morbidity and mortality in the last century: acute infections and trauma. The experts in this model are the various organ-system specialists, including cardiologists, pulmonologists, endocrinologists, neurologists, orthopedic surgeons and many others. Inherently, this approach to care minimizes the involvement of the patient, who functions mostly as a passive recipient of a procedure or prescription.[2] It is not a model that reimburses the practitioner for looking into the origins of the patient's illness(es) or for determining whether those illnesses can be ameliorated by understanding original causes and developing treatments to re-establish homeostatic balance. Instead, it prioritizes immediate solutions to the most pressing problems,[3] an approach that is absolutely essential in emergency and hospital-based care. Unfortunately, difficulties arise when this model is applied to ongoing community-based care for the non-acute chronic conditions that represent 80% of the daily work of present-day clinicians.[4]

*Case Studies in Integrative and Functional Medicine* vividly illustrates, in comprehensive detail, the shift that will be required to transform 21st-century medicine into patient-centered, personalized, systems-based medicine. A core principle of functional medicine maintains that diagnosis is just the starting point for clinical care, not the last step before procedural or prescriptive interventions. *Clinical decision making,* particularly in the context of chronic complex illnesses with multiple comorbidities, requires a commitment to explore the scientific evidence, a willingness to allow that evidence to be tempered by knowledge and judgment derived from clinical experience, and dedication to creating a real partnership *with* the patient. *Effective clinical decision making* drills deeply into the "why" of every diagnosis, pursuing an understanding of each patient's unique terrain, influenced by genetics, environmental exposures and lifestyle patterns.

This textbook presents difficult clinical cases from the medical practices of highly skilled clinicians who understand how to achieve more satisfying outcomes through a robust, integrated, functional clinical assessment and treatment program. In the appendix, you will find selected case studies that illustrate the use of the *Functional Medicine Matrix Model* for evaluation and treatment.

Moving from conventional poly-pharmacy and procedure-based interventions into the robust approaches afforded by 21st-century breakthroughs in personalized medicine and systems biology *re-enchants and illuminates* the practice of clinical medicine. The blending of the foundational sciences of genomics (unique genes in a unique environment) with the intellectual architecture of functional medicine in a systems-based model will help each clinician create a more comprehensive portfolio of clinical services. The case studies in this volume illustrate how skills learned through rigorous training in functional medicine can successfully bring to the therapeutic relationship real patient-centered answers for chronic complex illnesses.

A powerful motivator for changes in our behavior as physicians is listening attentively to compelling stories brought to the clinic by our patients—stories that illustrate the terrible cost of living with chronic pain and functional disability. The intense satisfaction of finally resolving a patient's unanswered questions by applying a different lens for evaluation and assessment is transformative. Functional, integrative, systems medicine provides such a lens, and the stories in this book are both evocative and educational. This is why *Case Studies in Integrative and Functional Medicine* will prove to be a most important publication about functional and integrative medicine. I hope you enjoy the exploration of a new approach to clinical decision making, as exemplified by these case studies, as much as I have.

David S. Jones, MD
President of and Director of Medical Education, IFM

## References

1 Ely JW, Osheroff JA, Gorman PN, et al. A taxonomy of generic clinical questions: classification study. *BMJ. 2000;321:429-32.*

2 Holman H. Chronic disease—The need for a new clinical education. *JAMA. 2004;292(9):1057-1059.*

3 American College of Physicians. The Impending Collapse of Primary Care Medicine and its Implications for the State of the Nation's Health Care: A Report from the American College of Physicians. January 30, 2006.

4 Holman H. Chronic disease—The need for a new clinical education. *JAMA. 2004;292(9):1057-1059.*

# Preface

*Case Studies in Integrative and Functional Medicine* is a clinical reference for physicians and health professionals and a teaching tool for medical students and those in related disciplines who are interested in the practice of integrative and functional medicine. It also serves as a contribution to the field, citing the best-available research and open to examination by scientists and clinicians. As an Institutional Review Board and HIPAA compliant collection of case studies, the book is a first step in research, providing clinical reports of the efficacy of the approach for many conditions, while identifying questions in need of further investigation.

This book is the companion volume to the reference textbook, *Laboratory Evaluations for Integrative and Functional Medicine*, which provides the scientific rationale behind the laboratory tests used in these cases. For instance, in the case of the 66-year-old male with depression and sarcoidosis, a central finding is a high urinary level of quinolinic acid, a potent neuroinflammatory compound. A detailed discussion of the compound and its metabolic effects, exceeding the scope of the *Case Studies* book, may be found in the reference textbook. An additional companion text, the *Metametrix Handbook,* is a list-format reference designed for clinical practice that includes a brief overview of the laboratory analyte of concern, causes of imbalances and treatment considerations.

The cases here presented range in complexity from a multisystem analysis involving a 2.5-year-old male with autism to the straightforward case of a 54-year-old female with chronic asthma in need of essential fatty acids. We believe the difference in complexity reflects what we see in clinical practice and demonstrates that clinicians at every level of experience in functional medicine may readily incorporate integrative treatments and laboratory evaluations in practice.

The assessment and treatments used in the cases reflect the clinician's own judgment. In some instances, details determined to be less pertinent to the case as a whole were omitted. Also, we occasionally chose to narrow the focus of a case to a few key points of interest, such as the use of fatty acids in the 50-year-old male with amyotrophic lateral sclerosis, or the mitochondrial lesions noted in a 57-year-old male with statin-induced myopathy.

The process of narrowing our choices to the final 20 cases from those submitted was daunting. We realize that *Case Studies in Integrative and Functional Medicine* is, in fact, just a beginning; our intention is to host a growing web-based library of case studies and discussion for clinicians worldwide. The library will be available to all clinicians and researchers interested in depositing new cases, participating in discussion or accessing the database for educational and research purposes. We invite you to visit www.metametrix.com/casestudies for information on this and other educational projects sponsored by Metametrix Institute.

Kara Fitzgerald, ND

# The Editors

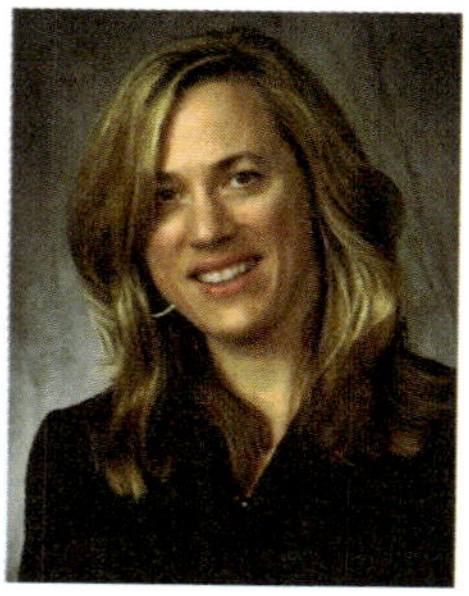

**Kara Fitzgerald, ND,** received her doctorate of naturopathic medicine from National College of Natural Medicine in Portland, Oregon. She completed the first CNME-accredited post-doctoral position in nutritional biochemistry and laboratory science at Metametrix Clinical Laboratory and a residency at Progressive Medical Center, a large, integrative medical practice in Atlanta, Georgia. Dr. Fitzgerald is a contributing author to *Laboratory Evaluations for Integrative and Functional Medicine* and the Institute for Functional Medicine's *Textbook of Functional Medicine.* Dr. Fitzgerald is an adjunct faculty and Curriculum Advisory Committee member at the Institute for Functional Medicine. She lectures internationally on the clinical application of functional laboratory interpretation for several organizations, including Metametrix. She maintains a clinical practice focused on complex chronic conditions at Advanced Diagnostic at Yale-New Haven at Long Wharf, in New Haven, Connecticut.

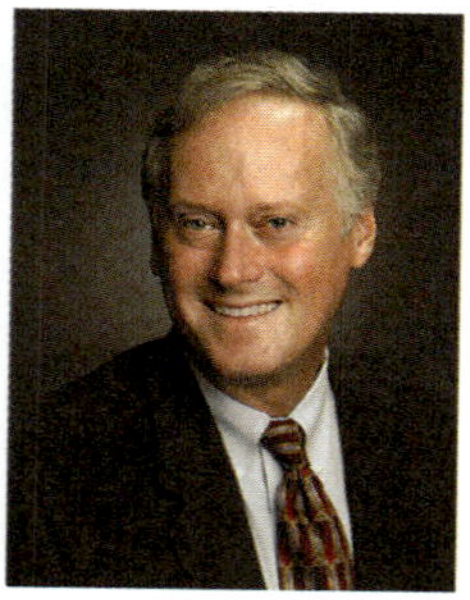

**J. Alexander Bralley, PhD,** Founder and CEO of Metametrix Clinical Laboratory, received his B.S. in biology from the University of Illinois in 1975 and his Ph.D. in medical sciences, specializing in neuroscience, from the University of Florida College of Medicine in 1980. He has worked and published in the area of nutritional biochemistry since then. For the past 26 years, he has been CEO and Laboratory Director of Metametrix Clinical Laboratory in Atlanta, Georgia, an internationally recognized clinical laboratory specializing in nutritional, metabolic, toxicologic and stool microbiome testing. He has been instrumental in developing testing and interpretation guidelines for innovative nutritional and metabolic analyses. Dr. Bralley has extensive experience in the use of nutritional therapies to treat chronic illnesses through consulting with physicians, reviewing the medical literature, and attending and speaking at conferences, where he is widely sought after to lecture on the use of laboratory testing to define nutrient needs for individuals. He is a member of several professional organizations for nutrition and clinical laboratory science. He is on the editorial review boards for *Alternative Medicine Review, the Journal of Applied Nutrition,* and *Integrative Medicine: A Clinicians Journal.* Dr. Bralley's ongoing research interests lie in examining the relationship between nutritional, metabolic, and toxic factors, how they affect chronic disease processes and influence health.

# Acknowledgments


## Clinician Contributors

- John Cline, MD
- Kara Fitzgerald, ND
- Cathryn Harbor, MD
- Mark Hyman, MD – Chairman, Institute for Functional Medicine
- Kathleen Janel, ND
- Stephanie Kaplan, ND
- Kathy Keipura, MD
- Todd LePine, MD
- Alane Palmer
- Kathleen Power, DC
- Adrienne Sprouse, MD
- Kathie Swift, MS, RD
- Stephanie Tuss

## Additional Contributors

- Editors
  - Kara Fitzgerald, ND
  - J. Alexander Bralley, PhD
  - Sheila Quinn
- Reviewers
  - Carolyn Bralley, MS
  - Jim Kirby
  - Todd LePine, MD
  - Rachel Marynowski, ND
  - Elizabeth Redmond, PhD
- Writers
  - Christie Egeston, MS
  - Kara Fitzgerald, ND
  - Cass Nelson-Dooley, MS
  - Terry Pollock, MS
  - Elizabeth Redmond, PhD
- Editorial assistance
  - Stephanie W. Kissel
  - Cathy Morris
- Book design and layout
  - Philip Gómez
- Laboratory graphics
  - Sue Kelly
- Acknowledgements
  - Eve Bralley, PhD
  - Winston Cardwell, ND
  - Martha R. Herbert, MD, PhD
  - Richard Lord, PhD

# Introduction

Functional medicine is fundamentally aligned with systems medicine. Systems medicine evolved out of the recognition that mapping the human genome would not provide the one gene/one disease answer that was anticipated. Rather, a radically more complex and elegant understanding emerged from the Genome Project, demonstrating that multiple, subtle mutations, or single nucleotide polymorphisms, could become pertinent in the face of certain lifestyle habits, nutrient insufficiencies, toxicant exposures, or psychosocial stressors, resulting in the chronic diseases we see today. Thus, the understanding that many modifiable factors inform an individual's disease risk was a central conclusion of the Human Genome Project, and from it, systems medicine was born.

Systems medicine suggests that other "omes" are as significant as our genome. That is: our epigenome, or the variables "above the gene" such as methylation or acetylation that impact DNA protein expression; the metabolome, which describes the metabolic end products generated by the genome; the proteome, which is specific to the proteins produced at the direction of nucleic acids; the human microbiome, which describes the microbial DNA belonging to the organisms that share residence with us; the nutrigenome, or how our nutrient intake impacts genetic/epigenetic expression; and finally, the exposome. The latter term describes the totality of an individual's environmental exposures from the prenatal period onward and how they impact genetic/epigenetic expression and disease risk.

As is suggested in systems medicine, optimal nutrition, the level of nutrient intake that maintains the best possible health, is highly variable from person to person[1] and is based on a combination of "omic" impacts. These recent concepts confirm the biochemical individuality and the genetotrophic theory of disease, first described by Roger Williams, the discoverer of pantothenic acid (vitamin $B_5$). Thus, each patient's biochemical individuality exerts a major influence on this emergent model of human health and the development of integrative, functional medicine. Their individuality influences not only the individual need for nutrients, but also the clinical presentation of nutrient insufficiency.[2] Although these concepts have been recognized for centuries, they are only recently gaining recognition in the current medical model as a result of the Genome Project.

The cases in CSIFM reflect Williams' observation and systems medicine concepts: On one hand, the laboratory data and clinical history suggest that similar clinical presentations may include very different underlying imbalances and disease triggers, as seen in the two autoimmune cases (rheumatoid arthritis and psoriatic arthritis) and the depression cases (sarcoidosis and depression; migraine and depression). On the other hand, as the table in *Appendix B* illustrates, individuals with very different clinical presentation may share similar underlying eitiopathogenic factors. For example, many cases share food-specific IgG antibodies and intestinal hyperpermeability as key imbalances, including atopic dermatitis, parasitic gastroenteritis and pervasive developmental disorder. Organic acid imbalances suggestive of mitochondropathy are also a common finding in different clinical conditions.

Thus, lifestyle choices and environmental exposures filtered through genetic predisposition are fundamental factors in the expression of disease, and a successful treatment approach must include an investigation of these factors. Data capturing at this level of complexity requires organization. An effective system of organization has been created by the Institute of Functional Medicine (IFM). *Appendix A* includes an overview of the IFM approach and demonstrates the use of the Functional Medicine Matrix in four cases.

## Reference Interval and Quintile Ranking

Many of the laboratory tests used in these cases use a quintile ranking in addition to the standard 95% reference interval, because the quintile ranking may allow for earlier identification of imbalances, (increased sensitivity) thereby providing more meaningful information for treatment. See Figure 1 below.

## 95% Reference Interval

A laboratory reference interval allows the clinician to make a decision regarding the patient's level of health. Traditionally, the test result would indicate either the presence or absence of a disease regarding its own accuracy, precision, sensitivity, and specificity (refer to Basic Concepts in LEIFM for a discussion). In integrative and functional medicine, this becomes a more difficult decision to make, since many of the chronic illnesses treated in this type of medicine are not clearly defined diseases. Rather, the analysis of nutrient and metabolic compounds indicates levels of insufficiency or imbalance that can relate to health issues.

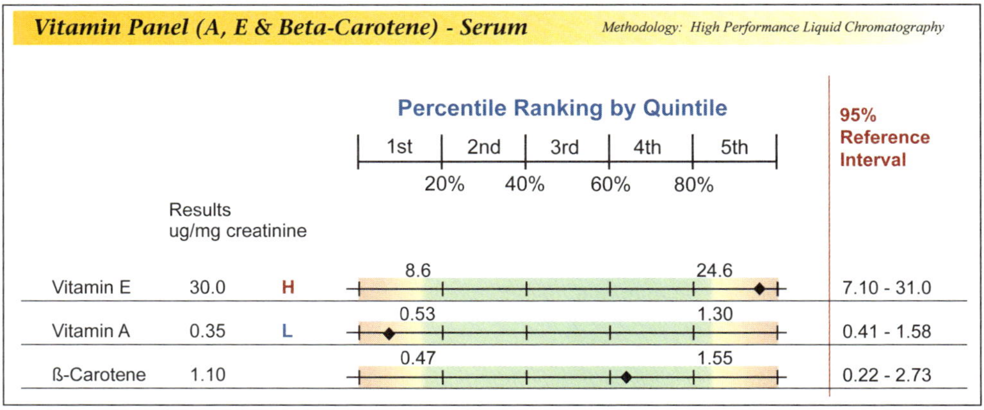


**Figure 1. An Example of Quintile and 95% Reference Interval Layout For Serum Vitamins.** Each result is printed with units displayed above the column and abnormality flags (H or L) are printed to the right of the quantitative value. Charts show the position of the result relative to quintiles (hash marks) that are further sub-divided into deciles of the reference population. Abnormality is indicated when results fall below the 1st or above the 9th decile. To the far right the broader 95% reference interval is displayed for examination of more extreme abnormalities.

Typically, an analyte in clinical chemistry is referenced by looking at population distributions of the test result, preferably in healthy individuals. For tests developed within a laboratory, the lab will usually draw from its database of test results over a period of time. The normal range is defined as that population within two standard deviations of the mean. In a normally distributed population, this would be 95% of the population, or the 95% reference or confidence interval. By definition, therefore, 5% of people tested would be abnormal.

Clearly, this is not the most useful way of evaluating whether a person may have marginal nutritional deficiencies. Take the example of magnesium: A recent government study showed 68% of Americans consumed less than the recommended daily allowance (RDA) for magnesium, and 19% consumed less than 50% of the RDA.[3] This would indicate that a large percentage of Americans are magnesium deficient. What, then, would be a useful reference interval for a clinician who wants to determine if their patient is magnesium deficient? Certainly, the typical two standard deviations from the mean would be relatively useless, since far more than 5% of the population should be magnesium insufficient.

# Quintile Ranking

A more reasoned approach is percentile ranking of the result. This has been particularly useful in assessing the measures of risk factors for certain disease states. High-sensitivity C-reactive protein (hs-CRP) measurements have been developed in this way to relate levels to risk of cardiovascular disease. By dividing the populations tested into quintile ranks, researchers were able to correlate risk of cardiovascular events with these rankings.[4] Those individuals falling in the highest or fifth quintile demonstrated significantly higher risk of cardiovascular events than those in the lowest quintile. In this way, hs-CRP has been shown to be a strong predictor of risk.

A similar approach can be taken with other analytes, whether nutrients, metabolites or toxic compounds. By arranging the test data by quintile, the clinician can easily determine where a patient falls relative to a population from which the reference data were obtained. This allows the clinician to more easily assess the significance of the finding, particularly as he gains experience using the test with patients.

## References

1. Ames BN, Elson-Schwab I, Silver EA. High-dose vitamin therapy stimulates variant enzymes with decreased coenzyme binding affinity (increased K(m)): relevance to genetic disease and polymorphisms. *The American journal of clinical nutrition.* Apr 2002;75(4):616-658.
2. Velazquez A. Biotin deficiency in protein-energy malnutrition: implications for nutritional homeostasis and individuality. *Nutrition (Burbank, Los Angeles County, Calif.* 1997;13(11-12):991-992.
3. King DE, Mainous AG, 3rd, Geesey ME, Woolson RF. Dietary magnesium and C-reactive protein levels. *Journal of the American College of Nutrition.* Jun 2005;24(3):166-171.
4. Rifai N, Ridker PM. High-sensitivity C-reactive protein: a novel and promising marker of coronary heart disease. *Clinical chemistry.* Mar 2001;47(3):403-411.

# 1 Atopic Disease

## Atopy

*Atopic disease (atopy) is defined as an allergic reaction for which there is a genetic predisposition. Atopic dermatitis (AD), asthma, allergic rhinitis (hay fever) and IgE-mediated gastroenteropathies all fall under the atopic designation if there is a pattern of inheritance. Interestingly, hay fever was not recognized until 1819. By 1875, hay fever had reached epidemic proportions, and was specifically attributed to urbanization. Thus, genetic, environmental and epigenetic (modification to the chromosome without changing DNA sequence) factors all play key roles in atopy, with the latter two factors possibly being stronger variables.[1, 2] Environmental factors involved in the pathogenesis of atopy include early exposure to antibiotics, vaccines and pollution, as well as excessive hygiene and antigens, such as viral infections and foods, including wheat, dairy and eggs.[3-6]*

*Atopy is epidemic in developed nations and is increasingly prevalent in developing nations. Indeed, research suggests that 80% of infants born with AD (20%), will go on to develop hay fever, asthma or allergy by age three.[8] In the US, direct and indirect costs of AD amount to an estimated 12 billion dollars annually.*

### 8-Year-Old Male with Atopic Dermatitis

| | |
|---|---|
| **Additional Symptoms and Conditions** | Severe, unremitting, atopic dermatitis covering face and upper and lower extremities. Secondary bacterial infections common. |
| **Medications** | Methotrexate, tacrolimus (Protopic®), hydrocortisone butyrate (Locoid®) pimecrolimus (Elidel®), triamcinolone, cetirizine (Zyrtec®),diphenhydramine (Benadryl®), Cetaphil, Eucerin. Multiple oral, IV and topical antibiotics. Medications were ineffective in controlling dermatitis this case. |
| **Tests Used** | Food specific IgG4 and IgE antibody panels, celiac panel, and serum vitamin D |
| **Imbalances Identified** | Moderate to high IgE antibody response to 29 foods; moderate to severe IgG4 antibody response to egg and dairy. IgA deficiency. |
| **Treatments** | Elimination and rotation diet, probiotics, essential and non-essential fatty acids, gastrointestinal medicinal food, zinc. |
| **Outcome** | Resolution of atopic dermatitis, although occasional flare-ups upon exposure to main antigenic foods (cow's dairy and egg) were noted. |

*Table continues on following page...*

## 8-Year-Old Male with Atopic Dermatitis

**Discussion/ Significance**

The 8-year-old male in this case suffered from severe, unremitting atopic dermatitis on his face and extremities. Embarrassment about his condition led to significant social anxiety. Potent immunosuppressive therapies , including corticosteroids and methotrexate, were not successful in mitigating the dermatitis. IgE and IgG4 antibody testing revealed a high number of severe reactions to commonly consumed foods, suggesting intestinal hyperpermeability. After twelve weeks of treatment designed to address intestinal hyperpermeability and dampen the allergic response, the AD resolved. One and one half years later, the child remained free of dermatitis, as long as cow's dairy and egg were avoided. Follow-up testing demonstrated improvement in IgE food-specific antibodies. IgG4 antibodies to egg and cow's dairy remained elevated, and may have been associated with the development of dermatitis upon ingestion of those foods, which occurred on occasion. Although it was virtually unknown in the 19th century, atopy is epidemic in the US and in most Western countries, and it is on the rise in developing nations. Clearly a product of environmental exposures, it results in an imbalance in gastrointestinal microbiota filtered through a vulnerable genetic and epigenetic predisposition. In this case, identifying and removing the main trigger foods led to a full resolution of atopy. Given the 12-billion dollar per year price tag of AD and the incidence of poor outcomes, further research into the safe, cost-effective approach used in this case is warranted.[9]

# CASE HISTORY

DE was 8 years old when he presented with severe atopic dermatitis (AD) characterized by pruritic, excoriated and scaly lesions on his face, including eye lids, and on the flexor surfaces of the feet, legs and arms, as well as on wrists and hands. Vesicles, exudates, and crusting were common findings. He was frequently on antibiotics for *Streptococcus* infections and required multiple hospital stays for intravenous antibiotic and steroidal treatments. He stated that his skin was very itchy, and that he scratched it often, sometimes waking up at night to do so. The medications he tried over time without significant effect included: triamcinolone, methotrexate, tacrolimus, hydrocortisone, pimecrolimus, cetirizine, and diphenhydramine. He also tried oatmeal baths, Cetaphil, Eucerin, again without benefit. DE was very embarrassed by his appearance and had few friends because of it. He refused to participate in summer camp or attend public school. His mother therefore enrolled him in private school. She stated that she "had flown him to doctors all over the country" without any apparent benefit. A previous skin-prick test demonstrated allergies to dust mites, pecans, and eggs. However, DE did not avoid those allergens. Rather, he ate a typical standard American diet (SAD) full of processed foods. DE's father had chronic, mild AD. No one else in the family had any atopic presentation. The mother pleaded at the first office visit to "please help my child."

> Atopy is epidemic in developed nations and is increasingly prevalent in developing nations. Interestingly, genetic, environmental and epigenetic factors all play key roles in atopy, with the latter two factors possibly being stronger variables given the rapid rise in its incidence.

# Initial Laboratory Results

**Laboratory tests ordered and rationale:**

1. **IgE food antibody testing**: Specific IgE antibody elevation characterizes atopy. IgE reaction to foods, particularly milk, egg, wheat, soy, and peanut, accounts for 75% of the cases of food-induced AD.[10]
2. **Food-specific IgG4 antibody testing**: IgG4 is considered an IgE blocking antibody. Its elevation might be associated with a reduced IgE response and might therefore be part of immune tolerance.[11] However, IgG4 antibody/antigen complexes might elicit an immune response and be associated with delayed type hypersensitivity reactions.
3. **Celiac panel**: Atopy has been associated with increased incidence of celiac disease.
4. **Serum vitamin D**: Hypovitaminosis D has been associated with atopic dermatitis.[12] However, DE's serum D level was normal.

**0077 IgE Food Antibody Assay (30 Antigens)** *Methodology: EIA*

| | Results (units) | Class | Response |
|---|---|---|---|
| Almond | 613 | +3 | High |
| Aspergillus | 170 | +2 | Moderate |
| Beef | 201 | +2 | Moderate |
| Cantaloupe | 552 | +3 | High |
| Cashew | 140 | +2 | Moderate |
| Chicken | 182 | +2 | Moderate |
| Corn | 200 | +2 | Moderate |
| Crab | 196 | +2 | Moderate |
| Egg, Whole | 1528 | +4 | Very High |
| Garlic | 851 | +4 | Very High |
| Lobster | 182 | +2 | Moderate |
| Milk | 1538 | +4 | Very High |
| Mustard | 370 | +3 | High |
| Oat | 586 | +3 | High |
| Orange | 151 | +2 | Moderate |
| Pea, Green | 205 | +2 | Moderate |
| Peanut | 1113 | +4 | Very High |
| Pinto Bean | 699 | +3 | High |
| Pork | 842 | +4 | Very High |
| Rice | 411 | +3 | High |
| Salmon | 1051 | +4 | Very High |
| Shrimp | 199 | +2 | Moderate |
| Soybean | 689 | +3 | High |
| Strawberry | 200 | +2 | Moderate |
| Sunflower | 65 | +1 | Mild |
| Tomato | 205 | +2 | Moderate |
| Tuna | 179 | +2 | Moderate |
| Turkey | 196 | +2 | Moderate |
| Walnut | 379 | +3 | High |
| Wheat | 187 | +2 | Moderate |

| Reference Ranges: (units) | | | | |
|---|---|---|---|---|
| | Class 0 | < 24 | Class 3 | 210 - 701 |
| | Class 0/1 | 24 - 45 | Class 4 | 702 - 3984 |
| | Class 1 | 46 - 87 | Class 5 | > 3984 |
| | Class 2 | 88 - 209 | | |

**Figure 1. IgE food antibody assay.** DE showed specific IgE antibodies to every food on the profile. Many antibody levels were moderate to very high.

**0270 IgG4 Food Antibodies (90 Antigens)** *Methodology: ELISA*

| | Results ng/mL | Response | Class |
|---|---|---|---|
| **Dairy/Meat/Poultry** | | | |
| Beef | <10 | | |
| Casein | >2000 | Severe | +5 |
| Chicken | <10 | | |
| Egg, White | 777 | Mod | +4 |
| Egg, Yolk | 521 | Mod | +4 |
| Lamb | <10 | | |
| Milk | >2000 | Severe | +5 |
| Pork | <10 | | |
| Turkey | <10 | | |
| **Fish/Shellfish** | | | |
| Clam | <10 | | |
| Codfish | <10 | | |
| Crab | <10 | | |
| Flounder | <10 | | |
| Halibut | <10 | | |
| Lobster | <10 | | |
| Mackerel | <10 | | |
| Oyster | <10 | | |
| Salmon | <10 | | |
| Shrimp | <10 | | |
| Trout | <10 | | |
| Tuna | <10 | | |
| **Fruits** | | | |
| Apple | <10 | | |

| | Results ng/mL | Response | Class |
|---|---|---|---|
| Apricot | <10 | | |
| Banana | <10 | | |
| Blueberry | <10 | | |
| Cantaloupe | <10 | | |
| Cranberry | <10 | | |
| Grape | <10 | | |
| Grapefruit | <10 | | |
| Honeydew | <10 | | |
| Lemon | <10 | | |
| Orange | 14 | | |
| Peach | <10 | | |
| Pear | <10 | | |
| Pineapple | <10 | | |
| Strawberry | <10 | | |
| Watermelon | <10 | | |
| **Grains** | | | |
| Barley | <10 | | |
| Corn | <10 | | |
| Oat | <10 | | |
| Rice | <10 | | |
| Rye | <10 | | |
| Wheat | 65 | Mild | +1 |
| **Legumes** | | | |
| Bean, String | 9 | | |
| Lentil | <10 | | |

**0270 IgG4 Food Antibodies (90 Antigens)** *Methodology: ELISA*

| | | | |
|---|---|---|---|
| Lima Bean | <10 | | |
| Navy Bean | <10 | | |
| Pea, Green | <10 | | |
| Peanut | 477 | Mod | +3 |
| Pinto Bean | 8 | | |
| Soybean | 58 | Mild | +1 |
| **Miscellaneous** | | | |
| Aspergillus | <10 | | |
| Black Pepper | <10 | | |
| Chocolate | <10 | | |
| Cinnamon | <10 | | |
| Coffee | <10 | | |
| Ginger | <10 | | |
| Malt | 9 | | |
| Tea | <10 | | |
| Vanilla | <10 | | |
| Yeast, Baker's | <10 | | |
| Yeast, Brewer's | <10 | | |
| **Nuts/Seeds** | | | |
| Almond | 29 | | |
| Cashew | <10 | | |
| Coconut | <10 | | |
| Pecan | <10 | | |
| Pistachio | <10 | | |
| Sesame | <10 | | |
| Sunflower | <10 | | |
| Walnut | <10 | | |

| | | | |
|---|---|---|---|
| **Vegetables** | | | |
| Asparagus | <10 | | |
| Avocado | <10 | | |
| Broccoli | <10 | | |
| Cabbage | <10 | | |
| Carrot | <10 | | |
| Cauliflower | 43 | Mild | +1 |
| Celery | <10 | | |
| Cucumber | <10 | | |
| Garlic | <10 | | |
| Lettuce | <10 | | |
| Mushroom | <10 | | |
| Mustard | <10 | | |
| Olive | <10 | | |
| Onion | <10 | | |
| Pepper, Green | <10 | | |
| Potato | <10 | | |
| Spinach | 25 | | |
| Sweet Potato | <10 | | |
| Tomato | <10 | | |
| Zucchini | <10 | | |

**Class Definitions:**

| Class | Cutoffs |
|---|---|
| Negative | 0-40 |
| Mild (+1/+2) | 80/150 |
| Moderate (+3/+4) | 500/900 |
| Severe (+5) | > 900 |

**Figure 2. Food-specific IgG4 antibodies.** DE had a number of mild, moderate, and severe IgG4 food antibodies in serum.

**0078 Celiac Panel** *Methodology: Immunoturbidimetric, ELISA*

| | Results | | |
|---|---|---|---|
| Total Immunoglobulin A | 71 L | | 104 - 522 mg/dL |
| Anti-Gliadin IgA II | <6 | Negative | |
| Transglutaminase antibody (IgA) | 6 | Negative | |

| | | |
|---|---|---|
| Negative | < 20 | Units |
| Weak Positive | 20 - 30 | |
| Moderate to Strong Positive | > 30 | |

**Figure 3. Celiac panel.** Low serum IgA levels were identified, compromising the validity of the negative celiac antibody findings.

# Initial Assessment

- Atopic dermatitis
- Intestinal hyperpermeability
- Multiple elevated IgE and IgG4 food antibodies
- IgA deficiency

# Initial Plan

- Diet: remove all foods with +2 IgG4 and IgE antibody levels or greater and rotate dietary substitutions (e.g., deer, bison, quail, pheasant) once every four days. Follow plan for 12 weeks.
- GI healing formula containing bovine serum-derived immunoglobulins, beneficial growth factors, and L-glutamine, 1 scoop daily
- Combination omega-6 and omega-3 fatty acids including flax, evening primrose oils, 1 tablespoon PO BID
- Zinc citrate 10 mg, 1 capsule PO QD
- Lactobacillus species probiotic 20 billion CFU, 2 capsules PO QD
- Include organic canola and olive oil in diet
- Apply topical olive oil to skin daily

**Treatment plan rationale:** Elimination of highly reactive foods is standard practice, and strict adherence to this regimen for a period of time may be required for resolution of symptoms. In this case, while very challenging to implement, it was deemed necessary by the clinician that DE not eat any foods associated with a +2 reaction or greater for 12 weeks. Thus, for a time, DE's diet was markedly limited. Concurrently, he was given a GI medicinal food containing bovine immunoglobulins, glutamine and zinc. In animal trials, supplementation with oral immunoglobulins has been shown to reduce inflammation and improve intestinal hyperpermeability and humoral immunity in the GI tract.[13-15] Zinc and glutamine have both been demonstrated to improve intestinal hyperpermeability.[16, 17] Flax and evening primrose oils, both effective in treating atopy,[18-20] were also used. Microbiota imbalance, strongly implicated in atopy and a likely factor in this case, given the history of chronic antibiotic use, was addressed with a lactobacillus species probiotic formula.[3] It was suggested that DE increase olive and canola oil in his diet, presumably to assist with providing sufficient lipids for skin health and cell regeneration.

## Six-Week Follow-up

Within 6 weeks after starting the treatment protocol, DE's skin was healing and there was no sign of infection. He did not require antibiotics between visits—unusual for him. DE was instructed to continue to follow the treatment plan as directed.

## Twelve-Week Follow-up

DE's skin showed remarkable improvement. The lesions were healing, and no new ones were forming. Follow-up IgE and IgG4 food antibody profiles were ordered after 12 weeks of treatment.

### Twelve-Week Follow-up Laboratory Results

**0077 IgE Food Antibody Assay (30 Antigens)** *Methodology: EIA*

| | Results (units) | Class | Response |
|---|---|---|---|
| Almond | 21 | | |
| Aspergillus | 11 | | |
| Beef | 15 | | |
| Cantaloupe | 22 | | |
| Cashew | 1 | | |
| Chicken | 5 | | |
| Corn | 11 | | |
| Crab | 10 | | |
| Egg, Whole | 23 | | |
| Garlic | 10 | | |
| Lobster | 20 | | |
| Milk | 44 | +0/1 | Borderline |
| Mustard | 34 | +0/1 | Borderline |
| Oat | 5 | | |
| Orange | 4 | | |
| Pea, Green | 8 | | |
| Peanut | 11 | | |
| Pinto Bean | 9 | | |
| Pork | 10 | | |
| Rice | 43 | +0/1 | Borderline |
| Salmon | 20 | | |
| Shrimp | 41 | +0/1 | Borderline |
| Soybean | 10 | | |
| Strawberry | 12 | | |
| Sunflower | 20 | | |
| Tomato | 15 | | |
| Tuna | 14 | | |
| Turkey | 22 | | |
| Walnut | 12 | | |
| Wheat | 14 | | |

**Figure 4. IgE food antibody assay.** DE showed no clinically relevant IgE antibodies after treatment. Class definitions are the same as in Figure 1.

**0075 IgG4 Food Antibodies (90 Antigens)** *Methodology: ELISA*

| | Results ng/mL | Response | Class |
|---|---|---|---|
| **Dairy/Meat/Poultry** | | | |
| Beef | <10 | | |
| Casein | >2000 | Severe | +5 |
| Chicken | <10 | | |
| Egg, White | >2000 | Severe | +5 |
| Egg, Yolk | 1410 | Severe | +5 |
| Lamb | <10 | | |
| Milk | 1244 | Severe | +5 |
| Pork | <10 | | |
| Turkey | <10 | | |
| **Fish/Shellfish** | | | |
| Clam | 9 | | |
| Codfish | <10 | | |
| Crab | <10 | | |
| Flounder | <10 | | |
| Halibut | <10 | | |
| Lobster | <10 | | |
| Mackerel | <10 | | |
| Oyster | 20 | | |
| Salmon | <10 | | |
| Shrimp | <10 | | |
| Trout | <10 | | |
| Tuna | <10 | | |
| **Fruits** | | | |
| Apple | <10 | | |
| Apricot | 12 | | |
| Banana | <10 | | |
| Blueberry | 22 | | |
| Cantaloupe | <10 | | |
| Cranberry | <10 | | |
| Grape | <10 | | |
| Grapefruit | 36 | | |
| Honeydew | <10 | | |
| Lemon | <10 | | |
| Orange | <10 | | |
| Peach | <10 | | |
| Pear | <10 | | |
| Pineapple | 41 | Mild | +1 |
| Strawberry | <10 | | |
| Watermelon | <10 | | |
| **Grains** | | | |
| Barley | <10 | | |
| Corn | 11 | | |
| Oat | <10 | | |
| Rice | <10 | | |
| Rye | <10 | | |
| Wheat | 9 | | |
| **Legumes** | | | |
| Bean, String | 20 | | |
| Lentil | 22 | | |
| Lima Bean | <10 | | |
| Navy Bean | <10 | | |
| Pea, Green | 14 | | |
| Peanut | 274 | Mod | +3 |
| Pinto Bean | <10 | | |
| Soybean | 1377 | Severe | +5 |

**0075 IgG4 Food Antibodies (90 Antigens)** *Methodology: ELISA*

| | Results ng/mL | Response | Class |
|---|---|---|---|
| **Miscellaneous** | | | |
| Aspergillus | <10 | | |
| Black Pepper | 18 | | |
| Chocolate | <10 | | |
| Cinnamon | <10 | | |
| Coffee | <10 | | |
| Ginger | 447 | Mod | +3 |
| Malt | 11 | | |
| Tea | <10 | | |
| Vanilla | <10 | | |
| Yeast, Baker's | <10 | | |
| Yeast, Brewer's | <10 | | |
| **Nuts/Seeds** | | | |
| Almond | 15 | | |
| Cashew | 13 | | |
| Coconut | 8 | | |
| Pecan | <10 | | |
| Pistachio | <10 | | |
| Sesame | <10 | | |
| Sunflower | 14 | | |
| Walnut | 12 | | |
| **Vegetables** | | | |
| Asparagus | 8 | | |
| Avocado | <10 | | |
| Broccoli | 9 | | |
| Cabbage | <10 | | |
| Carrot | <10 | | |
| Cauliflower | 30 | | |
| Celery | <10 | | |
| Cucumber | <10 | | |
| Garlic | <10 | | |
| Lettuce | <10 | | |
| Mushroom | <10 | | |
| Mustard | 21 | | |
| Olive | <10 | | |
| Onion | <10 | | |
| Pepper, Green | <10 | | |
| Potato | <10 | | |
| Spinach | 22 | | |
| Sweet Potato | <10 | | |
| Tomato | <10 | | |
| Zucchini | <10 | | |

**Class Definitions:**

| Class | Cutoffs |
|---|---|
| Negative | 0-40 |
| Mild (+1/+2) | 80/150 |
| Moderate (+3/+4) | 500/900 |
| Severe (+5) | > 900 |

**Figure 5. Food-specific IgG4 antibodies.** DE still had moderate to severe IgG4 food antibodies in serum. His reaction to egg worsened with follow-up testing (see Figure 2).

## Twelve-Week Follow-up Plan

- Continue elimination of problematic foods with +3 to +5 antibodies
- Reintroduce foods with +2 antibody reactions and if asymptomatic, rotate food every four days
- Continue GI healing formula

# DISCUSSION

Atopy is an inherited type-1 IgE-mediated hypersensitivity reaction described as being "Th2 dominant." Early triggers stimulating Th2 dominance and associated disruption in GI microflora include, but are not limited to, antibiotic use, vaccines, food allergy and excessive hygiene.[3-5] There is also a genetic and epigenetic predisposition to atopy.

Atopic dermatitis is a common manifestation of atopy, particularly in early childhood.[21] A key genetic mutation associated with AD involves a protein needed for normal epidermal barrier function, called filaggrin. The null filaggrin mutation is found in about 9% of those of European descent.[22] In one study 42% of AD patients, particularly those presenting with severe hand eczema,[23] showed positive for one or more of the filaggrin mutations.[22]

The food-specific IgE serologic test is one standard diagnostic tool for food allergy in AD, along with skin prick testing and the atopy patch test.[21] Specific elimination diets and double-blind, placebo-controlled food challenge remain the gold standard for diagnosing food allergy.[24-26] IgE reactions in cases of AD have been clearly established in the literature.[25, 27-29] IgG antibodies have been detected in cases of atopy[30, 31] and have been seen to be elevated in cases of increased barrier permeability.[32-34] The IgG4 food-specific antibody has been referred to as a tolerance-inducing IgE blocking antibody[35] and, therefore, considered protective. In this case, however, IgG4 elevations appeared associated with the dermatitis. Symptomology associated with IgG4 has been noted and attributed to an IgG1-generated immune response to the IgG4 antibody/antigen complex.[36, 37]

DE's food allergy tests confirmed IgE and IgG4 antibody reactions. As seen in Figure 1, DE showed very high IgE reactions to: egg, garlic, milk, pork, and salmon. He showed moderate to high IgE antibodies to: almond, cantaloupe, mustard, oat, pinto bean, rice, and walnut. DE had severe IgG4 antibodies to milk and moderate IgG4 antibodies to egg (Figure 2).

> The 8-year-old male in this case suffered from severe, unremitting atopic dermatitis on his face and extremities. Embarrassment about his condition led to significant social anxiety.

DE had low serum IgA and tested negative for tissue transglutaminase (tTG) and anti-gliadin antibody (AGA) as shown in Figure 3. DE's low serum IgA may have contributed to his dermatitis. Low IgA has been associated with allergic manifestations[38] including atopic dermatitis.[39] Additionally, the lower total IgA level may have influenced the celiac antibody testing, causing a false-negative finding. Further investigation into celiac disease using IgG antibody testing would be prudent to conclusively rule-out the condition. DE had normal vitamin D levels (results not shown). His omega-3 fatty acid levels were low-normal (results not shown).

The mother reported that a previous skin-prick test (SPT) showed that DE had allergies to dust mites, pecans, and eggs. SPT is considered a sensitive method and relatively correlative with some IgE methodologies.[40] It is unknown whether other foods were tested and found negative. Nor is it known whether an elimination of these foods was undertaken for any length of time. At the time of his initial presentation above, he was not avoiding eggs or pecans.

Moderate-to-high levels of IgE antibody to rice was an unusual finding revealed by DE's food antibody tests. It is a reminder that foods commonly regarded as "low allergen" can be allergenic in certain persons. Rice is a food that would not have been suspected as allergenic in this country or withdrawn from DE's diet using standard elimination and rotation diets. Rice has been implicated in atopic dermatitis in Japan,[41] however, presumably on account of the high dietary intake, and thus allergenicity, of rice in that country.

**The medications he tried over time without significant effect included: triamcinolone, methotrexate, tacrolimus, hydrocortisone, pimecrolimus, cetirizine, and diphenhydramine.**

After 12 weeks of a rigorous elimination and rotation diet, fatty acids, probiotics, zinc and a GI healing formula, DE's skin showed dramatic improvement. Follow-up food antibody tests showed no moderate, high, or very high levels of IgE antibodies to foods (Figure 4). DE did, however, continue to have severe IgG4 antibodies to dairy and eggs, peanut and soy (Figure 5). When he was periodically exposed to egg or dairy, he developed pruritis. His exposure was always brief, and may explain why his symptoms did not escalate to AD.

The dramatic and rapid improvement of DE's IgE lab results was a unique aspect of this case. Elimination diets frequently reduce the severity of atopic dermatitis, but there are mixed reports about the behavior of serum IgE food antibodies upon removal of the allergens. [24,42] In one study of young children with atopic dermatitis, 16 months of food elimination did not lower levels of specific food IgE antibodies in serum.[24] In contrast, another study showed specific food IgE antibodies (measured by radioallergosorbent test) significantly decreased upon elimination of the allergenic foods in patients with atopic dermatits.[42] Similarly, challenge meals have been reported to significantly increase levels of specific food IgE antibodies in patients with atopic dermatitis.[43] The elimination diet and GI healing formula may have been instrumental in DE's improvement on the laboratory test, with the latter treating intestinal hyperpermeability and the former reducing antibody burden.

At 12 weeks, DE was able to reintroduce foods that originally invoked a +2 IgE response but he continued to avoid those foods with a +3 and above antibody response. Almost one and one half years later, he remained free of dermatitis and was generally healthy.

A key part of DE's success was that his mother followed the treatment plan diligently, incorporating alternative meats such as deer, bison, quail, and pheasant for DE's diet. However, when DE visited his grandmother, who didn't follow the protocol, DE began to develop pruritis. The clinician suspected that dairy and egg were probably the chief allergenic foods for DE. She stated that it was the "most amazing turn-around I've seen in all my years."

# CONCLUSION

Atopy is epidemic in Western countries and is strongly associated with many environmental exposures. Historically, the rise of atopy is closely correlated with urbanization. Interestingly, atopy is an inherited complex of conditions, although the rapidly increasing prevalence demonstrates that a classic Mendelian inheritance pattern is not responsible for the condition alone. Rather, a complex interplay among genes, environmental exposure and epigenetic modifications are likely at issue in this, and many other, complex chronic diseases.

**Laboratory analysis of IgE and IgG4 food antibodies suggested that a core pathogenic mechanism of this case was intestinal hyperpermeability, significant GI-mediated immune dysregulation and foods that were potently antigenic, including egg and dairy.**

Fortunately, laboratory analysis of IgE and IgG4 food antibodies suggested that a core pathogenic mechanism of this case was intestinal hyperpermeability, significant GI-mediated immune dysregulation—likely confounded by chronic antibiotic use—and foods that were potently antigenic, including egg and dairy. An initial restrictive diet with supportive nutrients resolved the AD. Continued avoidance of dairy and egg allowed for a lasting cure.

Further investigation into this safe and cost-effective approach for AD is warranted.

---

**Authors: Kara Fitzgerald, ND; Cass Nelson-Dooley, MS**
**Case Clinician: Alane Palmer**

## References

1. Diaz-Sanchez D. Pollution and the immune response: atopic diseases--are we too dirty or too clean? *Immunology.* Sep 2000;101(1):11-18.
2. Williams HC. Is the prevalence of atopic dermatitis increasing? *Clin Exp Dermatol.* Nov 1992;17(6):385-391.
3. Ehlers S, Kaufmann SH. Infection, inflammation, and chronic diseases: consequences of a modern lifestyle. *Trends Immunol.* May 2010;31(5):184-190.
4. Hon KL, Chan IH, Chow CM, et al. Specific IgE of common foods in Chinese children with eczema. *Pediatr Allergy Immunol.* Jul 1 2010.
5. Kay AB. Allergy and allergic diseases. First of two parts. *N Engl J Med.* Jan 4 2001;344(1):30-37.
6. Sly PD, Kusel M, Holt PG. Do early-life viral infections cause asthma? *J Allergy Clin Immunol.* Jun 2010;125(6):1202-1205.
7. NIH. Atopic Dermatitis. http://www.niams.nih.gov/Health_Info/Atopic_Dermatitis/default.asp. Accessed 10/12/2010, 2010.
8. Kapoor R, Menon C, Hoffstad O, Bilker W, Leclerc P, Margolis DJ. The prevalence of atopic triad in children with physician-confirmed atopic dermatitis. *J Am Acad Dermatol.* Jan 2008;58(1):68-73.

9. Chisolm SS, Taylor SL, Balkrishnan R, Feldman SR. Written action plans: potential for improving outcomes in children with atopic dermatitis. *J Am Acad Dermatol.* Oct 2008;59(4):677-683.

10. Greenhawt M. The role of food allergy in atopic dermatitis. *Allergy Asthma Proc.* Sep 2010;31(5):392-397.

11. Jarvinen KM, Beyer K, Vila L, Chatchatee P, Busse PJ, Sampson HA. B-cell epitopes as a screening instrument for persistent cow's milk allergy. *J Allergy Clin Immunol.* Aug 2002;110(2):293-297.

12. Hata TR, Kotol P, Jackson M, et al. Administration of oral vitamin D induces cathelicidin production in atopic individuals. *J Allergy Clin Immunol.* Oct 2008;122(4):829-831.

13. Dickinson EC, Gorga JC, Garrett M, et al. Immunoglobulin A supplementation abrogates bacterial translocation and preserves the architecture of the intestinal epithelium. *Surgery.* Aug 1998;124(2):284-290.

14. Pierce JL, Cromwell GL, Lindemann MD, Russell LE, Weaver EM. Effects of spray-dried animal plasma and immunoglobulins on performance of early weaned pigs. *J Anim Sci.* Dec 2005;83(12):2876-2885.

15. Tjellstrom B, Stenhammar L, Magnusson KE, Sandqvist T. Oral immunoglobulin treatment in Crohn's disease. *Acta Paediatr.* Feb 1997;86(2):221-223.

16. Maes M, Leunis JC. Normalization of leaky gut in chronic fatigue syndrome (CFS) is accompanied by a clinical improvement: effects of age, duration of illness and the translocation of LPS from gram-negative bacteria. *Neuro Endocrinol Lett.* Dec 2008;29(6):902-910.

17. Sturniolo GC, Di Leo V, Ferronato A, D'Odorico A, D'Inca R. Zinc supplementation tightens "leaky gut" in Crohn's disease. *Inflamm Bowel Dis.* May 2001;7(2):94-98.

18. Foster RH, Hardy G, Alany RG. Borage oil in the treatment of atopic dermatitis. *Nutrition.* Jul-Aug;26(7-8):708-718.

19. Ross SM. An integrative approach to eczema (atopic dermatitis). *Holist Nurs Pract.* Jan-Feb 2003;17(1):56-62.

20. Wright S. Atopic dermatitis and essential fatty acids: a biochemical basis for atopy? *Acta Derm Venereol Suppl (Stockh).* 1985;114:143-145.

21. Ricci G, Dondi A, Patrizi A. Useful tools for the management of atopic dermatitis. *Am J Clin Dermatol.* 2009;10(5):287-300.

22. Palmer CN, Irvine AD, Terron-Kwiatkowski A, et al. Common loss-of-function variants of the epidermal barrier protein filaggrin are a major predisposing factor for atopic dermatitis. *Nat Genet.* Apr 2006;38(4):441-446.

23. Thyssen JP, Carlsen BC, Menne T, et al. Filaggrin null mutations increase the risk and persistence of hand eczema in subjects with atopic dermatitis: results from a general population study. *Br J Dermatol.* Jul;163(1):115-120.

24. Niggemann B, Celik-Bilgili S, Ziegert M, Reibel S, Sommerfeld C, Wahn U. Specific IgE levels do not indicate persistence or transience of food allergy in children with atopic dermatitis. *J Investig Allergol Clin Immunol.* 2004;14(2):98-103.

25. Werfel T. Food allergy. *J Dtsch Dermatol Ges.* Jul 2008;6(7):573-583.

26. Niggermann B. When is an oral food challenge positive? *Allergy* 2010;65(1):2-6.

27. Leonardi S, Rotolo N, Vitaliti G, Spicuzza L, La Rosa M. IgE values and T-lymphocyte subsets in children with atopic eczema/dermatitis syndrome. *Allergy Asthma Proc.* Sep-Oct 2007;28(5):529-534.

28. Hon KL, Lam MC, Leung TF, et al. Are age-specific high serum IgE levels associated with worse symptomatology in children with atopic dermatitis? *Int J Dermatol.* Dec 2007;46(12):1258-1262.

29. Tokura Y. Extrinsic and intrinsic types of atopic dermatitis. *J Dermatol Sci.* Feb 16.

30. Eysink PE, De Jong MH, Bindels PJ, et al. Relation between IgG antibodies to foods and IgE antibodies to milk, egg, cat, dog and/or mite in a cross-sectional study. *Clin Exp Allergy.* May 1999;29(5):604-610.

31. Berrens L, Homedes IB. Relationship between IgE and IgG antibodies in type I allergy. *Allerg Immunol (Leipz).* 1991;37(3-4):131-137.

32. Kemeny DM, Urbanek R, Amlot PL, Ciclitira PJ, Richards D, Lessof MH. Sub-class of IgG in allergic disease. I. IgG sub-class antibodies in immediate and non-immediate food allergy. *Clin Allergy.* Nov 1986;16(6):571-581.

33. Paganelli R, Fagiolo U, Cancian M, Scala E. Intestinal permeability in patients with chronic urticaria-angioedema with and without arthralgia. *Ann Allergy.* Feb 1991;66(2):181-184.

34. White JF. Intestinal pathophysiology in autism. *Exp Biol Med (Maywood).* Jun 2003;228(6):639-649.

35. Tomicic S, Norrman G, Falth-Magnusson K, Jenmalm MC, Devenney I, Bottcher MF. High levels of IgG4 antibodies to foods during infancy are associated with tolerance to corresponding foods later in life. *Pediatr Allergy Immunol.* Feb 2009;20(1):35-41.

36. Lord RS, Bralley JA. Laboratory Evaluations for Integrative and Functional Medicine. Atlanta: Metametrix Institute; 2008:435.

37. Larsson PH. Purification of antibodies. *Methods Mol Med.* 2008;138:197-207.

38. Ludviksson BR, Eiriksson TH, Ardal B, Sigfusson A, Valdimarsson H. Correlation between serum immunoglobulin A concentrations and allergic manifestations in infants. *J Pediatr.* Jul 1992;121(1):23-27.

39. Ludviksson BR, Arason GJ, Thorarensen O, Ardal B, Valdimarsson H. Allergic diseases and asthma in relation to serum immunoglobulins and salivary immunoglobulin A in pre-school children: a follow-up community-based study. *Clin Exp Allergy.* Jan 2005;35(1):64-69.

40. Mullin GE, Swift KM, Lipski L, Turnbull LK, Rampertab SD. Testing for food reactions: the good, the bad, and the ugly. *Nutr Clin Pract.* Apr;25(2):192-198.

41. Ikezawa Z, Miyakawa K, Komatsu H, et al. A probable involvement of rice allergy in severe type of atopic dermatitis in Japan. *Acta Derm Venereol Suppl (Stockh).* 1992;176:103-107.

42. Agata H, Kondo N, Fukutomi O, Shinoda S, Orii T. Effect of elimination diets on food-specific IgE antibodies and lymphocyte proliferative responses to food antigens in atopic dermatitis patients exhibiting sensitivity to food allergens. *J Allergy Clin Immunol.* Feb 1993;91(2):668-679.

43. Ionescu G, Radovici D, Negoescu A, Preda I, Mahal H. [Circulating immune complexes, specific IgE against food and inhalation allergens, serum histamine levels and disorders of intestinal permeability in atopic patients before and after test meals]. *Immun Infekt.* Jul 1985;13(4):147-155.

# 2 Autoimmune Conditions

## Psoriatic Arthritis

*Autoimmune diseases (ADs) are chronic, often debilitating and potentially life-threatening conditions that collectively affect up to 23.5 million Americans, and their incidence is rising.[1] They are heterogeneous in pathology but share common etiopathogenic factors such as intestinal hyperpermeability.[2] Although up to 100 ADs have been identified, there are likely more.[1] Genetics plays a clear role in the predisposition for the development and phenotype of AD, but various combinations of factors, such as toxins, endogenous hormone imbalances, microbes (including of GI origin), infections, stress and food antigens, are involved in disease expression.[2-5] Standard treatments include NSAIDs, steroids, anti-neoplastic agents and tumor necrosis factor-alpha antagonists. These tools have potentially devastating side effects and are often applied regardless of the diagnosis. Frequently, they are only modestly effective in relieving symptoms and limiting the advancing disease process. Direct healthcare costs of AD are estimated at around 100 billion dollars per year in the United States. By comparison, cancer care costs about 57 billion dollars per year.[1] The rising incidence of this debilitating and costly group of conditions dictates that safe, alternative approaches to treatment be considered now.*

### 56-Year-Old Male with Psoriatic Arthritis*

| | |
|---|---|
| **Additional Symptoms and Conditions** | Psoriasis and psoriatic nails, constipation, esophageal reflux, aphthous stomatitis, blepharitis, migraines, and depression |
| **Medications** | Etodolac (Lodine®), methotrexate, and adalimumab (Humira®) |
| **Tests Used** | IgG food-specific antibodies, celiac panel with genes, inflammatory markers, and a multiprofile panel assessing nutrients, fatty acids, amino acids, organic acids, oxidative stress, and whole blood toxic metals. DNA-based stool analysis, complete blood count, and comprehensive metabolic panel with insulin and A1C |
| **Imbalances Identified** | Multiple IgG food sensitivities, intestinal hyperpermeability, gastrointestinal candidiasis, hypovitaminosis D, low red blood cell magnesium, elevated arachidonic acid, subclinical hypothyroidism, metabolic syndrome, suspected fatty liver |
| **Treatments** | Diet: 100% gluten and dairy free; avoid yeast and eggs; discontinue alcohol, caffeine, sugar; fluconazole; gastrointestinal anti-inflammatory medicinal food; probiotics; vitamin D; EPA/DHA; methyl donors ($B_{12}$, folic acid, $B_6$); amino acids (taurine, glycine, N-acetyl-cysteine, methionine); high-dose multivitamin and mineral without iron; daily meditation practice |

* This case was modified with permission by Kara Fitzgerald, ND, and Mark Hyman, MD, and published by The Institute for Functional Medicine in its *Textbook of Functional Medicine*, 2010.

*Table continues on following page...*

## 56-Year-Old Male with Psoriatic Arthritis*

| | |
|---|---|
| **Outcome** | 80% reduction in pain with improved mobility; stiffness and swelling resolved; discontinued NSAID and adalimumab (Humira®); reduced methotrexate; improved mood; resolved reflux and constipation; weight loss |
| **Discussion/ Significance** | Using a systems medicine approach, including a comprehensive history, laboratory analysis and treatment, allowed the underlying imbalances of this case to be successfully identified and treated. A systems research model, able to capture and analyze complexity, would be well-suited to assess the efficacy of this type of multi-variable and individualized approach. If deemed effective on a larger scale, such an approach may be a logical solution for those suffering from complex, chronic diseases including AD. |

# CASE HISTORY

At age 56, MP presented with a diagnosis of psoriatic arthritis that was progressively worsening despite aggressive medication therapy. He experienced severe pain, decreased range of motion, and swelling in his feet, ankles, knees, and hands. He walked with a limp. His left shoulder was also frequently painful. All symptoms became worse in the morning. He had been taking etodolac and methotrexate for the past 3 years, and adalimumab for the past 6 months. The onset of psoriatic arthritis occurred with the development of pain and redness in his right great toe, for which he was treated unsuccessfully with antibiotics. Shortly thereafter, he developed psoriasis behind his knees, on his feet, and behind his ears. He had psoriatic nails for most of his life.

> Autoimmune diseases (ADs) are chronic, often debilitating and potentially life-threatening conditions that collectively affect up to 23.5 million Americans, and their incidence is rising.

Just prior to receiving the diagnosis of psoriatic arthritis, he had a left knee arthroscopy that was negative for degenerative disease but positive for synovitis. He also developed a hemorrhagic Baker's cyst, causing severe swelling and pain in his left foot and knee. MP also complained of esophageal reflux, a recent 15-pound weight gain, and intermittent depression.

MP's past medical history included migraine headaches and disc protrusion with sciatica at L5-S1. His mother, at age 82, was diagnosed with congestive heart failure, malnutrition, rheumatoid arthritis, depression, and schizophrenia. MP's father died at age 62; he had suffered from cancer, obesity, and alcoholism. His brothers were diagnosed with cancer, inflammatory arthritis, inflammatory bowel disease, alcoholism, and depression and his sisters with alcoholism, depression, and bipolar disorder. MP's son was diagnosed with schizophrenia and his daughter with ADHD. There was hypertension, diabetes, heart disease, and depression on both sides of the extended family.

In addition to etodolac, methotrexate, and adalimumab, MP took aspirin, omega-3 fatty acids, and a multivitamin and mineral. His past history included multiple courses of antibiotics.

MP led a stressful life with a highly demanding job. His schedule had little time for relaxation, although he reported meditating daily. MP was married with two children, including one who had been diagnosed with schizophrenia and lived at home.

MP's usual dietary intake included oatmeal with milk and sugar for breakfast; tuna with soup and cookies for lunch; fish or meat with vegetables and potato or pasta for dinner. He snacked on cookies and protein bars. He avoided chocolate and fatty foods. He ate out more than 5 times per week and craved sweets and caffeine, consuming 3 to 4 cups of coffee and one diet soda per day (357 to 464 mg caffeine). MP drank about 12 alcoholic beverages per week, including wine and the occasional scotch. He reported that his liver enzymes had been elevated, and he showed some concern about his drinking. Because of his schedule, he didn't exercise regularly, but he was interested in starting. He had a history of mold exposure and his teeth contained many mercury amalgams.

In his systems review, it was found that he was sensitive to loud noises, had dry eyes with crusty secretions, was intolerant of perfumes and auto exhaust, and had canker sores, esophageal reflux, and chronic constipation. He also had some difficulty with concentration and irritability. His blood pressure was 138/87, height 70.5", weight 204 pounds and body mass index was 28.85.

## Initial Laboratory Results

**Laboratory tests ordered and rationale:**

1. **IgG foods**: Food reactions have been associated with psoriatic arthritis pathogenesis, and may contribute to inflammation. Many IgG reactions demonstrate intestinal hyperpermeability, also a factor in inflammatory arthritis. Removing offending foods, if present, will reduce systemic inflammation.
2. **DQ genotype (celiac genes) and celiac panel**: Celiac disease and psoriatic arthritis have been linked, and share common inflammatory etiopathogenic features.
3. **Inflammatory markers**: Monitoring general inflammatory markers is standard practice for assessment of treatment efficacy.
4. **Multiprofile panel**: A comprehensive assessment including fatty acids, amino acids, organic acids, oxidative stress markers, and whole blood toxic metals. These tests assist in finding individual etiopathogenic factors that can affect treatment considerations. (Not all findings are discussed below. Panel results not grouped together)
5. **Metabolic panel and lipids**: General assessment of metabolic imbalances associated with inflammation
6. **Thyroid panel**: Subclinical hypothyroidism is frequently found in those with complex, chronic disease.
7. **DNA microbial stool profile**: Assessment of GI microbial status and GI function. GI imbalances are a common finding in inflammatory conditions.

### IgG (TOTAL) Reactive Foods*

| | | | |
|---|---|---|---|
| Almond (+2) | Chili Pepper (+2) | Lobster (+1) | Sesame (+1) |
| Amaranth (+1) | Clam (+2) | Milk, Cow's (+2) | Shrimp (+1) |
| Barley (+1) | Corn (+1) | Onion (+1) | Tomato (+1) |
| Bean, Kidney (+1) | Crab (+1) | Oyster (+2) | Wheat (+2) |
| Cantaloupe (+1) | Cranberry (+1) | Pineapple (+1) | Yeast, Baker's (+3) |
| Cashew Nut (+1) | Egg (+3) | Potato, White (+1) | Yeast, Brewer's (+4) |
| Cheese (+1) | Garlic (+1) | Scallops (+2) | |

** Results range from 0 (no reaction) to +5 (severe reaction).*

| Celiac Disease Panel | Results | Reference Interval |
|---|---|---|
| Immunoglobulin A | 438 | 82–453 mg/dl |
| Transglutaminase IgA | < 20 | < 20 Units |

| Test | Results |
|---|---|
| DQ Genotype | Allele Detected: HLA DQA1*0501 |

**Figure 1. Food-specific IgG antibodies, celiac panel, and DQ Genotype.** IgG food sensitivities demonstrated multiple reactions consistent with intestinal hyperpermeability. Celiac genes revealed a single allele that may be associated with increased risk of gluten intolerance.

| Inflammatory Markers | | Results | Reference Interval |
|---|---|---|---|
| Iron | | 80 | 50–150 µg/dL |
| Transferrin | | 246 | 201–336 mg/dL |
| TIBC | | 308 | 255–450 mg/dL |
| Iron saturation | | 26 | 20–50% |
| Ferritin | HN | 322 | 23–336 ng/mL |
| ESR Westergren | | 7 | 0–20 mm/hr |
| CRP High Sensitivity | HN | 2.9 mg/L | Relative Cardiovascular Risk:<br>Low < 1.0; Average 1.0–3.0; High 3.1–10.0 |
| Rheumatoid Factor | | < 20 | < 30 IU/mL |
| ANA Screen | | Negative | Negative |

| Test | | Results | Reference Interval |
|---|---|---|---|
| Vitamin D 25 OH | L | 21 ng/mL | < 20 ng/mL: Insufficiency<br>20–40 ng/mL: Hypovitaminosis D<br>40–100 ng/mL: Sufficiency<br>> 100 ng/mL: Toxicity |

| | | | | | |
|---|---|---|---|---|---|
| Magnesium * | 25 | L | 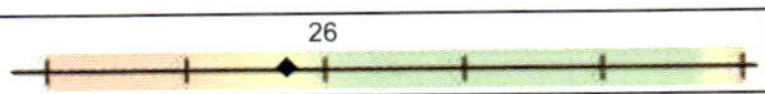 | 18 - 40 | ppm packed cells |



**Figure 2. Inflammatory markers, vitamin D, and RBC magnesium.** Significant findings revealed a high-normal ferritin level. Medications may have been dampening the other inflammatory markers. He also had hypovitaminosis D and low magnesium. Deficiencies of both may contribute to inflammation.

## ■ PSORIATIC ARTHRITIS

| | Results | | | Reference |
|---|---|---|---|---|
| ***Polyunsaturated Omega-3*** | uM | | | |
| Alpha Linolenic (18:3n3) | 35 | | 20 | 13 - 80 |
| Eicosapentaenoic (20:5n3) | 55 | | 17 | 5 - 210 |
| Docosapentaenoic (22:5n3) | 23 | | 16 | 11 - 50 |
| Docosahexaenoic (22:6n3) | 132 | | 59 | 31 - 213 |
| ***Polyunsaturated Omega-6*** | | | | |
| Arachidonic (20:4n6) | 502 | H | 201 … 451 | 158 - 521 |
| ***Saturated*** | | | | |
| Palmitic (16:0) | 1,810 | H | 792 … 1,794 | 667 - 2,526 |
| ***Monounsaturated*** | Results uM | | | |
| Palmitoleic (16:1n7) | 260 | H | 40 … 155 | 30 - 256 |
| Vaccenic (18:1n7) | 125 | H | 48 … 93 | 40 - 122 |
| Oleic (18:1n9) | 1,480 | H | 555 … 1,182 | 466 - 1,470 |
| | Results nmol/mL | | | |
| Lipid Peroxides | 1.6 | H | 1.5 | <= 2.0 |

**Figure 3. Plasma fatty acids and lipid peroxides.** Omega-3 fatty acids were at normal levels, probably as a result of MP's supplementation. However, the pro-inflammatory fatty acid arachidonic acid (AA) was high-normal and much more abundant than the anti-inflammatory eicosapentaenoic acid (EPA). The plasma saturated and monounsaturated fatty acids demonstrated elevations consistent with hypertriglyceridemia and dysinsulinemia. Serum lipid peroxide elevation indicated increased oxidative damage to lipid membranes.

| **Metabolic Panel** | | **Results** | **Reference Interval** |
|---|---|---|---|
| Glucose | H | 106 | 70–99 mg/dL |
| Insulin | HN | 21 | 6–27 uIU/mL |
| Glycohemoglobin A1C | | 5.5 | 4.4–6.8% |
| ALT | H | 44 | 0–40 IU/L |
| **Lipids** | | **Results** | **Reference Interval** |
| Cholesterol, Total | H | 218 | < 200 mg/dL |
| Triglycerides | H | 431 | < 150 mg/dL |
| Cholesterol, HDL | LN | 43 | 40–59 mg/dL |
| Cholesterol, LDL | | *Not analyzed due to interference of elevated triglycerides* | < 130 mg/dL |

**Figure 4. Metabolic panel and lipids.** MP's metabolic panel demonstrated findings consistent with metabolic syndrome, including a mild elevation of ALT, which may indicate early hepatosteatosis.

NOTES

| Thyroid Panel | Results | Reference Limits |
|---|---|---|
| TSH | HN 2.39 | 0.28–3.89 mIU/L |
| T4, Free | LN 0.58 | 0.58–1.64 ng/dL |
| T3, Free | LN 2.9 | 2.5–3.9 pg/mL |
| Thyroglobulin Ab | < 20 | < 40 IU/mL |
| Thyroid Peroxidase Ab | < 20 | < 35 IU/mL |

**Figure 5. Thyroid panel.** The thyroid panel demonstrated subclinical hypothyroidism. Current thinking on thyroid stimulating hormone (TSH) is that an optimal level may be 2.5mIU/L or less.[6]

| Yeast/Fungi | | Reference Range |
|---|---|---|
| Candida sp. | +3 => 10000 pg DNA/g specimen | Neg |

**Figure 6. Microbial stool analysis using DNA identification.** An elevated amount of *Candida* DNA was identified in the stool.

### Pertinent Negative Laboratory Results

Given MP's high number of amalgams, there was concern about mercury. According to the CDC, up to 75% of an individual's mercury exposure may be from amalgams.[7] MP's whole blood toxic metals were within normal limits, ruling out significant current toxic release from amalgams. A DMPS-challenged urine toxic element test was also ordered to assess body burden, but MP had not completed the test at the time of this publication.

## Initial Assessment

- Psoriatic arthritis
- Psoriasis
- Psoriatic nails
- Blepharitis
- Aphthous stomatitis
- Gastroesophageal reflux disease
- Chronic constipation
- Migraine headaches
- Depression
- Intestinal hyperpermeability
- Gluten sensitivity
- Multiple IgG food sensitivities
- Hypovitaminosis D
- Inflammation and oxidative stress

### PSORIATIC ARTHRITIS

- Suspected fatty liver
- Metabolic syndrome
- Subclinical hypothyroidism
- GI yeast overgrowth
- Mercury toxicity (multiple amalgams)
- Family history of heart disease, hypertension, psychiatric disorders, diabetes, autoimmunity

# Initial Plan

- Dietary changes: 100% gluten and dairy free; avoid yeast and eggs; discontinue alcohol, caffeine, sugar; eat whole, low glycemic-index foods, good fats, and proteins. Recommend prepared hypoallergenic meals.
- Anti-inflammatory medicinal food, 2 scoops QD
- 450 billion CFU probiotic, 1 packet BID
- Vitamin $D_3$ 5000 IU, 2 caps QD
- EPA/DHA 6:1, 1 cap BID
- Methyl donors ($B_{12}$, folic acid and $B_6$), 1 cap BID
- Amino acids (taurine, glycine, N-acetyl-cysteine, methionine), 3 caps BID
- High-dose multivitamin and mineral without iron, 4 tabs BID
- Fluconazole 100 mg, 1 tab QD × 30 days
- Continue daily meditation practice

**Treatment plan rationale:** Treatment for MP was focused on removing the antigenic foods and GI yeast, reducing inflammation, restoring GI mucosa, and providing needed nutrients. It was expected that thyroid and metabolic imbalances would normalize with these general interventions. Given his busy lifestyle, MP benefited from hypoallergenic, low glycemic-index prepared meals. Fluconazole was given for the *Candida*, followed by a mucosal-restoring medicinal food and high-dose probiotic.

Omega-3 fatty acids were given to support production of anti-inflammatory eicosanoids. Vitamin D (10,000 IU/day) was given to increase serum D levels to within 55 to 70 ng/mL, which is considered an optimal range in complex chronic disease. A supplement containing methyl donors was given to improve methylation and sulfuration activity based on the understanding that increased activity in these pathways may help with mood, metabolic imbalances, cardiovascular health and hepatic detoxification. The amino acid combination of taurine, glycine, N-acetyl-cysteine (NAC), and methionine was also prescribed to support hepatic methylation and sulfuration.[8-11] Taurine, glycine, and NAC are also known to have anxiolytic properties.[12-14] A high-dose multivitamin and mineral supplement was given for general micronutrient support, and to ensure adequate availability of cofactors and coenzymes. Metabolic polymorphisms can result in a lowered affinity of an enzyme for its coenzyme; thus, increased levels may be needed for optimal (or even adequate) functioning.[15,16] MP was encouraged to continue with his meditation practice, as meditation has been shown to improve well-being by reducing stress, inflammation and depression.[17-20]

## Five-Month Follow-up

MP arrived pain-free the day of the office visit, stating that he hadn't felt so good in years. He reported an 80% reduction in pain on average with improved mobility. He could climb stairs more quickly and was no longer limping. Morning pain and stiffness were gone. Previously, his hands were swollen and difficult to open. Now, the swelling was resolved and movement was normal. MP had not used any non-steroidal anti-inflammatory or adalimumab for two months. He reduced his usage of methotrexate from 15 to 5 mg per week.

**MP stated he was pain-free and that he hadn't felt so good in years. He was more mobile, and swelling and stiffness in his hands were gone. He had not required an NSAID or adalimumab for two months.**

His reflux and migraines were gone. His mood had improved and he was less irritable. He was no longer constipated. He reported having a single, well-formed bowel movement daily. He was still under a great deal of stress, working 80 hours a week, but meditation continued to be helpful. He reported that he was still getting occasional canker sores.

He quit caffeine and reduced alcohol intake considerably. He started hypoallergenic, gluten-, yeast-, dairy-, and soy-free prepared meals, which were perfect for his busy lifestyle, enabling him to follow the dietary suggestions. He was taking his supplements regularly. He was losing weight, his clothes fit much better and he was satisfied with his dietary changes. Overall, he was pleased with his progress.

- Blood pressure: 118/73 LAS (5 months ago: 138/87)
- Pulse: 58 BPM
- Weight: 190 pounds (5 months ago: 204 lbs)

# DISCUSSION

MP was taking a powerful combination of commonly prescribed medications for autoimmune conditions, including etodolac, methotrexate and adalimumab. Unfortunately, MP's symptoms continued to worsen. Laboratory analysis helped to reveal the etiology of MP's condition, enabling an effective treatment plan to be designed.

In Figure 1, ELISA testing for total IgG response to 90 different foods demonstrated a strong positive reaction to eggs and yeast, and mild positive reactions (+1 or +2) to 25 other foods, including gluten-containing wheat and barley. Food sensitivities generate significant inflammation, and as such are both a cause and effect of intestinal hyperpermeability.[21-23] Other factors contributing to MP's intestinal hyperpermeability included alcohol and NSAID use.[24,25] Intestinal hyperpermeability has been demonstrated to be a significant etiopathogenic mechanism in inflammatory arthritis and celiac disease.[2]

MP's genetic test for celiac disease demonstrated the presence of the DQ2 allele DQA1*0501 (Figure 1). Psoriatic arthritis is associated with celiac disease and subclinical gluten enteropathy.[26] HLA DQ is a heterodimer cell surface type protein found on antigen-presenting cells. HLADQ2 is encoded by the DQA1*0501 and the DQB1*0201 alleles. Approximately 90% of celiac patients express the DQ2 heterodimer serotype. Interestingly, more than 3% of celiac patients present with only half the DQ2 heterodimer, as did MP. In one study looking at 1008 European celiac patients, 57 encoded only half of the DQ2 heterodimer.[27] Because MP's test results demonstrated the presence of half the DQ2 heterodimer—specifically, the HLA DQA1*05 allele—celiac disease could not be ruled out. However, IgA tissue transglutaminase antibodies (tTG) were undetectable (Figure 1), which significantly reduced the likelihood of celiac disease.

Despite the equivocal celiac panel, a gluten-free trial was suggested because of the positive IgG reaction to wheat and barley and the presence of the DQ2 allele. It was also recommended that he eliminate dairy and those foods with reactivity of +3 and above, and limit intake of the +2 foods.

**Intestinal hyperpermeability has been demonstrated to be a significant etiopathogenic mechanism in inflammatory arthritis and celiac disease.**

Figure 2 showed reported levels of inflammatory markers, vitamin D and red blood cell magnesium. With the exception of a high-normal ferritin and elevated hs-CRP, none of the inflammatory markers were abnormal. Methotrexate and adalimumab attenuate markers of inflammation, and may have been responsible for these negative findings.[28-30]

MP's vitamin D level of 21ng/mL (Figure 2) may have contributed to the severity of his symptoms. The pathophysiology of psoriatic arthritis includes upregulation of Th1-driven inflammation. Vitamin D specifically regulates T-helper and dendritic cell function while inducing regulatory T-cells, causing a decrease in Th1 activity.[31,32] The optimal serum vitamin D range is now thought to be 40 to 70 ng/mL. It is suggested that individuals with chronic disease maintain levels between 55 and 70 ng/mL.[33] Hypovitaminosis D may have been a factor in MP's depression.[34] Sub-optimal magnesium (Figure 2) is found in a large percentage of the population, and is a common finding in those with chronic disease.[35]

In Figure 3, the omega-3 fatty acids (ALA, EPA and DHA) were all within normal limits, probably because MP was supplementing with them. However, the omega-6 fatty acid AA was high normal, supporting the production of pro-inflammatory cytokines. The 2- and 4-series eicosanoids, produced from AA, stimulate the up regulation of TNF-alpha, a Th1 cytokine strongly implicated in psoriatic arthritis pathogenesis.[36] MP was taking the drug adalimumab, which binds TNF-alpha directly, blocking its ability to bind certain receptors.[37] Reducing AA availability through diet and nutrients could similarly assist in modulating the inflammatory effects of psoriatic arthritis by reducing AA-derived eicosanoids.

Figure 3 showed elevated saturated and monounsaturated fatty acids, which represent a pattern seen in metabolic syndrome with hypertriglyceridemia, where insulin stimulates the liver enzyme fatty acid synthase to produce saturated fatty acids. Insulin also stimulates delta-9 desaturase which converts saturated to monounsaturated fatty acids, primarily palmitoleic, vaccenic and oleic.[38] Lipid peroxidation was also high, indicating increased oxidative damage to the lipid-rich cellular membranes.[39]

The metabolic assessment shown in Figure 4 demonstrated insulin resistance. It has been suggested that insulin stimulates the production of AA,[40] and AA elevation has been associated with insulin resistance.[41, 42] These findings suggested a possible mechanistic link between psoriatic arthritis and metabolic syndrome through the common pathway of eicosanoid-driven inflammation. An elevated AA/EPA ratio has been shown to positively correlate with depression.[43] MP had more than 7 times the amount of AA relative to EPA in his plasma, despite supplementation with omega-3 fatty acids.

MP's thyroid panel was within normal limits, including antibodies (Figure 5). Optimal TSH is now considered to be 2.5, but may be as low as 1.18 mIU/L.[6] Free T3 and free T4 were low normal. These results suggested that the thyroid should be monitored, particularly given the association of hypothyroidism with rheumatologic conditions. Nutrients involved with thyroid function, including red blood cell zinc, whole blood selenium and plasma tyrosine, were within normal limits.

As was suspected, DNA stool analysis demonstrated a significant quantity of *Candida* species in the gastrointestinal tract (Figure 6). *Candida* species in particular have been found in significant amounts relative to controls in the saliva, skin, and stool of psoriatic patients.[44]

As discussed above in the treatment rationale, a straightforward approach involving removing yeast and antigentic foods was used to address the imbalances found, reducing inflammation, restoring GI mucosa and providing the needed nutrients. It was expected that thyroid and metabolic imbalances would be normalized with these general interventions.

# CONCLUSION

Autoimmune diseases are debilitating conditions that affect millions of individuals.[1] Current standard-of-care therapies come with high risk profiles and may not slow the progression of the disease significantly.[45] Despite the extensive categorization of autoimmune diseases into diagnoses such as lupus, rheumatoid arthritis, psoriatic arthritis, inflammatory bowel disease, multiple sclerosis, nephritis, and scleroderma, the treatments are based on pathology, not etiology. The conventional approach to autoimmune disease seeks to answer the question of *what* disease the patient has, not *why* the patient has the disease, suggesting only small variations in treatment.

---

NOTES

Systems-based, or functional, medicine considers the diagnosis, of course, but also seeks to answer the question *why*. The etiology of a disease may vary among people with the same diagnosis or pathology. Conversely, the etiology may be the same in patients with very different pathologies—for example, mercury toxicity is found in both multiple sclerosis and Crohn's disease. Approaches to treatment, therefore, will vary according to the particular upstream causes and downstream effects present in each patient. Treating only the downstream effects (such as nutrient deficiencies or food sensitivities due to malabsorption and intestinal hyperpermeability) without treating the upstream causes (such as gluten sensitivity, gastrointestinal yeast, or mercury toxicity) will often result in treatment failure.

**The conventional approach to autoimmune disease seeks to answer the question of *what* disease the patient has, not *why* the patient has the disease, suggesting only small variations in treatment. Systems-based, or functional, medicine considers the diagnosis, of course, but also seeks to answer the question *why*.**

Focusing on the patient's individual etiology of autoimmune disease provides a personalized framework for diagnosis and treatment. Five primary etiologic factors have been identified that give rise to nearly all disease (including autoimmune disease) through their effects on gene expression: toxins, allergens, infections (or microbial imbalances), poor diet, and stress.

MP, a highly successful, educated physician had access to the latest medications and technologies to address his psoriatic arthritis. Unfortunately, however, his condition continued to deteriorate despite aggressive interventions. He was in constant pain, with limited mobility and use of his hands. Using a systems approach with MP including laboratory analysis and thorough history allowed the variables involved in the etiopathogenesis of his illness to be successfully identified and addressed. His pain was alleviated, his movement restored and his quality of life immeasurably improved. Associated complaints such as reflux, constipation, migraines and depression were all resolved in the process, as they all shared pathogenic mechanisms with PA. He was able to reduce the dosage or eliminate all of his medications. As MP became versed in understanding the environmental role in his condition, he was able to identify and avoid his disease triggers, allowing him to take charge of his health.

Employing a systems research model to explore multivariable treatment approaches, such as the one used with MP, will allow for a non-biased assessment of the efficacy of such approaches. Following this model of care, if demonstrated to be broadly efficacious, may be beneficial for addressing the rising incidence of complex, chronic disease.

---

**Authors: Kara Fitzgerald, ND; Mark Hyman, MD**

**Case Clinicians: Mark Hyman, MD, Chairman, Institute for Functional Medicine; Kathie Swift, MS, RD**

## References


1. AARDA. Autoimmune Disease Fact Sheet. http://www.aarda.org/autoimmune_statistics.php. Accessed 01-14-10, 2010.
2. Fasano A. Surprises from celiac disease. *Sci Am.* Aug 2009;301(2):54-61.
3. de Carvalho JF, Pereira RM, Shoenfeld Y. The mosaic of autoimmunity: the role of environmental factors. *Front Biosci (Elite Ed).* 2009;1:501-509.
4. Molina V, Shoenfeld Y. Infection, vaccines and other environmental triggers of autoimmunity. *Autoimmunity.* May 2005;38(3):235-245.
5. Mizokami T, Wu Li A, El-Kaissi S, Wall JR. Stress and thyroid autoimmunity. *Thyroid.* Dec 2004;14(12):1047-1055.
6. Wartofsky L, Dickey RA. The evidence for a narrower thyrotropin reference range is compelling. *J Clin Endocrinol Metab.* Sep 2005;90(9):5483-5488.
7. Registry AfTSaD. Public Health Statements: Mercury. http://www.atsdr.cdc.gov/phs/phs.asp?id=112&tid=24. Accessed 01-15-10.
8. Liska DJ. The detoxification enzyme systems. *Altern Med Rev.* Jun 1998;3(3):187-198.
9. Kelly GS. Clinical applications of N-acetylcysteine. *Altern Med Rev.* Apr 1998;3(2):114-127.
10. Birdsall TC. Therapeutic applications of taurine. *Altern Med Rev.* Apr 1998;3(2):128-136.
11. N-acetylcysteine. *Altern Med Rev.* Oct 2000;5(5):467-471.
12. Grant JE, Odlaug BL, Kim SW. N-acetylcysteine, a glutamate modulator, in the treatment of trichotillomania: a double-blind, placebo-controlled study. *Arch Gen Psychiatry.* Jul 2009;66(7):756-763.
13. Berk M, Jeavons S, Dean OM, et al. Nail-biting stuff? The effect of N-acetyl cysteine on nail-biting. *CNS Spectr.* Jul 2009;14(7):357-360.
14. Sahley. Amino acids are key for anxiety disorders. *Townsend Letter for Doctors and Patients.* Jan. 19 2010.
15. Ames BN. A role for supplements in optimizing health: the metabolic tune-up. *Arch Biochem Biophys.* Mar 1 2004;423(1):227-234.
16. Ames BN. The metabolic tune-up: metabolic harmony and disease prevention. *J Nutr.* May 2003;133(5 Suppl 1):1544S-1548S.
17. Oke SL, Tracey KJ. The Inflammatory Reflex and the Role of Complementary and Alternative Medical Therapies. *Ann N Y Acad Sci.* Sep 28 2007.
18. Maunder RG, Levenstein S. The role of stress in the development and clinical course of inflammatory bowel disease: epidemiological evidence. *Curr Mol Med.* Jun 2008;8(4):247-252.
19. Huynh TV, Gotay C, Layi G, Garrard S. Mindfulness meditation and its medical and non-medical applications. *Hawaii Med J.* Dec 2007;66(12):328-330.
20. Deyo M, Wilson KA, Ong J, Koopman C. Mindfulness and rumination: does mindfulness training lead to reductions in the ruminative thinking associated with depression? *Explore (NY).* Sep-Oct 2009;5(5):265-271.
21. DeMeo MT, Mutlu EA, Keshavarzian A, Tobin MC. Intestinal permeation and gastrointestinal disease. *J Clin Gastroenterol.* Apr 2002;34(4):385-396.
22. Atkinson W, Sheldon TA, Shaath N, Whorwell PJ. Food elimination based on IgG antibodies in irritable bowel syndrome: a randomised controlled trial. *Gut.* Oct 2004;53(10):1459-1464.
23. Macdonald TT, Monteleone G. Immunity, inflammation, and allergy in the gut. *Science.* Mar 25 2005;307(5717):1920-1925.
24. Farhadi A, Banan A, Fields J, Keshavarzian A. Intestinal barrier: an interface between health and disease. *J Gastroenterol Hepatol.* May 2003;18(5):479-497.
25. Mielants H, Goemaere S, De Vos M, et al. Intestinal mucosal permeability in inflammatory rheumatic diseases. I. Role of antiinflammatory drugs. *J Rheumatol.* Mar 1991;18(3):389-393.
26. Lindqvist U, Rudsander A, Bostrom A, Nilsson B, Michaelsson G. IgA antibodies to gliadin and coeliac disease in psoriatic arthritis. *Rheumatology (Oxford).* Jan 2002;41(1):31-37.

27. Karell K, Louka AS, Moodie SJ, et al. HLA types in celiac disease patients not carrying the DQA1*05-DQB1*02 (DQ2) heterodimer: results from the European Genetics Cluster on Celiac Disease. *Hum Immunol.* Apr 2003;64(4):469-477.

28. Caramaschi P, Biasi D, Tonolli E, et al. Antibodies against cyclic citrullinated peptides in patients affected by rheumatoid arthritis before and after infliximab treatment. *Rheumatol Int.* Nov 2005;26(1):58-62.

29. Emad Y, Ragab Y, Shaarawy A, Raafat H, El-Kiki HA, Rasker JJ. Enhanced MRI in early undifferentiated oligoarthritis of the knee joints: Improvements already visible after 2 months of DMARDs treatment. *Clin Rheumatol.* Jun 18 2008.

30. Arvidson NG, Larsen A, Aaseth J, Larsson A. Short-term effects of the TNFalpha antagonist infliximab on the acute phase reaction and activities of daily life in patients with rheumatoid arthritis. *Scand J Clin Lab Invest.* 2007;67(3):337-342.

31. Cantorna MT, Mahon BD. Mounting evidence for vitamin D as an environmental factor affecting autoimmune disease prevalence. *Exp Biol Med (Maywood).* Dec 2004;229(11):1136-1142.

32. Myers WA, Gottlieb AB, Mease P. Psoriasis and psoriatic arthritis: clinical features and disease mechanisms. *Clin Dermatol.* Sep-Oct 2006;24(5):438-447.

33. Cannell JJ, Hollis BW. Use of vitamin D in clinical practice. *Altern Med Rev.* Mar 2008;13(1):6-20.

34. Check your vitamin D intake to avoid multiple health consequences. Three 2008 studies link low vitamin D levels to depression, hip fractures, and increased risk of death. *Duke Med Health News.* Nov 2008;14(11):9-10.

35. Sales CH, Pedrosa Lde F. Magnesium and diabetes mellitus: their relation. *Clin Nutr.* Aug 2006;25(4):554-562.

36. Calder PC. n-3 polyunsaturated fatty acids and cytokine production in health and disease. *Ann Nutr Metab.* 1997;41(4):203-234.

37. Complete Prescribing Information - Humira. http://www.rxabbott.com/pdf/humira.pdf. Accessed October 24, 2008.

38. Attie AD, Krauss RM, Gray-Keller MP, et al. Relationship between stearoyl-CoA desaturase activity and plasma triglycerides in human and mouse hypertriglyceridemia. *J Lipid Res.* Nov 2002;43(11):1899-1907.

39. Nayak CD, Nayak DM, Raja A, Rao A. Erythrocyte indicators of oxidative changes in patients with graded traumatic head injury. *Neurol India.* Jan-Mar 2008;56(1):31-35.

40. Das UN. Is obesity an inflammatory condition? *Nutrition.* Nov-Dec 2001;17(11-12):953-966.

41. Aldamiz-Echevarria L, Prieto JA, Andrade F, Elorz J, Sanjurjo P, Rodriguez Soriano J. Arachidonic acid content in adipose tissue is associated with insulin resistance in healthy children. *J Pediatr Gastroenterol Nutr.* Jan 2007;44(1):77-83.

42. Galgani JE, Aguirre CA, Uauy RD, Diaz EO. Plasma arachidonic acid influences insulin-stimulated glucose uptake in healthy adult women. *Ann Nutr Metab.* 2007;51(5):482-489.

43. Adams PB, Lawson S, Sanigorski A, Sinclair AJ. Arachidonic acid to eicosapentaenoic acid ratio in blood correlates positively with clinical symptoms of depression. *Lipids.* Mar 1996;31 Suppl:S157-161.

44. Waldman A, Gilhar A, Duek L, Berdicevsky I. Incidence of Candida in psoriasis--a study on the fungal flora of psoriatic patients. *Mycoses.* May 2001;44(3-4):77-81.

45. Bissonnette R, Ho V, Langley RG. Safety of conventional systemic agents and biologic agents in the treatment of psoriasis. *J Cutan Med Surg.* Sep-Oct 2009;13 Suppl 2:S67-76.

# Arthritis and Other Rheumatic Conditions

*One-in-five adult Americans (46 million) have been diagnosed with some form of arthritis.[2] The most common is osteoarthritis, followed by rheumatoid arthritis (RA) and systemic lupus erythematosis (SLE). The death rate from arthritis and other rheumatic conditions (AORC) rose almost 70% between 1979 and 1998, with significant contribution from autoimmune arthropathies, including RA and SLE. The total cost attributed to AORC was $128 billion in 2003, up almost 48% since 1997.[2] RA, in particular, can be a debilitating condition associated with a potentially devastating progression and a high cost to society. The female-to-male ratio of RA is 3:1, and associated comorbidities include cardiovascular disease, cancer, infection, and osteoporosis. Although the medications used for treatment have improved the quality of life in some RA patients, they are associated with a high risk of complications that include infection, cancer, liver and renal toxicity and bone marrow suppression. Indeed, while the morbidity of RA may be lowered by the new class of biological medications, mortality may be higher.[3, 4]*

## 53-Year-Old Female with Rheumatoid Arthritis and Osteoporosis

| | |
|---|---|
| **Additional Symptoms and Conditions** | Raynaud's phenomenon, fatigue, IBS-constipation, GERD, menopausal symptoms, chronic urinary tract and upper respiratory infections, weight gain |
| **Medications** | Diclofenac and misoprostol (Arthrotec 75®), alendronate with $D_3$ (Fosamax Plus D®), clonidine (Catapres®). Note: Hydroxychloroquine (Plaquenil®), methotrexate, and prednisone had been discontinued by the patient prior to the initial visit. |
| **Tests Used** | Food-specific IgG4 antibodies; multiprofile with plasma amino acids, fatty acids, essential elements and urinary organic acids; antinuclear antibodies, rheumatoid factor, thyroid panel, bone resorption marker, high-sensitivity c-reactive protein |
| **Imbalances Identified** | Multiple food sensitivities, fatty acid imbalances, essential element and amino acid insufficiency, oxidative stress, inflammation, autoimmunity, increased bone resorption, subclinical hypothyroidism |
| **Treatments** | Oligoantigenic anti-inflammatory diet, proteolytic enzymes, essential fatty acids, nutrient IV therapy, GI support therapies, nutrients, thyroid hormone, homeopathic remedy, psychotherapy |
| **Outcome** | Significant improvement in arthritis and all other complaints; medications discontinued; ANA and RF negative; 7.5% improvement in left trochanteric bone density (osteoporotic to osteopenic) |
| **Discussion/ Significance** | This patient presented with multiple, inflammation-driven conditions, of which RA was central. She had developed intolerable side effects from the prescribed RA medication protocol and, against medical advice, had discontinued all but an NSAID. A comprehensive battery of tests was completed to identify underlying imbalances that might have contributed to her condition. Treatment included dietary, nutritional, hormonal and mind/body support. After one year of therapy, the patient experienced significant improvement in, or resolution of, all her symptoms. She discontinued her medications and became proficient in identifying and avoiding the environmental triggers of her disease. Her inflammatory biomarkers were normalized and she experienced a 7.5% improvement in left trochanteric bone density. Further research into this low-risk, effective approach to treating autoimmune arthropathy and osteoporosis is warranted. |

# CASE HISTORY

NV was 53 years old when she presented with a diagnosis of inflammatory arthritis (IA). She complained of nearly constant swelling, stiffness, and pain, with occasional numbness and tingling in her hands, wrists and elbows. At the visit, she reported her pain as 8 (0 = no pain; 10 = greatest pain) and stated that the morning pain was frequently unbearable, rating it as 9 to 10. She was using diclofenac and misoprostol twice a day for pain with minimal relief. Because of the swelling in her fingers, she was unable to wear her wedding ring. Although she noted a worsening of IA symptoms when she ate dairy products, she continued to consume them.

The onset of her IA about 6.5 years earlier coincided with the development of mold in her home's basement after flooding. NV did not know what type of mold it was. She and her husband moved from the home shortly after the start of her symptoms, and she experienced a full remission. Two years later, after the loss of a close aunt, NV experienced a return of all symptoms and was prescribed hydroxychloroquine, methotrexate, and prednisone. She was unable to tolerate the side effects of the medications—effects that she indicated were reflux, photosensitivity, and alopecia. She discontinued the medications against medical advice and refused new medications. NV reported that laboratory results from her last rheumatology appointment showed a pronounced elevation of antinuclear antibodies (ANA) and erythrocyte sedimentation rate (ESR); the rheumatoid factor (RF) was negative. She stated that her ANA had been consistently positive for 4 years.

**The onset of her IA about 6.5 years earlier coincided with the development of mold in her home's basement after flooding. She and her husband moved from the home shortly after the start of her symptoms, and she experienced a full remission.**

NV also reported severe fatigue and rated her energy level at 1 on a scale of 0 to 10, with the afternoons being the most difficult time of day. She awoke feeling tired and unrefreshed, a situation that she attributed to IA and insomnia secondary to hot flashes. Although NV took clonidine for her menopausal hot flashes, which she only experienced at night, it was only mildly helpful. After the onset of her IA, Raynaud's phenomenon developed in both hands and occasionally in the feet upon exposure to cold temperatures.

Additional medical history showed chronic urinary tract infections (UTIs); a recent diagnosis of osteoporosis for which she just started the bisphosphonate medication alendronate with $D_3$; irritable bowel syndrome (IBS) with severe constipation (1 to 2 bowel movements per week); and gastroesophageal reflux disease (GERD). She had gained 30 pounds over the past four years. She had undergone a radical hysterectomy (uterus, ovaries, fallopian tubes, and cervix) due to severe uterine fibroids when she was 32 years old, at which time the hot flashes and insomnia developed. NV had taken multiple antibiotics over the years for UTIs and upper respiratory tract infections.

NV's father, who was alive at age 86, had type 2 diabetes and had experienced two myocardial infarctions in the past. Her mother had died at age 85. Prior to her death, she had undergone three hip replacements to treat severe osteoporosis. Her mother had had a complete thyroidectomy, the need for which NV could not explain.

NV had retired from nursing after 20 years. Training dogs in her spare time was her primary form of exercise. Her father was living in her home, and she was his primary caregiver. While they were very close, she found the caregiving highly stressful. She had a strong marriage and a number of good, supportive friends.

**Although the medications used for treatment have improved the quality of life in some RA patients, they are associated with a high risk of complications that include infection, cancer, liver and renal toxicity and bone marrow suppression.**

NV skipped breakfast, drank black tea daily, and frequently had double cheeseburgers from a fast food restaurant for lunch. Dinner was frequently eaten out, and most recently had included Mexican chicken with rice, chips, and salsa. NV craved salty and sweet foods and drank diet soda daily.

Significant physical examination findings included a blood pressure reading of 112/72. She was was 5'6" tall and weighed 170 lbs. Her body mass index was 27.4. There was marked edema, warmth, and tenderness in her metacarpal phalangeal joints and her proximal interphalangeal joints bilaterally. There was decreased digital flexion due to edema. Her capillary refill rate was normal, and there was no evidence of digital cyanosis or ulceration. Her wrists and elbows were warm, with mild edema and tenderness to palpation; active and passive range of motion was intact, but painful. Her neck was supple, with no masses. Her thyroid was of normal size, smooth, without masses and not tender. Her heart demonstrated a regular rate and rhythm, with no murmurs or rubs noted; her lungs were clear to auscultation bilaterally.

A recent bone densitometry demonstrated left trochanter osteoporosis, with a T-score of -2.7 (a score below -2.5 is indicative of osteoporosis).

## Initial Laboratory Results

**Laboratory tests ordered and rationale:**

1. **Complete blood count, metabolic panel with lipids, and thyroid panel**: Routine laboratory assessments.
2. **Antinuclear antibodies (ANA)**: ANA testing is directed toward nuclear material. ANAs are frequently elevated in inflammatory arthritis and indicate level of disease activity. Useful for tracking treatment efficacy.
3. **Hs-C-reactive protein (hs-CRP)**: hs-CRP is a standard acute phase reactant protein used to monitor general inflammation.
4. **Bone resorption marker (deoxypyridinoline)**: Urine biomarker tracking bone resorption—useful for tracking osteoporosis treatment efficacy
5. **Vitamin D**: Low levels are associated with increased inflammation and with increased incidence of numerous diseases.[5]
6. **Food-specific IgG4 antibodies**: Food reactions have been associated with inflammatory arthritis.[6,7] Multiple IgG4 reactions suggest

intestinal hyperpermeability, also a factor in inflammatory arthritis. Removing offending foods may reduce pain and inflammation.

7. **Multiprofile panel**: A comprehensive assessment including fatty acids, amino acids, organic acids, and oxidative stress markers; assists in detecting individual etiopathogenic factors and in individualizing treatment plans. (Only significant findings are discussed below.)
8. **Stool test**: Assessment of GI microbial status and GI function. GI imbalances have been identified as involved in the pathogenesis of rheumatoid arthritis.[8]

| Test | Results | Reference Limits |
|---|---|---|
| Antinuclear Antibodies | H ANA 1:2860 | < 1:40 titers |
| Hs-CRP | H 5 mg/dL | < 1 mg/dL |
| Rheumatoid Factor | < 14 | < 14 IU/mL |
| 25-Hydroxyvitamin D | 27 | 10–64 ng/mL |
| Thyroid Stimulating Hormone | 1.48 | 0.40–5.50 mIU/L |
| Free T3 | 2.5 | 2.0–4.4 pg/mL |

| | | | |
|---|---|---|---|
| Bone Collagen Peptide (DPD) | 4.9 | 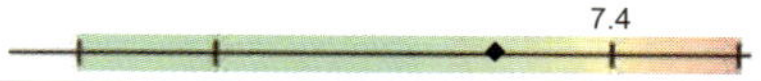 | <= 7.4 |



**Figure 1. Antinuclear antibodies, hs-CRP, rheumatoid factor, vitamin D, deoxypyridinoline (DPD), and thyroid panel.** Results showed elevated antinuclear antibodies and hs-CRP with a suboptimal vitamin D level. (It is recommended that vitamin D levels in complex disease be maintained at 55–70 ng/mL.[9]) Thyroid and urine DPD results were within normal limits. (DPD units: nM/mM creatinine)

| Food-specific IgG antibodies | Results |
|---|---|
| Eggs, casein, milk, rye | Severe (+5) |
| Wheat, malt | Moderate (+3/+4) |
| Yeast, chocolate, broccoli | Mild (+1/+2) |

**Figure 2. Food-specific IgG antibodies.** Test demonstrated multiple reactions suggesting mild intestinal hyperpermeability.

NOTES

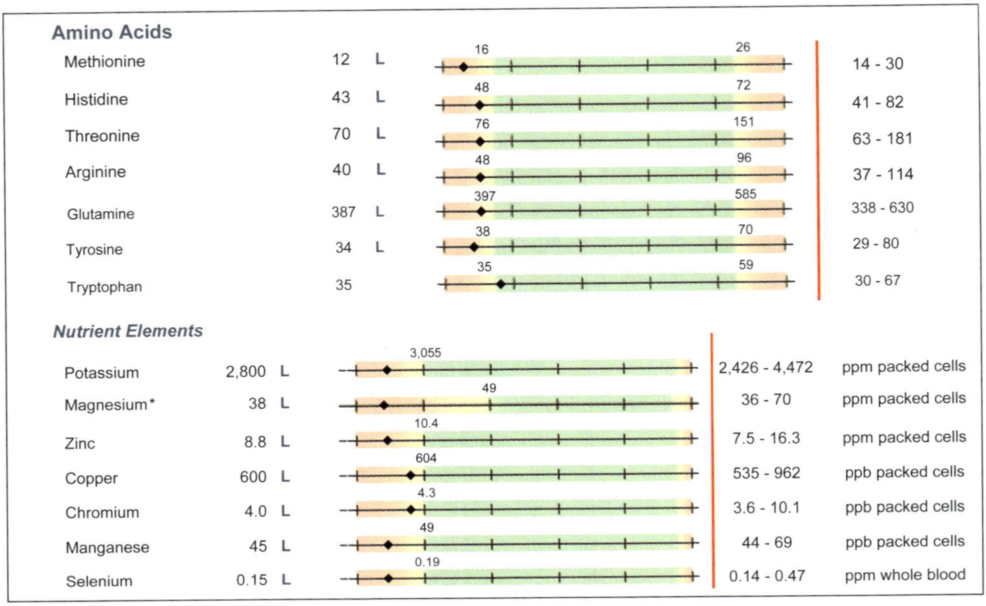


**Figure 3. Amino acids and essential elements.** Low essential and non-essential amino acids and low essential elements. Taken together, these findings can indicate maldigestion and/or malabsorption or poor diet. (Amino acid units: µmol/L)

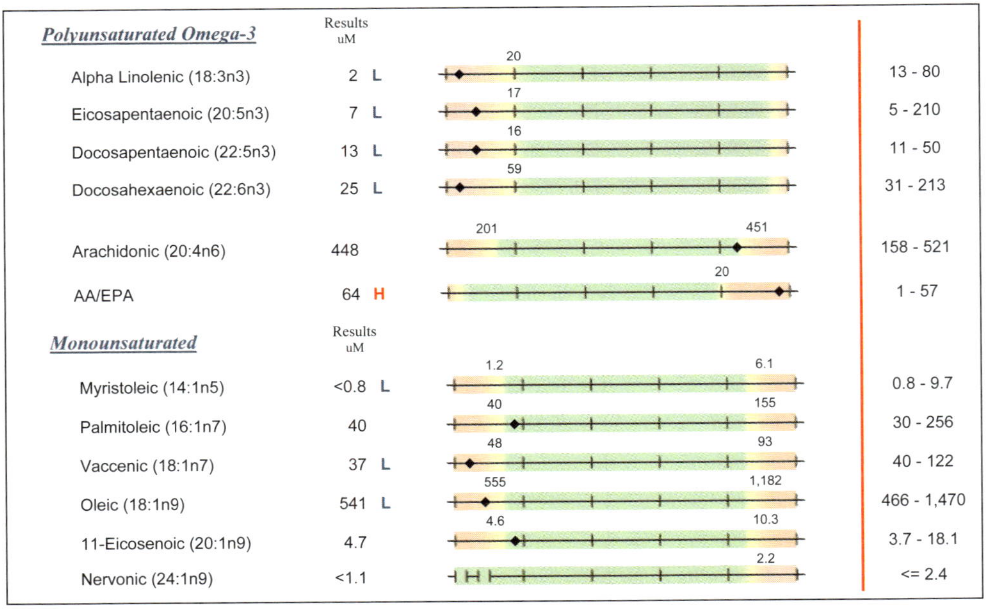


**Figure 4. Plasma fatty acids.** Low omega-3 fatty acids with a relative elevation of the pro-inflammatory omega-6 fatty acid arachidonic acid (AA), which is in the fifth quintile. Imbalance was reflected in the very elevated AA/EPA ratio. The monounsaturated fatty acids were all in the first quintile (low to low normal).

| | | | | |
|---|---|---|---|---|
| Quinolinate | 5.0 | H | 4.0 | <= 5.8 |
| 5-Hydroxyindoleacetate | 2.1 | | 2.1 / 5.6 | 1.6 - 9.8 |
| 8-Hydroxy-2-deoxyguanosine ** | 6.3 | H | 5.3 | <= 7.6 |
| ** Units for 8-Hydroxy-2-deoxyguanosine are ng/mg creatinine | | | | |
| Sulfate | 941 | L | 958 / 2,347 | 690 - 2,988 |
| Pyruvate | 6.2 | H | 3.9 | <= 6.4 |
| a-Ketoglutarate | 23.0 | H | 19.0 | <= 35.0 |
| Succinate | 15.1 | H | 11.6 | <= 20.9 |
| Fumarate | 1.52 | H | 0.59 | <= 1.35 |
| Adipate | 12.0 | H | 5.2 | <= 8.3 |

**Figure 5. Urinary organic acids.** High levels of quinolinate and 8-OHdG with a low level of sulfate suggested increased oxidation and inflammation. 5-Hydroxyindoleacetate, a serotonin metabolite, was low. Both quinolinate and serotonin are derived from tryptophan. Under inflammatory conditions, quinolinate is produced preferentially over serotonin. Fifth quintile elevations of citric acid cycle intermediates (pyruvate, α-ketoglutarate, succinate, fumarate) suggested a mild mitochondropathy, which may be treated with CoQ10. A fifth quintile level of adipate suggested a functional need for carnitine. (Units: µg/mg creatinine; 8OH2-DG: ng/mg cr)

| Stool Test | | Results | Range |
|---|---|---|---|
| Opportunistic aerobic bacteria: | | | |
| Bacillus sp. | | Rare | Negative |
| Enterococcus sp. | | Abundant | Negative |
| Yeast | | +1 Candida sp. | |
| Total sIgA | L | 130 | 400–800 mg% dry weight |
| Chymotrypsin | L | 3 | 4–9 U/10 g |

**Figure 6. Stool analysis and chemistries.** Stool test results demonstrated microbial imbalances consistent with dysbiosis; low secretory IgA and low chymotrypsin.

### Pertinent Negative Laboratory Results

Comprehensive metabolic panel (CMP), lipids, and complete blood count (CBC) were within normal limits.

## Initial Assessment

- Rheumatoid arthritis (RA)
- Osteoporosis
- Raynaud's phenomenon
- Fatigue
- IBS-constipation
- GERD

- Menopausal symptoms
- Chronic urinary tract infections
- Intestinal hyperpermeability
- Multiple food sensitivities
- Inflammation and oxidative stress
- Dysbiosis

**Assessment rationale:** NV's condition had previously been given the less-specific diagnosis of inflammatory arthritis, but her clinical and laboratory findings were consistent with a diagnosis of rheumatoid arthritis as defined by the American Rheumatism Association, even though rheumatoid factor was found negative.[10]

## Initial Plan

- Anti-inflammatory medicinal food, 2 scoops PO QAM
- EPA/DHA concentrate 3000 mg, 1 tsp PO QD
- Vitamin D 1000 IU, 1 cap PO QD
- Proteolytic enzymes, 3–6 tablets PO TID between meals as needed for pain (includes pancreatin, bromelain, papain, trypsin, chymotrypsin, lipase, rutin)
- CoQ10 100 mg, 1 tab PO QD
- L-Carnitine 500 mg, 2 tabs PO QD
- Antimicrobial botanicals, 3 capsules PO BID (includes wormwood, oleuropein, berberine, grapefruit seed extract, thyme, uva ursi extract, black walnut hull extract, oregano extract)
- Plant-based digestive enzymes, 2 tabs with meals
- Nutrient intravenous therapy, 1×/week for 2 months (copper, magnesium, zinc, calcium, selenium, manganese, chromium, essential amino acids, B complex, glutathione, vitamin C)
- Diet: eliminate all moderate to severe food sensitivities; follow anti-inflammatory diet; add green tea, nuts, seeds (raw, organic), olive oil, canola oil, fresh fatty fish including wild-caught salmon and sardines. Eat organic as much as possible. Avoid processed foods.

**Treatment plan rationale:** The initial focus was on reducing inflammation and treating nutrient deficiencies (as identified on laboratory and clinical assessment) specific to the patient. This was achieved by using an anti-inflammatory medicinal food (including antioxidants, vitamins and minerals, hypoallergenic rice protein, glutamine, anti-inflammatory botanicals and active constituents), omega-3 fatty acids EPA and DHA, vitamin D, a proteolytic enzyme compound, which may reduce inflammatory mediators in rheumatic diseases,[11] and an anti-inflammatory oligoantigenic diet based on IgG4 findings. Stool test identified dysbiosis and poor digestion, which were addressed with a botanical antimicrobial compound and digestive enzymes. Nutrients were delivered by IV to achieve rapid repletion. Nutrient IVs may be effective at improving fatigue, a chief complaint of the patient.[12]

## Two-Month Follow-up

After initiating the protocol, NV noted an immediate improvement in energy and pain. Her energy, which had been at 1 on a scale of 0 to 10, was now at 8. Pain level in her hands and elbows, previously reported at 8, was now at 4. She no longer required diclofenac and misoprostol. The swelling of her hands and elbows also diminished and she was able to wear her wedding ring. She reported increased episodes of Raynaud's phenomenon, however, with the onset of winter weather.

**After initiating the protocol, NV noted an immediate improvement in energy and pain...She no longer required diclofenac and misoprostol.**

NV reported that the dietary changes were very hard to make, but that she noticed the benefit of staying off antigenic foods, since her energy, pain, and weight all improved. She reported temporary pain and swelling in her hands after eating take-out Chinese food for dinner one night, although the symptoms abated after one day.

NV also noted a significant reduction in hot flashes with a corresponding improvement in her sleep. She stopped taking clonidine. She was also having a formed bowel movement daily.

NV discontinued her osteoporosis medication alendronate after developing jaw pain three weeks previously. The jaw pain resolved with cessation of the medication.

Although reflux was generally improved, since the GI anti-inflammatory medicinal food caused significant reflux, she stopped taking it. She tolerated the other supplements, however, and enjoyed relaxing while receiving the IV nutrient therapy.

Significant exam findings included reduced swelling in her hands and elbows, with reduced pain during active and passive range of motion. The temporomandibular joints were nontender to palpation with full range of motion intact. Blood pressure read 102/72, left arm seated; temperature 97.9 F; pulse 72 beats per minute; weight 156 lbs (was 170); height 5'6"; BMI 25.2 (it was 27.4).

## Two-Month Follow-up Plan

Continue plan as directed with the following changes:

- Discontinue the anti-inflammatory medicinal food
- For osteoporosis:
  - Add calcitonin 200 IU, 1 spray intranasally QD, alternating nostrils
  - Begin gentle weight-bearing exercise

**Laboratory tests ordered:** Urinary bone collagen peptide (deoxypyridinoline) follow-up

# Five-Month Follow-up

One month previously, NV's father died suddenly from a massive myocardial infarction. He had been living at her house, and she was his primary caregiver. She was in very deep grief at the time of this office visit.

Soon after his death, NV first developed a severe urinary tract infection and then pneumonia. She was treated for both by her primary care physician. She was inconsistent with supplements and dietary changes. Her hands and elbows became painful and swollen and she was once again unable to wear her wedding ring. She also reported a new symptom of joint pain in her left shoulder, which improved with motion. She did not recollect overusing or injuring the area. Her constipation returned. She had difficulty falling asleep at night. She was taking Excedrin PM® for sleep and pain. Her energy level was once again very low.

Significant physical exam findings: EENT and lung exams were unremarkable. Hands and elbows were swollen, tender to palpation and slightly warm. Digital flexion was limited and painful. Left shoulder active range of motion was intact, but painful; there was no swelling or warmth, but area was tender to palpation.

## Five-Month Follow-up Laboratory Results

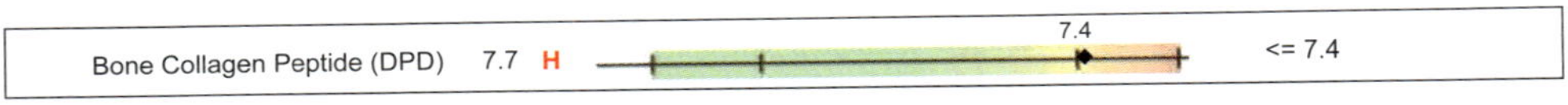


**Figure 7. Deoxypyridinoline (DPD).** DPD was elevated, demonstrating increased bone turnover. This finding was not surprising, because NV had discontinued the alendronate after developing jaw pain. (Units: nM/mM creatinine, urine)

# Five-Month Follow-up Plan

Continue the plan as directed with the following changes:

- Bone health formula, 4 caps PO BID (includes: calcium, magnesium, vitamin D, vitamin $K_2$, strontium, boron, silicon, phosphorus, essential trace minerals, B vitamins, and vitamin C)
- Melatonin 3 mg, 1 tab PO QHS PRN for insomnia
- Homeopathic remedy Ignatia Amara 30c, 3 pellets under tongue away from food, as needed for pain
- Counselor referral
- Laboratory tests ordered: ANA, hs- CRP, rheumatoid factor, CBC, CMP with fasting insulin, TSH, food-specific IgG4 antibodies, organic acids

**Treatment rationale:** In addition to the calcitonin spray, a general bone health nutrient supplement was introduced for the osteoporosis. Weight-bearing exercises were again encouraged. Melatonin was started for insomina, and Ignatia Amara, a homeopathic remedy with a historic use for illnesses related to grief, was initiated. (Ignatia Amara also has some demonstrated efficacy for emotionally-mediated symptoms associated with menopause.[13]) Because NV's emotional response had an immediate and marked impact on her physically, it was suggested that she consult a specialist in mind/body medicine.

## Phone Call

After some limited relief, NV reported a severe exacerbation of her arthritic symptoms. She suspected it resulted from the addition of the bone formula, which contained sodium caseinate as a preservative. She was becoming versed in identifying her triggers, and the milk protein casein was a significant one. She was learning that even very small exposures to the compounds she reacted to could be problematic. When she stopped the bone formula, her symptoms abated in about one day. She noticed a similar reaction to soy sauce. She was started on a caseinate-free bone formula, which she tolerated well.

NV reported a severe exacerbation of her arthritic symptoms. She suspected it resulted from the addition of the bone formula, which contained sodium caseinate as a preservative.

## Six-Month Follow-up

NV reported a general improvement in her arthritis and Raynaud's symptoms, although she stated that the fatigue and constipation continued. She noted that stress and dietary transgressions caused painful flare-ups, particularly in her hands and elbow. When she took the prescribed homeopathic remedy, Ignatia Amara, she experienced hours-long resolution of the pain. The melatonin helped with sleep.

NV continued to grieve the loss of her father. She stated that she was interested in the previously recommended referral to a mind/body therapist, but had not yet pursued it.

### Six-Month Follow-up Laboratory Results

| Test | | Results | Reference Limits |
|---|---|---|---|
| Antinuclear Antibodies | H | 1:2560 | < 1:40 titers |
| Hs-CRP | H | 5.6 | < 1 mg/dL |
| Rheumatoid Factor | H | 24 | < 14 IU/mL |
| Thyroid Stimulating Hormone | | 3.45 | 0.40–5.50 mIU/L |
| Free T3 | | 2.1 | 2.0–4.4 pg/mL |
| IgG food antibodies: | | Severe reactions to: eggs, casein, milk | |

**Figure 8. Antinuclear antibodies (ANA), rheumatoid factor (RF), thyroid stimulating hormone (TSH), free triiodothyronine (free T3), and food- specific IgG4 antibodies.** ANA and hs-CRP were elevated; RF was modestly high for the first time; TSH was above the optimal range of 2.5.[14] These findings reflected IA flare-up. IgG antibodies to eggs and dairy protein continued to be severe.

| Analyte | Result | Flag | Graph markers | Reference range |
|---|---|---|---|---|
| Quinolinate | 2.8 | | 4.0 | <= 5.8 |
| 5-Hydroxyindoleacetate | 2.8 | | 2.1 / 5.6 | 1.6 - 9.8 |
| 8-Hydroxy-2-deoxyguanosine ** | 10.3 | H | 5.3 | <= 7.6 |
| ** Units for 8-Hydroxy-2-deoxyguanosine are ng/mg creatinine | | | | |
| Sulfate | 1,230 | | 958 / 2,347 | 690 - 2,988 |
| Pyruvate | 6.2 | H | 3.9 | <= 6.4 |
| Succinate | 15.1 | H | 11.6 | <= 20.9 |
| Fumarate | 1.32 | H | 0.59 | <= 1.35 |
| Malate | 2.1 | H | 1.4 | <= 3.1 |
| Hydroxymethylglutarate | 5.7 | H | 3.6 | <= 5.1 |

**Figure 9. Urinary organic acids.** Findings showed improved quinolinate and 5-hydroxyindoleacetate, suggesting a reduction in inflammation and improvement in serotonin production. A significant increase in 8-OHdG indicated aggressive oxidative stress. Sulfate and adipate were improved. Citric acid cycle intermediates were still elevated, suggesting a continued need for CoQ10. (Units: ug/mg creatinine except as stated above)

**Pertinent Negative Laboratory Results:**

- CMP, lipids, CBC, and insulin were within normal limits.

# Six-Month Follow-up Plan

Continue supplements with the following changes:

- Resume nutrient intravenous therapy, 1×/week for 2 months
- High-dose probiotic blend 100 billion CFU, ¼ tsp PO QD
- GI botanical and fiber support, 1 scoop per day with water
- Magnesium powder (600 mg elemental magnesium), 1 tsp PO QD
- Armour thyroid 30 mg, 1 tab PO QD taken away from food and other supplements
- Diet review: Continue all prior recommendations. Handout and web resources on hidden sources of food antigens given to patient.

**Laboratory tests ordered (to be completed in 4 to 6 months):** DXA scan (osteoporosis), X-ray series for wrists and hands, ANA, RF, CMP with lipids and fasting insulin, CBC, thyroid panel, and DPD were ordered.

**Treatment rationale:** Intensive nutrient therapy was once again started because of the considerable flare-up and laboratory findings. Fiber and probiotics were initiated for constipation. Low-dose Armour thyroid was introduced for the elevated TSH and clinical symptoms consistent with hypothyroidism.

# One-Year Follow-up Visit

NV spoke repeatedly about her gratitude for "having her life back." All of her symptoms were resolved or improved. She was able to wear her wedding ring most of the time. She was pleased with her 30-pound weight loss, which she attributed to eating the metabolically correct foods for her rather than any calorie restriction. She also stated that she hadn't yet started weight-bearing exercises for her osteoporosis.

NV spoke repeatedly about her gratitude for "having her life back." . . . All of her symptoms were resolved or improved. She was pleased with her 30-pound weight loss, which she attributed to eating the metabolically correct foods for her rather than any calorie restriction.

She was aware of her disease triggers, including foods (eggs, dairy, gluten, and soy); emotions (particularly grief and stress); and physical demands (including overwork).

She visited the therapist who specialized in mind/body medicine, and connected two severe arthritic flare-ups to the loss of her relative and then her father. She hadn't previously realized the extent of the impact of these events on her medical condition.

Because NV recognized many of her arthritis triggers, she felt in control of, rather than a victim of, her RA.

Significant physical exam findings: weight 140 (was 170); BMI 22.6.

She was advised to continue her treatment plan with no changes.

## One-Year Follow-up Laboratory Results

| Test | Initial | Five-Month F/U | One-Year F/U | Reference Range |
|---|---|---|---|---|
| Bone Collagen Peptide (deoxypyridinoline) | 4.9 | H 7.7 | 5.7 | ≤ 7.4 nm/millimole creatinine |
| DXA scan T score (left trochanter) | -2.7 | N/A | -2.5 | +1 to -1 Normal<br>-1 to -2.5 Osteopenia<br>< -2.5: Osteoporosis |

**Figure 10. Bone density and bone resorption results over time.** Initial results were at the initiation of alendronate; five-month follow-up was after cessation of alendronate. The one-year follow-up occurred after seven months of an integrative intervention program of calcitonin, bone support nutrients, general nutrients, and dietary changes. At one year, NV reported that she had not yet followed through with weight-bearing exercises. BMD showed improvement from baseline by 7.5%, which is comparable to the results of a three to four year course of alendronate therapy.[15, 16]

NOTES

| Test | Initial | Six-Month F/U | One-Year F/U | Reference Range |
|---|---|---|---|---|
| Antinuclear Antibodies | H 1:2860 | H 1:2560 | < 1:40 | < 1:40 |
| Rheumatoid Factor | N/A | H 24 | < 14 | < 14 IU/mL |
| Thyroid Stimulating Hormone | 1.48 | 3.45 | 0.85 | 0.40–5.50 mIU/L |
| Free T3 | 2.5 | 2.1 | 2.7 | 2.0–4.4 pg/mL |

**Figure 11. Antinuclear antibodies, rheumatoid factor, thyroid stimulating hormone and free triiodothyronine (T3) over time.** Values were normal or improved at one-year follow-up. The patient noted that it was the first time ANA had been normal in six years.

### Additional Laboratory Results

- X-ray series of wrists and hands were unremarkable, except both wrists were noted to be osteopenic.
- Comprehensive metabolic panel (CMP), lipids, insulin, and complete blood count (CBC) were within normal limits.

## DISCUSSION

The pathophysiology of RA has been suggested to involve an initiation phase of nonspecific inflammation caused by a variety of stimuli, followed first by an amplification phase caused by Th1 cell activation, and then by a chronic inflammatory stage with active tissue injury.[17] Recent research suggests RA shares a trio of key pathogenic mechanisms with celiac disease and other autoimmune conditions. The trio includes: a genetic predisposition, exposure to environmental antigen(s), and intestinal hyperpermeability (IP). IP is caused in part by the protein zonulin, production of which is induced by the environmental antigen.[8] RA candidate genes include *HLA DRB1, PTPN22, CTLA4,* and *PADI4.*[18]

Recent research suggests RA shares a trio of key pathogenic mechanisms with celiac disease and other autoimmune conditions. The trio includes: a genetic predisposition, exposure to environmental antigen(s), and intestinal hyperpermeability.

In this case, NV's family medical history and her own complaints (RA, IBS, Raynaud's phenomenon, GERD, osteoporosis) all shared a strong inflammatory component. Her mother had thyroid disease, which is most commonly autoimmune, although the clinical specifics were unknown. The mother also had severe osteoporosis and the father had heart disease. RA patients have increased risk of both cardiovascular disease and osteoporosis.[19] Inflammation-mediated osteoclastic activity in RA induces osteoporosis.[20] Autoimmune thyroiditis and Raynaud's phenomenon have been associated with RA, and may all involve eicosanoid dysregulation.[21-25]

There were a number of environmental exposures that NV experienced that likely contributed to RA pathogenesis. Most prominent were mold and high emotional stress, both recognized as RA triggers.[26,27] Others include foods, smoking,[28] toxins,[29] obesity[30] and infection.[31] Long-standing gastrointestinal inflammation is often antecedent to RA. NV had a history of chronic antibiotic use, which is associated with altered intestinal flora[32] and thought to be an etiologic factor in inflammatory arthritis.[33] Food sensitivities, of which NV had many, are associated with IBS[34] and intestinal hyperpermeability. Both have been proposed as factors contributing to the pathogenesis of RA.[8, 35, 36]

Laboratory evaluation in this case was broad, reflecting the molecular complexity of the conditions and the web of metabolic interactions. In addition to standard autoimmune biomarkers, investigation was made into gastrointestinal function, microbiota imbalances, food-specific IgG4 antibodies, organic and fatty acids, and micronutrient status.

In Figure 1, the initial battery of testing demonstrated that antinuclear antibody (ANA) levels were elevated, which was to be expected; NV had discontinued hydroxychloroquine, methotrexate, and prednisone, and she was in an active disease phase. Elevated ANAs indicate that damage was occurring in the joint space, an indication reflected clinically in the pain and swelling of her hands and elbows. Her vitamin D level was shown to be suboptimal. (Vitamin D insufficiency is associated with inflammatory arthropathies.[9, 37]) Some suggest that vitamin D levels in complex disease be maintained at 55 to 70 ng/mL.[9] The level of deoxypyridinoline (DPD), a well-regarded biomarker demonstrating bone resorption, has been shown to be correlated with increased bone turnover in RA.[38, 39] In this case, however, it appeared that NV's treatment with alendronate was sufficient to inhibit excess turnover, as her DPD level was within normal limits. Thyroid stimulating hormone (TSH) and free triiodothyronine (fT3) levels were within normal limits. Because of the known association of thyroid disorders and RA, regular assessment was indicated.[21, 40]

As discussed, NV had a number of food-specific IgG4 antibodies (Figure 2), which have been identified in RA and which suggest intestinal hyperpermeability.[8, 35, 36] Given the association with celiac disease,[8, 23] a celiac panel would have been a reasonable assessment to consider in this patient, particularly given the severe IgG4 reaction to wheat.

NV's amino acid panel (Figure 3) demonstrated a number of low values that may have had a negative impact on important metabolic activities. Methionine (met), the only essential sulfur-containing amino acid, was well below normal limits, suggesting deficiency. In one animal study, it was demonstrated that met deficiency limited the production of sulfur-containing compounds including glutathione and sulfate, particularly during high detoxification demand.[41] The impact of low met in NV was suggested by the low urinary sulfate and the increased oxidative stress marker, 8-OHdG (Figure 5). Taken together, these imbalances suggested insufficient glutathione, possibly due to increased utilization. Glutathione also requires glycine and glutamate, which may be derived from threonine and glutamine, which were also low. (Glutamine is a potent anti-inflammatory amino acid, modulating systemic and gastrointestinal cytokines, and increasing production of glutathione.[42]) Tyrosine was in the first quintile. (Derived from phenylalanine, tyrosine is the precursor to thyroid hormones and catecholamines.) Given the importance of these hormones in energy production, tyrosine insufficiency may have been contributing to NV's fatigue. The tryptophan level was also in the first quintile, whereas the tryptophan derivative quinolinate (Figure 5) was elevated. Chronic elevation of quinolinate, an IFNγ-induced CNS inflammatory mediator with significant neurotoxic potential[43], has been associated with tryptophan and serotonin depletion.[44]

NV's red blood cell essential element levels were uniformly low normal (Figure 3). Toxic exposure, malabsorption, maldigestion, or insufficient intake may be causal factors.[45] Inadequate essential element status can have far-reaching effects, compromising optimal physiological function system-wide. Indeed, Table 1 on page 90 shows essential element involvement to be among the top causes of death in the United States. Specific to NV, an inverse association between erythrocyte (and plasma) magnesium levels and superoxide dismutase was found in inflammatory arthritis, increasing oxidative stress.[46]

The pathogenesis of RA is closely associated with the pro-inflammatory eicosanoids derived from arachidonic acid (AA) including prostaglandins, thromboxanes and leukotrienes.[47, 48] High-dose fish oil containing adequate amounts of eicosapentaenoic (EPA) and docosahexaenoic (DHA) acids has been shown to inhibit the AA-derived eicosanoids, thereby diminishing inflammation.[48] AA-derived inflammatory mediators are also implicated in NV's other complaints, including osteoporosis, Raynaud's phenomenon, and IBS.[22, 23, 49-51] NV's AA was high relative to the omega-3 fatty acids, particularly EPA (Figure 4); that elevated AA/EPA ratio reflects the imbalance between the pro- and anti-inflammatory fatty acids.

**Laboratory evaluation in this case was broad, reflecting the molecular complexity of the conditions and the web of metabolic interactions.**

The monounsaturated fatty acids (MUFA) were low to low normal (Figure 4). Benefits of MUFA intake include improved membrane fluidity, reduced cardiovascular risk, and reduced inflammation. The Mediterranean diet, which is rich in MUFAs, was shown to reduce pain, early morning stiffness, and systolic blood pressure in a small pilot study of women with RA.[52] Intake of oleic acid, the main constituent in olive oil, is inversely correlated with the level of C-reactive protein (CRP).[53]

As mentioned above, quinolinate was elevated in NV (Figure 5). Quinolinate is a neuroinflammatory compound, produced in response to the Th1-derived cytokine IFN$\gamma$, which is in turn stimulated by tumor necrosis factor-alpha (TNF-$\alpha$). Both of these cytokines are elevated in the synovium of RA patients, and participate in the pathogenesis of the disease.[54] Quinolinate agonizes glutamatergic NMDA receptors in the central nervous system. Chronic elevation is considered excitotoxic and oxidative, and is associated with a number of neurodegenerative conditions, including Alzheimer and Parkinson diseases and amyotrophic lateral sclerosis.[43, 55] Chronic elevation of quinolinate is also associated with depression because excessive tryptophan catabolism leads to reduced serotonin availability.[56] This scenario is suggested in the case of NV, where, in addition to the quinolinate elevation, the serotonin metabolite 5-hydroxyindoleacetate (Figure 5) and plasma tryptophan (Figure 3) were low. Given the level of inflammatory activity, it isn't surprising that the 8-OHdG is elevated, indicating oxidative stress. In RA patients, 8-OHdG has been shown to be correlated with the inflammatory marker CRP.[57] Increased glutathione utilization secondary to oxidative stress may result in depleted sulfate and methionine, as shown in Figures 3 and 5.

Adipate is produced when there is a compromise in mitochondrial $\beta$-oxidation of fatty acids (Figure 5). Its elevation may indicate a need for carnitine, which shuttles fatty acids into the mitochondria in the form of carnitine acyltransferase for the production of metabolic energy. At her initial visit, NV reported a 30-pound weight gain and fatigue, both of which may have been due, in part, to compromised fatty acid metabolism. Organic acid assessment also revealed an accumulation of citric acid cycle (CAC) intermediates, providing functional evidence for a CoQ10 deficiency. Accumulation of the CAC intermediates, adipate, and 8OHdG suggested subclinical mitochondropathy.

Gastrointestinal bacterial overgrowth was evidenced by the presence of opportunistic organisms in NV's stool test (Figure 6). Low stool IgA suggested either a genetic deficiency or protracted GI inflammation. GI inflammation was also reflected in the food sensitivities, of which NV had many (Figure 2). Chymotrypsin insufficiency suggested poor pancreatic output, leading to compromised macronutrient digestion.[58] Maldigestion may have contributed to insufficiency in amino acids and essential elements (Figure 3).

The initial plan was designed to treat systemic and GI inflammation and support nutrient repletion, using EPA and DHA, a gastrointestinal anti-inflammatory medicinal food, vitamin D, and a nutrient-dense oligoantigenic diet with MUFA. Additionally, proteolytic enzymes were given to help reduce the inflammatory proteins associated with RA.[11] Nutrients were given as indicated in the initial evaluation: CoQ10, carnitine, and high-dose nutrient IV therapy with minerals, amino acids, B vitamins, vitamin C and glutathione. Antimicrobial botanicals were used to reduce the number of opportunistic bacteria in the lower GI.

**Quinolinate is a neuroinflammatory compound, produced in response to the Th1-derived cytokine INFγ, which is in turn stimulated by tumor necrosis factor-alpha (TNF-α). Both of these cytokines are elevated in the synovium of RA patients, and participate in the pathogenesis of the disease.**

After two months of therapy, NV noticed a remarkable improvement in pain, stiffness, and swelling in her hands, elbows and wrist. Her pain level, previously 8 out of 10, was now 4. She stopped using the NSAID. Her energy, hot flashes, sleep and IBS had improved. She was having a normal bowel movement daily. Her GERD was greatly improved. She reported a 14-pound weight loss. NV had started to experience temporomandibular pain with the alendronate and chose to stop taking the medication. The Raynaud's phenomenon continued.

A follow-up DPD was ordered at the two-month visit to establish bone resorption activity after cessation of the alendronate, and its level was found to be high (Figure 7). Intranasal calcitonin was introduced for initial osteoporosis therapy.

At five months, NV reported a significant increase in symptoms thought to be due to the death of her father one month previously. NV had experienced a similar health crisis with the death of another close relative 4.5 years before. Emotional grief was a powerful trigger in her disease process. In addition to an RA flare-up, she also developed a urinary tract infection and pneumonia. Both were treated with antibiotics. Because of overwhelming grief, she was inconsistent with her diet and supplements during this time. Her sleep was very poor. NV's revised treatment plan included a homeopathic remedy, Ignatia Amara, which has been used successfully in the treatment of emotionally-mediated symptoms associated with menopause.[13] A referral to a mind/body counselor was also made for support. She was started on a bone health nutrient formula for osteoporosis and melatonin as needed for insomnia. A battery of laboratory tests was ordered.

NV called to report that an initial improvement in symptoms was offset shortly thereafter by a flare-up. She suspected the probable cause to be the bone nutrient formula, which contained sodium caseinate. A supplement elimination and reintroduction trial confirmed her suspicion. A similar, casein-free bone support product was started and was tolerated well.

Figure 8 showed elevated ANA and a positive rheumatoid factor (RF). NV reported that she had never been RF+. TSH had increased to 3.45. Optimal TSH is considered to be 2.5; and may be as low as 1.18.[14] Free T3 remained low normal. Food sensitivities had diminished, although she continued to have severe reactions to eggs, casein, and cow's milk. The laboratory results reflected the decline in NV's health following the death of her father.

A significant increase in 8-OHdG indicated aggressive oxidative stress (Figure 9). 8OHdG levels are correlated with the inflammatory marker CRP in RA patients. The elevation also corroborated her clinical decline. Interestingly, however, the QUIN level was now within normal limits, and, as a consequence, tryptophan was available for serotonin production, as reflected in the normalized 5-HIAA. Sulfate and adipate had normalized. Citric acid cycle intermediates were still elevated, suggesting a continued need for CoQ10. Treatment was revised to improve antioxidant and nutrient status by means of IV nutrient therapy, GI function with fiber, high-dose probiotics, and magnesium powder, and to improve thyroid function by means of Armour thyroid. Dietary restrictions and previously prescribed supplements were continued. Laboratory tests were ordered for completion in 4 to 6 months.

BMD improved from baseline level by 7.5%, which is comparable to a result gained from three to four years of alendronate therapy.

At her one-year follow-up visit, NV's symptoms were largely resolved. She was aware of her disease triggers, including foods (eggs, dairy, gluten, and soy); emotions (particularly grief and stress); and physical demands (including overwork). She had experienced a total weight loss of 30 pounds, with which she was pleased. In general, she felt in control of, rather than a victim of, her condition.

Figure 10 shows improvement in DXA scan and DPD over time. Her bone density was now osteopenic (left trochanter T score -2.7 to -2.5) and her DPD level was normal. BMD improved from baseline level by 7.5%, which is comparable to a result gained from three to four years of alendronate therapy.[15, 16] It is interesting to note that her BMD level improved despite the fact that NV had never taken hormone replacement therapy, despite a radical hysterectomy, and did not follow through with the plan of weight-bearing exercises (WBE). It is likely that her BMD level would improve further if she engaged in WBE. ANA and RF were now undetectable; thyroid function was good (Figure 11). Figure 11 shows an impressive normalization of laboratory values over time.

---

NOTES

# CONCLUSION

In this case, the patient presented with inflammatory arthritis of almost seven years' duration. She described the pain in her hands, wrists and elbows as frequently unbearable, rating it 8 to 10 most of the time. However, she experienced intolerable side effects from the medications she was prescribed, including reflux, alopecia and severe photosensitivity. Thus, despite the extreme pain, swelling, and stiffness caused by the RA, she discontinued two of her medications, hydroxychloroquine and methotrexate, against medical advice. Her other complaints included osteoporosis, Raynaud's phenomenon, fatigue, IBS-constipation, GERD, menopausal symptoms, chronic urinary tract and upper respiratory infections, and weight gain.

A comprehensive laboratory evaluation identified multiple IgG4 food-specific antibodies, essential fatty acid and amino acid imbalances, nutrient and essential element deficiencies, and dysbiosis in addition to elevated antinuclear antibody, hs-CRP and rheumatoid factor levels. Clinical history identified the onset of RA as being associated with mold exposure. Significant RA flare-ups were associated with the loss of a loved one. Treatment based on laboratory findings included reducing inflammation, eliminating food sensitivities, restoring nutrient status and GI balance. Emotional support was also a significant aspect of treatment. Over time, the patient became versed in identifying and minimizing her RA triggers, which included foods, food preservatives, and emotional stress.

After one year of therapy, the patient experienced significant resolution of all symptoms and discontinued her medication. Her inflammatory biomarkers became normalized and she experienced improvement in bone density. This safe, cost-effective, systems-based approach to treating autoimmune arthropathy and osteoporosis may be effective for others with similar presentations.

---

**Author: Kara Fitzgerald, ND**
**Case Clinician: Kara Fitzgerald, ND**

## References

1. AARDA. Autoimmune Disease Fact Sheet. http://www.aarda.org/autoimmune_statistics.php. Accessed 01-14-10, 2010.
2. CDC. Arthritis. http://www.cdc.gov/arthritis/data_statistics/arthritis_related_stats.htm. Accessed 3/15/10.
3. Fauci AS. *Harrison's principles of internal medicine / editors, Anthony S. Fauci ... [et al.]. 17th ed. New York: McGraw-Hill Medical; 2008. p. 2083.*
4. Naz SM, Symmons DP. Mortality in established rheumatoid arthritis. *Best Pract Res Clin Rheumatol. Oct 2007;21(5):871-883.*
5. Holick MF. Vitamin D deficiency. *N Engl J Med. Jul 19 2007;357(3):266-281.*
6. Danao-Camara TC, Shintani TT. The dietary treatment of inflammatory arthritis: case reports and review of the literature. *Hawaii Med J. May 1999;58(5):126-131.*
7. Panush RS, Webster EM, Endo LP, Greer JM, Woodard JC. Food induced ("allergic") arthritis: inflammatory synovitis in rabbits. *J Rheumatol. Mar 1990;17(3):285-290.*
8. Fasano A. Surprises from celiac disease. *Sci Am. Aug 2009;301(2):54-61.*
9. Cannell JJ, Hollis BW. Use of vitamin D in clinical practice. *Altern Med Rev. Mar 2008;13(1):6-20.*

10. Rindfleisch JA, Muller D. Diagnosis and management of rheumatoid arthritis. *Am Fam Physician. Sep 15 2005;72(6):1037-1047.*

11. Leipner J, Iten F, Saller R. Therapy with proteolytic enzymes in rheumatic disorders. *BioDrugs. 2001;15(12):779-789.*

12. Gaby AR. Intravenous nutrient therapy. *Altern Ther Health Med. Jul-Aug 2007;13(4):14.*

13. Wasilewski BW. Homeopathic remedies as placebo alternatives--verification on the example of treatment of menopause-related vegetative and emotional disturbances. *Sci Eng Ethics. Jan 2004;10(1):179-188.*

14. Wartofsky L, Dickey RA. The evidence for a narrower thyrotropin reference range is compelling. *J Clin Endocrinol Metab. Sep 2005;90(9):5483-5488.*

15. Center JR, Nguyen TV, Schneider D, Sambrook PN, Eisman JA. Mortality after all major types of osteoporotic fracture in men and women: an observational study. *Lancet. Mar 13 1999;353(9156):878-882.*

16. Kado DM, Browner WS, Palermo L, Nevitt MC, Genant HK, Cummings SR. Vertebral fractures and mortality in older women: a prospective study. Study of Osteoporotic Fractures Research Group. *Arch Intern Med. Jun 14 1999;159(11):1215-1220.*

17. Fauci AS. *Harrison's principles of internal medicine / editors, Anthony S. Fauci ... [et al.]. 17th ed. New York: McGraw-Hill Medical; 2008. p.2086.*

18. Plenge RM, Padyukov L, Remmers EF, et al. Replication of putative candidate-gene associations with rheumatoid arthritis in >4,000 samples from North America and Sweden: association of susceptibility with PTPN22, CTLA4, and PADI4. *Am J Hum Genet. Dec 2005;77(6):1044-1060.*

19. McInnes IB, Gracie JA. Targeting cytokines beyond tumor necrosis factor-alpha and interleukin-1 in rheumatoid arthritis. *Curr Pain Headache Rep. Dec 2005;9(6):405-411.*

20. Korczowska I, Olewicz-Gawlik A, Trefler J, Hrycaj P, Krzysztof Lacki J. Does low-dose and short-term glucocorticoids treatment increase the risk of osteoporosis in rheumatoid arthritis female patients? *Clin Rheumatol. May 2008;27(5):565-572.*

21. Ginaldi L, Di Benedetto MC, De Martinis M. Osteoporosis, inflammation and ageing. *Immun Ageing. Nov 4 2005;2:14.*

22. Hata T, Kavanaugh A. Rheumatoid arthritis in dermatology. *Clin Dermatol. Sep-Oct 2006;24(5):430-437.*

23. Maksymowych WP, Brown MA. Genetics of ankylosing spondylitis and rheumatoid arthritis: where are we at currently, and how do they compare? *Clin Exp Rheumatol. Jul-Aug 2009;27(4 Suppl 55):S20-25.*

24. Cooke JP, Marshall JM. Mechanisms of Raynaud's disease. *Vasc Med. Nov 2005;10(4):293-307.*

25. Boilard E, Nigrovic PA, Larabee K, et al. Platelets amplify inflammation in arthritis via collagen-dependent microparticle production. *Science. Jan 29;327(5965):580-583.*

26. Stojanovich L, Marisavljevich D. Stress as a trigger of autoimmune disease. *Autoimmun Rev. Jan 2008;7(3):209-213.*

27. Luosujarvi RA, Husman TM, Seuri M, et al. Joint symptoms and diseases associated with moisture damage in a health center. *Clin Rheumatol. Dec 2003;22(6):381-385.*

28. Kallberg H, Padyukov L, Plenge RM, et al. Gene-gene and gene-environment interactions involving HLA-DRB1, PTPN22, and smoking in two subsets of rheumatoid arthritis. *Am J Hum Genet. May 2007;80(5):867-875.*

29. Khuder SA, Peshimam AZ, Agraharam S. Environmental risk factors for rheumatoid arthritis. *Rev Environ Health. Oct-Dec 2002;17(4):307-315.*

30. Pedersen M, Jacobsen S, Klarlund M, et al. Environmental risk factors differ between rheumatoid arthritis with and without auto-antibodies against cyclic citrullinated peptides. *Arthritis Res Ther. 2006;8(4):R133.*

31. Mehraein Y, Lennerz C, Ehlhardt S, Remberger K, Ojak A, Zang KD. Latent Epstein-Barr virus (EBV) infection and cytomegalovirus (CMV) infection in synovial tissue of autoimmune chronic arthritis determined by RNA- and DNA-in situ hybridization. *Mod Pathol. Jul 2004;17(7):781-789.*

32. Jernberg C, Lofmark S, Edlund C, Jansson JK. Long-term ecological impacts of antibiotic administration on the human intestinal microbiota. *Isme J. May 2007;1(1):56-66.*

33. Tlaskalova-Hogenova H, Stepankova R, Hudcovic T, et al. Commensal bacteria (normal microflora), mucosal immunity and chronic inflammatory and autoimmune diseases. *Immunol Lett. May 15 2004;93(2-3):97-108.*

34. Drisko J, Bischoff B, Hall M, McCallum R. Treating irritable bowel syndrome with a food elimination diet followed by food challenge and probiotics. *J Am Coll Nutr. Dec 2006;25(6):514-522.*

35. Hvatum M, Kanerud L, Hallgren R, Brandtzaeg P. The gut-joint axis: cross reactive food antibodies in rheumatoid arthritis. *Gut. Sep 2006;55(9):1240-1247.*

36. Nissinen R, Leirisalo-Repo M, Nieminen AM, et al. Immune activation in the small intestine in patients with rheumatoid arthritis. *Ann Rheum Dis. Oct 2004;63(10):1327-1330.*

37. Cantorna MT, Mahon BD. Mounting evidence for vitamin D as an environmental factor affecting autoimmune disease prevalence. *Exp Biol Med (Maywood). Dec 2004;229(11):1136-1142.*

38. Kameyama O, Nakahigashi Y, Nakao H, Uejima D, Tsuji H. Activity of rheumatoid arthritis and urinary pyridinoline and deoxypyridinoline. *J Orthop Sci. 2000;5(4):385-389.*

39. Yasunori K, Masaaki T, Tetsuyuki N, Hayato K, Akira N. Reduction of urinary levels of pyridinoline and deoxypyridinoline and serum levels of soluble receptor activator of NF-kappaB ligand by etanercept in patients with rheumatoid arthritis. *Clin Rheumatol. Sep 2008;27(9):1093-1101.*

40. Yazar M, Sarban S, Kocyigit A, Isikan UE. Synovial fluid and plasma selenium, copper, zinc, and iron concentrations in patients with rheumatoid arthritis and osteoarthritis. *Biol Trace Elem Res. Aug 2005;106(2):123-132.*

41. Reicks MM, Hathcock JN. Effects of methionine deficiency and ethanol ingestion on acetaminophen metabolism in mice. *J Nutr. Mar 1987;117(3):572-579.*

42. Wischmeyer PE. Can glutamine turn off the motor that drives systemic inflammation? *Crit Care Med. May 2005;33(5):1175-1178.*

43. Guillemin GJ, Smith DG, Smythe GA, Armati PJ, Brew BJ. Expression of the kynurenine pathway enzymes in human microglia and macrophages. *Adv Exp Med Biol. 2003;527:105-112.*

44. Muller N, Schwarz MJ. The immune-mediated alteration of serotonin and glutamate: towards an integrated view of depression. *Mol Psychiatry. Nov 2007;12(11):988-1000.*

45. Lord RS, Bralley JA. Laboratory Evaluations for Integrative and Functional Medicine. 2nd ed. Duluth, GA: Metametrix Institute; 2008:68.

46. Tuncer S, Kamanli A, Akcil E, Kavas GO, Seckin B, Atay MB. Trace element and magnesium levels and superoxide dismutase activity in rheumatoid arthritis. *Biol Trace Elem Res. May 1999;68(2):137-142.*

47. Sharma JN, Mohammed LA. The role of leukotrienes in the pathophysiology of inflammatory disorders: is there a case for revisiting leukotrienes as therapeutic targets? *Inflammopharmacology. Mar 2006;14(1-2):10-16.*

48. Calder PC. n-3 polyunsaturated fatty acids, inflammation, and inflammatory diseases. *Am J Clin Nutr. Jun 2006;83(6 Suppl):1505S-1519S.*

49. Werz O. Inhibition of 5-lipoxygenase product synthesis by natural compounds of plant origin. *Planta Med. Oct 2007;73(13):1331-1357.*

50. Imir AG, Lin Z, Yin P, et al. Aromatase expression in uterine leiomyomata is regulated primarily by proximal promoters I.3/II. *J Clin Endocrinol Metab. May 2007;92(5):1979-1982.*

51. Kilkens TO, Honig A, Maes M, Lousberg R, Brummer RJ. Fatty acid profile and affective dysregulation in irritable bowel syndrome. *Lipids. May 2004;39(5):425-431.*

52. McKellar G, Morrison E, McEntegart A, et al. A pilot study of a Mediterranean-type diet intervention in female patients with rheumatoid arthritis living in areas of social deprivation in Glasgow. *Ann Rheum Dis. Sep 2007;66(9):1239-1243.*

53. Yoneyama S, Miura K, Sasaki S, et al. Dietary intake of fatty acids and serum C-reactive protein in Japanese. *J Epidemiol. May 2007;17(3):86-92.*

54. Okamoto H, Cujec TP, Yamanaka H, Kamatani N. Molecular aspects of rheumatoid arthritis: role of transcription factors. *Febs J. Jul 24 2008.*

55. Guillemin GJ, Smythe G, Takikawa O, Brew BJ. Expression of indoleamine 2,3-dioxygenase and production of quinolinic acid by human microglia, astrocytes, and neurons. *Glia. Jan 1 2005;49(1):15-23.*

56. Maes M, Mihaylova I, Ruyter MD, Kubera M, Bosmans E. The immune effects of TRYCATs (tryptophan catabolites along the IDO pathway): relevance for depression - and other conditions characterized by tryptophan depletion induced by inflammation. *Neuro Endocrinol Lett. Dec 2007;28(6):826-831.*

57. Kageyama Y, Takahashi M, Ichikawa T, Torikai E, Nagano A. Reduction of oxidative stress marker levels by anti-TNF-alpha antibody, infliximab, in patients with rheumatoid arthritis. *Clin Exp Rheumatol. Jan-Feb 2008;26(1):73-80.*

58. Dominguez Munoz JE. Diagnosis of chronic pancreatitis: Functional testing. *Best Pract Res Clin Gastroenterol. Jun 2010;24(3):233-241.*

# 3 Behavioral and Neuro-developmental Conditions

## Autism Spectrum Disorders

*Autism spectrum disorders (ASDs) are collectively the most commonly diagnosed pediatric neurodevelopmental condition. ASDs include autism, pervasive developmental disorder–not otherwise specified (PDD-NOS), Rett syndrome and Asperger disorder. ASD is characterized by impaired communication and social interaction and may involve developmental delays and seizure disorders. Recent parent-reported diagnosis of ASD in the United States put it at higher levels (1:91) than previously thought, with its diagnosis in boys occurring four to five times more frequently than in girls (1:58).[1] CDC estimates are currently 1:110;[1] up from 1:150 in 2007.[2] Annual medical expenditures for those affected are generally four to six times greater than for those without ASD.[1] While twin studies demonstrate that genetics play a significant role in ASD, the impact of environment should not be underestimated, given the approximate 20-fold increase in incidence over the last 20 years.[3]*

### 2.5-Year-Old Male with Pervasive Developmental Disorder

| | |
|---|---|
| **Additional Symptoms and Conditions** | Irritable bowel syndrome, irritability, skin rash |
| **Tests Used** | Complete blood count and metabolic panel, food-specific IgE and IgG antibodies, multiprofile panel (fatty acids, amino acids, organic acids, essential and toxic elements, lipid-soluble vitamins, and oxidative stress markers), functional stool test, celiac panel, genetic testing, urinary polypeptides, urine toxic elements test |
| **Imbalances Identified** | Lactic acidosis, bacterial and fungal dysbiosis, GI inflammation, polypeptide elevations, anti-gliadin antibodies, IgG food reactions, intestinal hyperpermeability, fatty acid imbalance, oxidative stress, glutathione-s-transferase enzyme mutation, methylation and sulfuration lesions, subclinical mitochondropathy, essential element deficiencies |
| **Treatments** | High-dose probiotics, digestive enzyme, cod liver oil, multivitamin and mineral powder, zinc and magnesium, methylation support nutrients, rifaximin (Xifaxan®), nystatin; gluten and dairy-free diet, avoid IgG sensitivities |
| **Outcome** | At ten months, in mainstream nursery school, indistinguishable from the other children |
| **Discussion/ Significance** | This child's response to treatment, while remarkable, is not considered unusual among clinicians using what is described as a biomedical approach.[4-6] Given the rapidly rising incidence of this disorder,[3] research evaluating the efficacy of the biomedical approach to treating ASD is warranted. |

# CASE HISTORY

TL was 2.5 years old when he presented with a recent diagnosis of regressive pervasive developmental disorder-not otherwise specified (PDD-NOS). PDD-NOS falls into the autistic spectrum of disorders (ASD) and is sometimes referred to as atypical autism. According to his parents, TL's symptoms began at age 22 months, shortly after receiving the measles, mumps, and rubella (MMR) vaccine. TL was previously meeting normal developmental milestones and had a vocabulary of 20 words. He was a happy and responsive baby, who smiled regularly. Over the months since the vaccine, TL had developed aphasia, was irritable and intolerant of certain sensory stimuli, and had difficulty maintaining eye contact, interacting with others, or responding to his name. He developed foul-smelling bowel movements (BMs), itchy ears, dark circles under his eyes, and red blotchy skin. He refused all but soft-textured foods.

**It is believed by many clinicians and researchers that autism pathogenesis consists of a complex interplay between genetics (including polymorphisms in detoxification and biotransformation enzymes), environmental exposures, and imbalanced immune response.**

Comprehensive neuropsychiatric and developmental evaluations were conducted (listed below). Based on the results, full-time special education with speech and occupational therapy was recommended.

While pregnant with TL, his mother consumed tuna regularly and had two amalgams. They lived in a large east coast city, in an apartment building known to have lead paint. The building also required periodic insect exterminations, although never in the family's own unit.

TL's delivery was by emergency cesarean section at 36 weeks because of placental abruption. His birth weight was 6 lbs, 10 oz, and his Apgar score was normal. TL was breastfed for 3 months until he developed colic with severe bloating. He was switched to Enfamil. It was later determined that he was dairy intolerant. Gerber rice cereal was introduced at 6 months, followed by Cheerios (indicating possible gluten exposure). TL suffered from frequent colds and diaper rash and had a month-long stomach virus invoking much vomiting and diarrhea. TL followed a full pediatric vaccine schedule, and was reportedly irritable after receiving vaccines per administration.

TL's family was generally healthy, with no incidence of autism spectrum disorders, allergies, or autoimmune conditions.

TL's diet was limited, given his intolerance to many foods and food textures. He ate soy yogurt, berries, bananas, bread, rice, peanut butter, and limited fruits and vegetables.

NOTES

# Neuropsychiatric/ Developmental Evaluations and Initial Laboratory Results

**Comment:** TL underwent multiple neuropsychiatric and developmental evaluations to achieve the diagnosis of PDD-NOS. Significant findings or pertinent negative findings are listed under each assessment tool.

- Gross motor development and tone
  - TL's gross motor development and proximal and distal extremity muscle tone were determined to be within normal limits.
- Hearing Evaluation
  - TL's hearing evaluation was within normal limits.
- Bayley Scales of Infant Development II
  - Mental Development Index: < 50;<br>(> -2.0 standard deviation points (SD) below the mean.)
- Vinland Adaptive Behavior Scales
  - Communication: 73 (moderately low)
  - Socialization: 74 (moderately low)
- Sensory Caregiver Profile 7 to 36 months
  - Oral sensory processing: > -2.0 SD below the mean
- Childhood Autism Rating Scale (CARS): 32
  - **Comment:** In the CARS assessment, TL showed significant delay in social and play skills, listening, visual response, object use and verbal and non-verbal communication. A score of 32 was consistent with Autistic/PDD-NOS disorders
- Peabody Developmental Scale II:
  - > 25% delay fine and visual motor skills

### Developmental Assessment of Young Children

| Domain | TL's percentile ranking | z-score |
|---|---|---|
| Cognitive Development | 6 | -1.67 |
| Communication Development | 0.3 | -3.00 |
| Motor Development | 23 | -0.67 |
| Social/Emotional Development | 9 | -1.33 |
| Adaptive Skills | 7 | -1.33 |

### Preschool Language Scale-4

| | Auditory Comprehension | Expressive Communication | Total Language |
|---|---|---|---|
| Percentile Rank | 1 | 3 | 1 |
| Standard Score | 57 | 71 | 60 |
| Standard Deviation | > 2.5 SD below mean | 2.0 SD below mean | > 2.5 SD below mean |

**Laboratory tests ordered and rationale:**

It is believed by many clinicians and researchers that autism pathogenesis consists of a complex interplay between genetics (including polymorphisms in detoxification and biotransformation enzymes), environmental exposures and imbalanced immune response.[7] Significant food immunological reactions, gastrointestinal disturbances and nutrient imbalances are frequently found in ASD.[8] At the molecular level, oxidative stress, methylation lesions, inflammation and mitochondrial dysfunction are common findings.[9, 10] Successful treatment generally requires addressing multiple imbalances simultaneously. Because of these factors, clinicians treating autistic individuals from a functional or integrative approach tend to use laboratory testing broadly, evaluating numerous areas of potential imbalance:

Clinicians treating autistic individuals from a functional or integrative approach tend to use laboratory testing broadly, evaluating numerous areas of potential imbalance.

1. **Complete blood count and metabolic panel**: Routine laboratory assessments
2. **Food-specific IgE and IgG antibodies**: Food reactions are a common finding in ASD.[11]
3. **Multiprofile panel**: A comprehensive assessment including fatty acids, amino acids, organic acids, essential and toxic elements, lipid-soluble vitamins and oxidative stress markers; assists in detecting the individual etiopathogenic factors used to individualize treatment plans.
4. **Stool test**: Assessment of GI microbial status and GI function. GI imbalances are a common finding in many inflammatory conditions.[12]
5. **Celiac panel**: Gluten intolerance and gluten sensitivity have been found in ASD.[8, 11, 13-15]
6. **Genetic testing for mutations in glutathione and methylation enzymes**: Increased incidence of mutations in these enzyme systems has been identified in ASD.[16-18]
7. **Urinary polypeptides**: Elevation of specific polypeptides has been associated with ASD.[19]
8. **Urine toxic elements test with DMPS provocation**: Elevated toxic metals have been found in ASD.[20] Since the provocation agent may chelate essential as well as toxic elements, the test was to be completed after initial treatment had begun.

## Only significant findings are discussed below:

| | Result | | Graph marker | Reference |
|---|---|---|---|---|
| **Bacterial - general** | | | | |
| Benzoate | > 160.00 | H | 5.3 | <= 38.0 |
| Hippurate | 384 | | 582 | <= 2,105 |
| **L. acidophilus / general bacterial** | | | | |
| D-Lactate | 16.4 | H | 2.2 | <= 10.4 |
| **Yeast / Fungal** | | | | |
| D-Arabinitol | 52 | | 57 | <= 83 |

*Creatinine =44 mg/dl*

**Figure 1. Urinary organic acids—compounds of bacterial and fungal origin.** Elevations were consistent with bacterial overgrowth. The elevated benzoate relative to hippurate suggested phase II liver biotransformation pathway (glycine conjugation) insufficiency. D-arabinitol is specific for *Candida* species; though not frankly elevated, its level may be considered high-normal by some clinicians. (Units: µg/mg creatinine)

| | | Results | Reference Limits |
|---|---|---|---|
| Eosinophil protein X (EPX) | H | 19 | ≤ 7.0 µg/g |
| Calprotectin | | 46 | ≤ 50 µg/g |
| pH | L | 5.4 | 6.1–7.9 |
| Fungi | | Positive for Candida parapsilosis, Rhodotorula, and Trichosporon with microscopy and culture | |

**Figure 2. Functional Stool Testing.** EPX elevation indicated inflammation. Low pH indicated GI microbial imbalance and the fungi findings suggested GI fungal overgrowth.

| | | Results | Reference Limits |
|---|---|---|---|
| Indolyl-3-acrylolyglycine (IAG) | H | 161.8 µg/mg cr | 4.6–9.5 |
| Deltorphin II | H | 37.7 µg/mg cr | 0.9–25.5 |
| Dermorphin | H | 32.4 µg/mg cr | 2.0–15.5 |
| Leucine Enkephalin | H | 29.6 µg/mg cr | 0.7–16.0 |

**Figure 3. Urinary polypeptides.** Elevations have been found in ASD. IAG has been proposed as a potential diagnostic biomarker for ASD.

NOTES

| | Results | Reference Limits |
|---|---|---|
| IgG anti-gliadin | H 91 | normal 0–19 units |
| IgA tissue transglutaminase | < 2 | normal 0–19 units |
| IgA anti-gliadin | < 2 | normal 0–19 units |

**IgG (TOTAL) Reactive Foods (BLOOD)**

| | | | |
|---|---|---|---|
| Amaranth (+1) | Egg (+1) | Onion (+1) | Sage (+1) |
| Asparagus (+1) | Eggplant (+1) | Oregano (+1) | Sesame (+1) |
| Beef (+1) | Ginger (+1) | Peanut (+1) | Soybean (+1) |
| Cheese (+1) | Lamb (+1) | Pineapple (+1) | Sugar, Cane (+1) |
| Cinnamon (+1) | Milk, Cow's (+2) | Pumpkin (+1) | Wheat (+2) |
| Clove (+1) | Milk, Goat's (+1) | Rice (+1) | Yeast, Baker's (+1) |
| Cranberry (+1) | Nutmeg (+1) | Rye (+1) | Yeast, Brewer's (+2) |

**Figure 4. Celiac panel and food-specific IgG antibodies.** Elevated IgG antigliadin antibodies suggested gluten sensitivity, and possibly gluten enteropathy. The IgG food panel showed a mild reaction to 28 foods. Both the positive gliadin reaction and IgG panel results strongly suggested intestinal hyperpermeability. IgE food allergies test (not shown) was negative.

| | Result | Flag | Scale marks | Reference range |
|---|---|---|---|---|
| Eicosapentaenoic (20:5n3) | 5 | L | 6 | 3 - 247 |
| Arachidonic (20:4n6) | 585 | | 318; 690 | 234 - 856 |
| AA/EPA | 129.3 | H | 90.8 | 1.4 - 137.2 |
| Vitamin A | 0.45 | L | 0.53; 1.30 | 0.41 - 1.5 |

**Figure 5. Plasma fatty acids and serum fat-soluble vitamins.** Low EPA and normal AA. Taken together, these findings may be pro-inflammatory (the high AA/EPA ratio). Vitamin A level was low. Retinoid receptor imbalances have been linked to ASD pathogenesis and may be responsive to natural A supplementation.[21] (Fatty acid units: μM; vitamin A: mg/L)

| | Results |
|---|---|
| Glutathione S-Transferase P1 enzyme (*GSTP1*): | Homozygous single nucleotide polymorphisms (SNPs) identified at two positions on *GSTP1* gene: *I105V* and *A114V* |

| | Result | Flag | Scale marks | Reference range |
|---|---|---|---|---|
| Pyroglutamate | 122 | H | 60 | <= 135 |
| Sulfate | 179 | L | 211; 585 | 122 - 786 |
| 8-Hydroxy-2-deoxyguanosine * | 11.5 | H | 5.9 | <= 8.7 |

* Units for 8-Hydroxy-2-deoxyguanosine are ng/mg creatinine

**Figure 6. Markers relating to glutathione status and oxidative stress.** GST enzymes are involved in phase II biotransformation; they are critical for biotransforming xenobiotic exposures, including both metallo- and organotoxins. *GSTP1* is located in the brain and skin. Point mutations in GST enzymes have been found in ASD.[16, 18] Urinary organic acids pyroglutamate and sulfate imbalance may demonstrate glutathione insufficiency. Elevated urinary 8-OHdG indicated significant oxidative stress. (Organic acid units: μg/mg creatinine, except as stated above.)

| | Results |
|---|---|
| Methylenetetrahydrofolate reductase (*MTHFR*) enzyme: | Heterozygous single nucleotide polymorphism (SNP) identified on *MTHFR* gene: *C677T* |

| | | | Chart label | Reference |
|---|---|---|---|---|
| Homocysteine | 3.1 | L | 4.0 / 10.0 | 3.0 - 14.0 |
| Methylmalonate | 3.8 | H | 3.5 | <= 4.8 |

**Figure 7. Methylation markers.** The *MTHFR* heterozygous SNP may compromise methylation activity. Low serum homocysteine and a fifth quintile elevation of MMA (a functional marker indicating $B_{12}$ deficiency) also may indicate compromised methylation activity. (MMA units: µg/mg creatinine; homocysteine: µmol/L)

| | | Results | Reference Limits |
|---|---|---|---|
| Anion gap | H | 18 mmol/L | 8–16 mmol/L |

| | | | Chart label | Reference |
|---|---|---|---|---|
| Pyruvate | 4.8 | | 5.3 | <= 9.7 |
| Lactate | 101.9 | H | 22.2 | 3.1 - 113.0 |
| Citrate | 1,399 | H | 1,346 | 71 - 1,967 |
| Isocitrate | 185 | H | 162 | 57 - 257 |
| Succinate | 72.6 | H | 58.0 | 0.7 - 99.0 |
| Malate | 10.7 | H | 3.2 | <= 6.6 |

**Figure 8. Urinary organic acids assessing mitochondrial function.** The pattern of imbalance shown above (elevated citric acid intermediates) suggested a mild mitochondropathy requiring CoQ10 and a subclinical lactic acidosis. The elevated D-lactate in Figure 1 also contributed to lactic acidosis. (Units: µg/mg creatinine)

| | | | | Chart label | Reference | Units |
|---|---|---|---|---|---|---|
| 1 | Potassium | 685 | L | 1,414 | 1,062 - 2,184 | ppm packed cells |
| 2 | Magnesium* | 22 | L | 23 | 15 - 35 | ppm packed cells |
| 3 | Zinc | 4.4 | L | 4.7 | 3.6 - 8.0 | ppm packed cells |
| 4 | Copper | 432 | | 311 | 264 - 493 | ppb packed cells |
| 5 | Manganese | 31 | L | 32 | 27 - 52 | ppb packed cells |

**Figure 9. Erythrocyte essential elements.** Levels were mostly low. The low quantity of zinc relative to copper has been seen in ASD.

## Pertinent Negative Laboratory Results

- Comprehensive metabolic panel (CMP) and complete blood count (CBC) were within normal limits.

## Initial Assessment

- PDD-NOS
- Irritable bowel syndrome with microbial dysbiosis
- Intestinal hyperpermeability
- Gluten sensitivity
- IgG food sensitivities
- Nutrient deficiencies
- Detoxification/biotransformation impairments:
  - Methylation
  - Hypohomocysteinemia
  - Glutathione conjugation
  - Glycine conjugation
  - Mild methylmalonic aciduria ($B_{12}$ deficiency)
- Oxidative stress
- Mitochondropathy
- Mild lactic acidosis

## Initial Plan

- Dietary Intervention
  - Diet: avoid all gluten-containing foods; continue to avoid dairy; minimize IgG food sensitivities × 3 months.
- GI Treatment
  - Rifaximin 200 mg, 1 tab PO TID × 7 days
  - Nystatin 500,000 units, 2 caps PO BID × 3 months (after completion of antibiotic)
  - Charcoal capsules, 2 hours after medicine PRN
  - Probiotic combination 18 bill CFU, 1 packet PO QD
  - Digestive enzymes, 2 caps PO TID with meals
- Nutrient Support
  - Cod liver oil, 1 tsp PO BID
  - Multivitamin and mineral powder (specifically designed for ASD), 1 scoop PO QD
  - Zinc citrate 30 mg, 1 cap PO QD
  - Magnesium citrate 150 mg, 2 caps PO BID
  - Methylation support (folic acid, folinic acid, $B_{12}$, $B_6$, trimethylglycine, N-acetylcysteine, essential elements and nutrients), 1 cap PO QD

**Treatment plan rationale:** A variety of etiological factors (genetic and environmental) can contribute to the onset of ASD; laboratory assessment of children diagnosed with ASD often entails "casting a wide biochemical net" to capture the many possible imbalances contributing to the disorder.[11]

TL's food sensitivities required the elimination of gluten and a number of other foods. TL was also given Rifaximin, which is effective against small intestinal bacterial overgrowth.[22-24] Charcoal was offered as support if the bacterial die-off produced an increase in toxins and worsening of symptoms (Herxheimer reaction). Nystatin was used to eliminate TL's fungal overgrowth. Probiotics and digestive enzymes were initiated for the IBS, digestion and absorption.

Due to detection of the essential fatty acid, vitamin A and other nutrient deficiencies, cod liver oil (containing vitamin A) and a multivitamin mineral formula were started. Multivitamin and mineral formulas designed for children with ASD may be powdered, and frequently include higher doses of nutrients commonly found deficient, such as B vitamins and zinc. Normalizing methylation and sulfuration (methylation) was also a key step for TL, as it is for most autistic children. $B_{12}$, folinic acid, and trimethylglycine have been shown to improve a number of metabolic activities, including glutathione synthesis. TL was also given higher amounts of magnesium and zinc, as he required more than his multivitamin and mineral supplied.

**After starting treatment, TL began speaking with a limited vocabulary almost immediately, with regular attempts at new words.**

## Two-Month Follow-up

After starting treatment, TL began speaking with a limited vocabulary almost immediately, with regular attempts at new words. He began interacting with people and demonstrated increased eye contact. His mood improved and tantrums decreased. His energy was better. His bowel movements became larger and loose, but less odiferous. His skin rashes had worsened. TL didn't tolerate the dietary changes well. His parents stated that he craved the restricted foods like an addict. He started eating Play-Doh, which contains gluten.

## Two-Month Follow-up Plan

Continue with protocol and add:

- Fluconazole (Diflucan) 100 mg, 1 tab PO QD × 30 days
- *Saccharomyces boulardii* 250 mg, 1 packet PO QD
- Amino acid formula, 1 cap PO BID (contains glutamine, glycine, methylsulfonylmethane, N-acetylcysteine, taurine, glutathione, ornithine, and calcium-D-glucarate)
- CoQ10 100 mg, chew 1 tab BID

**Treatment plan rationale:** Because TL continued to present with signs and symptoms of fungal overgrowth, including behavioral episodes and rashes, fluconazole was initiated. *Saccharomyces boulardii* was also introduced, as it has been shown to reduce GI inflammation, normalize stool consistency, and (in animals) reduce fungal overgrowth.[25,26] An amino acid formula was introduced to improve toxicant mobilization. CoQ10 was given to stimulate metabolism and support mitochondrial activity (mitochondropathy was suspected because of the abnormal citric acid cycle intermediates and L-lactate elevation seen on organic acids).

**Laboratory tests ordered**

- Urine toxic elements (with oral DMPS provoking agent)
- Organic acids
- Stool test

# Four-Month Follow-up

TL experienced remarkable and immediate improvement in bowel movement consistency with the introduction of *Saccharomyces boulardii*. Potty training had been initiated. There was an increase in self-stimulatory behaviors, such as turning lights on and off and wheeling back and forth, but in general he was doing well. He was a well-liked child, enjoyed school, and was in a good mood most of the time. Parents noted that if probiotics were missed, TL's bowel movements immediately became large and loose. Parents requested a simpler supplement protocol, as he was taking 19 items per day.

## Four-Month Follow-up Laboratory Results

*(See Table 1 for baseline and follow-up laboratory comparison.)*

| | | Results | Reference Limits |
|---|---|---|---|
| Mercury | H | 14 µg/mg creatinine | ≤ 5 µg/g creatinine |

**Figure 10. Six-hour urine toxic elements (with oral DMPS).** Mercury was elevated.

| | Result | | Chart marker | Reference |
|---|---|---|---|---|
| **Bacterial - general** | | | | |
| Benzoate | 2.0 | | 5.3 | <= 38.0 |
| Hippurate | 1,163 | H | 582 | <= 2,105 |
| **L. acidophilus / general bacterial** | | | | |
| D-Lactate | 1.8 | | 2.2 | <= 10.4 |
| **Yeast / Fungal** | | | | |
| D-Arabinitol | 58 | H | 57 | <= 83 |

*Creatinine = 164 mg/dl*

**Figure 11. Urinary organic acids—compounds of bacterial or fungal origin.** Improvement from baseline in all markers except D-arabinitol, which was elevated, indicating fungal overgrowth. (Units: µg/mg creatinine)

| | | Results | Reference Limits |
|---|---|---|---|
| Eosinophil protein X (EPX) | | 1.6 µg/g | ≤ 7.0 µg/g |
| Calprotectin | H | 90 µg/g | ≤ 50 µg/g |
| pH | | 6.3 | 6.1–7.9 |
| Fungi | | Negative for Candida species, with microscopy and stool culture | |

**Figure 12. Functional Stool Testing.** Results demonstrated improvement in EPX, pH, and fungi, but calprotectin was elevated, demonstrating continued inflammation.

| | | Chart marker | Reference |
|---|---|---|---|
| Pyroglutamate | 30 | 64 | <= 122 |
| Sulfate | 196 | 154 – 554 | 107 - 693 |
| 8-Hydroxy-2-deoxyguanosine * | 5.8 | 5.9 | <= 8.7 |

* Units for 8-Hydroxy-2-deoxyguanosine are ng/mg creatinine

**Figure 13. Urinary organic acid markers relating to glutathione status and oxidative stress.** All markers were within normal limits. (Units µg/mg creatinine except as noted above)

| | | | | |
|---|---|---|---|---|
| Pyruvate | < 0.5 | | 5.3 | <= 9.7 |
| Lactate | 51.4 | H | 22.2 | 3.1 - 113.0 |
| Citrate | 780 | | 1,062 | 71 - 1,967 |
| Cis-Aconitate | 77 | | 135 | 43 - 224 |
| Isocitrate | 136 | | 162 | 57 - 257 |
| a-Ketoglutarate | 8.5 | | 57.9 | 3.1 - 127.0 |
| Succinate | 30.4 | | 38.0 | 0.7 - 99.0 |
| Fumarate | 0.22 | | 0.86 | <= 1.96 |
| Malate | 2.2 | | 3.2 | <= 6.6 |
| Hydroxymethylglutarate | 15.2 | | 18.6 | <= 27.2 |

**Figure 14. Urinary organic acids assessing mitochondrial function.** All markers had significantly improved on follow-up assessment. L-lactate was still mildly elevated, but it was greatly improved from the initial L-lactate level. (Units: µg/mg creatinine)

| | | | Chart marker | Reference |
|---|---|---|---|---|
| Methylmalonate | 4.4 | H | 3.5 | <= 4.8 |

**Figure 15. Urinary organic acids—methylmalonate.** MMA was higher than in previous testing, indicating a continued need for $B_{12}$ despite supplementation. (Units: µg/mg creatinine)

NOTES

## Four-Month Follow-up Plan

- Discontinue the following:
  - Probiotic 18 bill CFU
  - Amino acid formula
  - Zinc citrate
  - Magnesium citrate
- Continue the following:
  - Digestive enzymes
  - *Saccharomyces boulardii,* 1 packet QD
  - Methylation support
  - Multivitamin and mineral powder
  - Charcoal capsules 2 hours after medicine PRN (to combat negative reaction to microbial toxins)
  - Continue gluten- and dairy-free diet
- Add the following:
  - Probiotic combination 450 bill CFU, 1 packet PO QD
  - Ketoconazole 200 mg, 1 tab PO QD × 14 days
  - Nystatin 500,000 Units, 1 cap PO BID × 3 months, to be started after completing the ketoconazole
  - Dimercaptosuccinic acid (DMSA) 100 mg, 1 tab PO BID between meals, every other week on M, W, F. Ensure regular bowel movements and sufficient fluids while taking DMSA.
  - Methylcobalamin pre-filled syringes 64.5 μg/kg, SQ injection, three times a week
  - L-glutathione cream 1 gram, applied topically QD
  - Zinc sulfate cream 1 gram, applied topically QD
  - Magnesium sulfate cream 1 gram, applied topically QD

**Treatment plan rationale:** The four-month follow-up plan was designed to address the continued yeast presence with two weeks of ketoconazole followed by three months of Nystatin, with concurrent aggressive probiotics. Per the parent's request, TL's protocol was simplified with the introduction of topical glutathione, zinc, and magnesium. Subcutaneous $B_{12}$ was initiated, based on the continued elevation of methylmalonate.

## Seven-Month Follow-up Visit

The introduction of $B_{12}$ injections caused a remarkable change in TL. He became more focused, able to spend 20 to 30 minutes on the same task at one time. He used more words and started to pronounce C, K, and G. He was generally less mentally "stuck." At first, the changes only occurred on the days he received the shots; his therapists often asked, "Is it a $B_{12}$ day?" The changes eventually became constant. TL's therapists were reconsidering his diagnosis; whether he required a special needs school or could be mainstreamed. The plan was continued as directed.

**The introduction of $B_{12}$ injections caused a remarkable change in TL.**

## Ten-Month Follow-up Visit

TL began mainstream nursery school, and was indistinguishable from the "normal" children. He loved school, did very well socially, and liked his routine. Without probiotics, his stools continued to be massive and loose. His parents had taken before and after videos. They were very pleased with his progress *(see father's note below)*.

*"Up until two years of age, TL was developing at a normal level. His vocabulary was up to twenty words, but suddenly he started to regress. When we took him to see our pediatrician he was down to five words; three months later he couldn't say one.*

*After seeing a speech doctor and psychologists, he was diagnosed with pervasive development disorder or autism. We knew we had to do something because he wasn't getting any better. He was irritable and would throw tantrums all the time.*

*It wasn't until we discovered Dr. Hyman that we started to put the pieces of the puzzle together. After going through Dr. Hyman's program, we found that our son had several food allergies, heavy metal poisoning, severe gut inflammation, and imbalances in his gut bacteria as well as yeast overgrowth.*

*After learning about this we changed his diet right away and within days of removing dairy we saw immediate results. We saw more concentration. With the $B_{12}$ supplements our son developed more verbal skills and was able to focus. What's amazing is that we didn't know there was a fog until we started eliminating the heavy metals (by chelation). After TL went through chelation he became much more alive, responsive, and verbal."*

**~ TL's father**

**Figure 16. Father's comments.** Discription of TL's progress after 10 months of treating the underlying imbalances that were contributing to his ASD.

# DISCUSSION

Onset of ASD is in childhood, frequently seen by 18 to 24 months and is characterized by abnormalities in social interactions, significantly impaired communication skills, and restricted repetitive and stereotyped behaviors.[27] Current estimates place the incidence of ASD at 1:91 to 1:110, with boys being affected four to five times more frequently than girls.[1] The etiology of ASD is multifactorial, with toxic exposures, pre-, peri- and postnatal infections, maternal infections, genetic abnormalities, nutrient deficiencies and vaccines being some of the implicated factors. Comorbidities include gastroenteropathies, allergies, autoimmunity and various psychiatric conditions.[7,9,16,20,28-30]

According to his parents, TL was a normally developing infant with a growing vocabulary. He was meeting developmental milestones, physically and intellectually. He had no family history that suggested he could be vulnerable to ASD. His parents noted that he experienced irritability after receiving all vaccines, which is not an uncommon occurrence. However, his parents also noted that there was a temporal correlation between his first MMR shot and the onset of PDD-NOS. MMR vaccine has been associated with the onset of ASD and ASD-associated gastroenteropathy, although there has been a great deal of controversy with this observation.[31,32] TL apparently experienced a significant in utero exposure to mercury and possibly, as an infant, to lead and insecticide. He was intolerant of dairy products and had symptoms consistent with allergies and irritable bowel syndrome.

**TL began mainstream nursery school, and was indistinguishable from the "normal" children.**

Figure 1 demonstrated an elevation of D-lactate, accumulation of which can lead to systemic acidosis. Signs of acute toxicity include altered mental status, disorientation and irritability.[33] Other signs of acidosis include a low stool pH, an elevated anion gap and elevated L-lactate. The cause of TL's lactic acidosis may have been carbohydrate malabsorption from gluten intolerance or bacterial overgrowth.[34]

Elevated benzoate, a constituent of some fruits and preservatives, may be produced by intestinal bacteria.[35] Elevated benzoate but normal hippurate (Figure 1) pointed towards impaired conversion, suggesting a biotransformation pathway lesion.

D-Arabinitol is specific for the presence of *Candida* species. While not frankly elevated, its presence may provide some corroboration for the finding of *Candida* species in the stool test (Figure 2).

TL's stool analysis results (Figure 2) strongly indicated inflammation. EPX is elevated in a number of GI inflammatory conditions, including gluten enteropathy and food allergies.[12] EPX is directly cytotoxic to the gastrointestinal mucosa,[36] contributing to intestinal permeability.[37] Calprotectin assay is sensitive for GI inflammation of organic origin but nonspecific for disease.[38] A low stool pH is associated with dysbiosis and acidic bacterial metabolites, including short chain fatty acids. Bacterial D-lactate producers thrive in an acidic environment. Alkalinizing the GI pH may therefore inhibit the growth of D-lactate, reducing systemic acidosis.[39] Multiple *Candida* species were also found, suggesting a lower-GI fungal overgrowth. Gastrointestinal candidiasis has been found in ASD and has been an alleged contributing factor in ASD symptomatology.

Elevation of the neuroactive dietary peptides (Figure 3) has been associated with ASD neurological and gastrointestinal symptomatology, and it is also indicative of intestinal permeability.[19] Elevation of IAG has been specifically associated with ASD and has been recommended for consideration as a diagnostic indicator.[40, 41]

A marked elevation of antigliadin antibodies was shown in Figure 4. Anti-gliadin antibodies and gluten sensitivity have long been a concern with ASD patients, and gluten-free diets are often used with this population.[8, 11, 13-15] Research indicates that a gluten-free diet may reduce gastrointestinal inflammation in some ASD children.[42, 43] The placebo arm of a double-blind placebo-controlled trial of a gluten-free casein-free diet for autism had to be discontinued due to the extent of improvement of the diet arm of the study.[62] Interestingly, while TL's IgG anti-gliadin antibodies (AGA) were markedly elevated, his IgA tissue transglutaminase and AGA were undetectable. Total IgA deficiency, a common finding among patients with celiac disease, has been observed in some ASD individuals.[32, 44] In the presence of inadequate total IgA, the specific IgA antibody tests may have shown falsely negative results. Clinically, TL responded favorably to the removal of gluten-containing foods from his diet. ELISA testing for total IgG response to 90 different foods demonstrated a mild positive reaction (+1 and +2) to 28 foods, including wheat and dairy (Figure 2). The positive IgG wheat reaction is consistent with IgG antigliadin antibodies. Food sensitivities are closely associated with GI inflammation[45] and intestinal permeability.[46]

EPA deficiency is implicated in inflammation-driven conditions, including numerous neuropsychiatric disorders (Figure 5). Evidence supports the benefit of omega-3 supplementation in ASD children.[47, 48] When EPA is in limited supply, enzyme and fatty acid substrate availability allows increased production of AA. Although TL's AA level was within normal limits, it exceeded the level of his EPA, resulting in an elevated AA/EPA ratio that can contribute to an inflammatory milieu.

**TL had positive, homozygous SNPs in two different locations on the glutathione-S-transferase P1 enzyme.**

TL had a very low vitamin A level (Figure 5). Autism may be linked to the disruption of the G-alpha protein, affecting retinoid receptors in the brain. Natural vitamin A may restore retinoid receptor function, which is involved in sensory perception, vision, language processing, and attention. The pertussis toxin found in the DPT vaccine may be involved in the G-alpha protein/retinoid receptor disruption.[21] TL's low vitamin A level may have been negatively affecting retinoid receptor activity, contributing to his autistic presentation.

TL had positive, homozygous SNPs in two different locations on the glutathione-S-transferase P1 enzyme (*GSTP1*) gene: *I105V* and *A114V* (Figure 6). It can therefore be concluded that both of TL's parents were at least heterozygous for the mutations. The GST family of enzymes catalyzes the conjugation of glutathione to various substrates for phase II biotransformation. SNPs in *GSTP1* may significantly impair the ability to biotransform toxicants in brain and skin, where this enzyme is located. Classes of compounds biotransformed by this enzyme (glutathione conjugation) include toxic metals, xenobiotics, solvents, pesticides, herbicides and polycyclic aromatic hydrocarbons. Point mutations in the gene coding for glutathione s-transferase enzymes have been associated with increased risk of autism.[16, 18]

Elevated 8-OHdG (Figure 6) indicated increased oxidative stress and identified the level of oxidative damage to the guanine residue of DNA. Guanine is the most easily oxidized of the DNA bases.[61] Given the *GSTP1* SNPs, inflammation and poor methylation (or methylation lesion) and nutrient imbalances, the increased oxidative damage was not a surprising result.

TL was positive for a heterozygous SNP (*C677T*) in the gene coding for methylenetetrahydrofolate reductase (*MTHFR*). *MTHFR* is the enzyme involved in the final methylation step of folic acid, producing 5-methyltetrahydrofolate from 5,10-methylenetetrahydrofolate. Impairment of this enzyme is most commonly evidenced by an accumulation of homocysteine, since 5-methyltetrahydrofolate is required to recycle homocysteine back to methionine. However, abnormal *MTHFR* function has been noted in autistic children, who may also present with low to normal, rather than high, homocysteine levels, as found here (Figure 7).

James and Neubrander demonstrated in 2004 that treating ASD children with methyl donors including $B_{12}$, folic acid, and trimethylglycine normalized glutathione and homocysteine levels,[9, 16] demonstrating the close relationship between methylation and sulfuration activity (Figure 17). Few laboratories consider low homocysteine to be alarming, despite its rate-limiting involvement in providing the cysteine residue for glutathione production. When oxidative stress increases, the enzymes involved in methylation are inhibited, thereby allowing homocysteine to be shunted into trans-sulfuration, producing glutathione. Homocysteine may be subject to depletion in chronic oxidative challenge, and low- to low-normal levels are common in ASD children.

**Methylation and sulfuration pathway lesions are a common finding in autistic children, and may be relieved with high-dose methyl-$B_{12}$ intramuscular injections.**

Furthermore, Deth et al. suggested that the increased incidence of genetic polymorphisms found in methylation and sulfuration in ASD subjects significantly impacts methionine synthase (MS). Folate and cobalamin-dependant MS are involved in dopamine-stimulated phospholipid methylation. This signaling process, which is mediated by the D4 dopamine receptor, which promotes neuronal synchronization and attention, is also impaired in autism.[49]

Figure 7 also showed a fifth quintile elevation of methylmalonate (MMA). MMA is a sensitive functional marker of $B_{12}$ (adenosylcobalamin) intracellular activity. Thus, methylmalonic aciduria is indicative of $B_{12}$ insufficiency. Methylation and sulfuration pathway lesions are a common finding in autistic children, and may be relieved with high-dose methyl-$B_{12}$ intramuscular injections.[7, 9] Specific elevation of urinary methylmalonate has been noted in children diagnosed with regressive ASD and gastrointestinal symptomatology post-MMR vaccinations.[32] $B_{12}$ therapy is generally considered to be a cornerstone intervention in ASD children.

Substantial laboratory evidence in this case for potential glutathione abnormalities included: (a) elevated pyroglutamate (Figure 6), which may be indicative of limited glutathione availability via increased glutathione utilization or glycine insufficiency;[50, 51] (b) low urinary sulfate, which indicated limited substrate availability for phase II sulfation and may also be correlated with low glutathione;[52] (c) the *GSTP1* and *MTHFR* mutations, which can cause increased glutathione need, and decreased synthesis, respectively; (d) low homocysteine—a glutathione substrate; (e) $B_{12}$ insufficiency also compromising glutathione synthesis; (f) low essential element cofactors, including $B_6$, potassium and magnesium—needed for glutathione synthesis; and (g) increased oxidative stress (8-OHdG) suggesting insufficient glutathione.

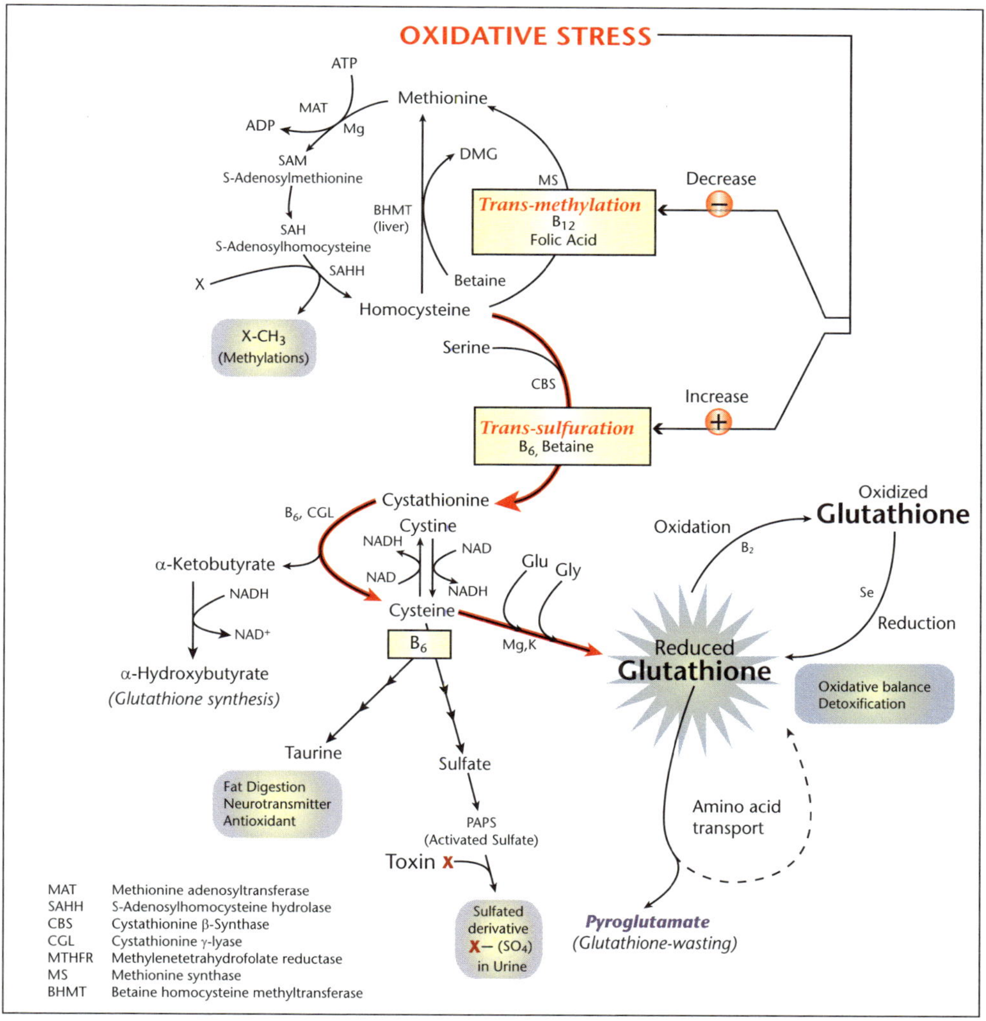


**Figure 17. Methylation, sulfuration and oxidative stress.** Under conditions of increased oxidative stress, enzymes involved in methylation are inhibited, allowing homocysteine to be trans-sulfurated to form glutathione. In ASD, there are documented genetic lesions in methylation and sulfuration, altering the normal physiologic response, resulting in lower glutathione and ineffectively controlled oxidative stress.

**Table 1. Select baseline and four-month follow-up laboratory result comparison.** Improvements were noted in oxidative stress, lactic acidosis, mitochondrial function, and glutathione status. Gastrointestinal inflammation continued, and $B_{12}$ deficiency had worsened. Improvements noted with (*).

| Compound | Pre test | Post-test | Ref Range | Percent Change |
|---|---|---|---|---|
| Benzoate* | >160 H | 2.0 | ≤ 38.0 µg/mg cr (fifth quintile < 5.3) | -99% |
| D-Arabinitol | 52 | 58 | ≤ 83 µg/mg cr (fifth quintile < 57) | +11.5% |
| D-lactate* | 16.4 H | 1.8 | ≤ 10.4 µg/mg cr (fifth quintile < 2.2) | -89% |
| Eosinophil Protein X* | 19 H | 1.6 | ≤ 7.0 µg/g | -92% |
| Calprotectin | 46 | 90 H | ≤ 50 µg/g | +96% |
| 8-OHdG* | 11.5 H | 5.8 | ≤ 8.7 µg/mg cr (fifth quintile < 5.9) | -50% |
| Pyroglutamate* | 122 HN | 30 | ≤ 135 µg/mg cr (fifth quintile < 60) | -75% |
| Sulfate* | 179 LN | 196 | 122-786 µg/mg cr (fifth quintile 211-585) | +9.5% |
| Methylmalonate | 3.8 HN | 4.4 HN | ≤ 4.8 µg/mg cr (fifth quintile < 3.5) | +15.8% |
| L-lactate* | 101.9 HN | 51.4 HN | 3.1-113.0 µg/mg cr (fifth quintile < 22.2) | -50% |

Elevations of citric acid cycle intermediates (Figure 8) and elevated L-lactate suggested mitochondropathy. There is a significant increased incidence of mitochondropathy in ASD children.[10, 63] One study demonstrated mitochondrial dysfunction in ASD children with an elevated blood L-lactate/pyruvate ratio.[53] Phenotypic expression of the mitochondrial disorders, genetic and secondary, have been known to occur after exogenous toxic exposures, including vaccines, organo- and metallotoxins, and drugs.[63] Taken together, TL's elevated urinary D-lactate and L-lactate probably contributed to the slight elevation in the anion gap, causing low-grade metabolic acidosis.

A general pattern of low RBC elements suggested poor digestion and absorption. When essential elements are in short supply, not only is metabolism compromised, but there may also be a risk of toxic metal uptake via essential element transporters in the GI tract and CNS.[54] TL's copper level was relatively high compared to his zinc. Low zinc availability will allow ready GI uptake of copper, because they share transport proteins. Abnormal copper metabolism with low zinc and increased oxidative stress has been found in autistic children.[55] Zinc, copper, and manganese are all required for superoxide dismutase (SOD) in the mitochondria (Mn) and cytosol (Zn, Cu). SOD quenches superoxide radicals, and inadequate cofactors will compromise enzyme activity. Magnesium is required for more than 375 enzymes because of its presence in ATP. Magnesium (in ATP) is required to activate $B_6$ via pyridoxal kinase to pyridoxal-5-phosphate. Supplementation with both magnesium and $B_6$ has been shown to improve ASD symptoms and normalize RBC Mg levels.[56]

At his two-month follow-up, TL was doing significantly better but continued to present with signs and symptoms of fungal overgrowth, including behavioral episodes and rashes, prompting the introduction of fluconazole. *Saccharomyces boulardii* was also introduced, as it has been shown to reduce GI inflammation, normalize stool consistency, and (in animals) reduce fungal overgrowth.[25, 26] An amino acid formula was introduced to improve toxicant mobilization. CoQ10 was given to stimulate metabolism and support mitochondrial resuscitation (normalize citric acid cycle intermediates and reduce the L-lactate elevation).

At his four-month follow-up, TL's urinary mercury levels were elevated (Figure 10), which was not unexpected given TL's in utero exposure to mercury via his mother's regular ingestion of tuna fish.

Figure 11 demonstrated a reduction in gastrointestinal microbial-produced organic acids. Particularly significant was the reduced benzoate and the improved conversion of benzoate to hippurate. The antimicrobials and dietary changes likely reduced the total benzoate load, while pantothenic acid (multivitamin and mineral) and glycine (amino formula) improved biotransformation to hippurate via glycine conjugation in the liver. The bacterial D-lactate producers were reduced, as reflected by the normal level of urinary D-lactate. This finding greatly eased concern about metabolic acidosis and encephalopathy, even though the L-lactate remained slightly elevated (Figure 14). Despite aggressive antifungal medication, the mild elevation of D-arabinitol (Figure 11) indicated the continued presence of *Candida albicans*.

Figure 12 demonstrated improvement in all stool markers, with the exception of calprotectin, which was now elevated. Calprotectin is derived from neutrophils and is a sensitive, but not disease specific, marker of inflammation throughout the gastrointestinal tract. In one study, fecal calprotectin was highest in children with organic bowel disease, versus controls and children with functional bowel disease.[38] Stool *Candida* culture was negative, despite the elevated D-arabinitol. It is possible that the *Candida* reservoir was extra-enteral, or in the upper bowel, and therefore not present in a stool specimen, which reflects lower bowel growth.

8-OHdG had previously been very elevated. As expected, with improved diet and nutrient intake, it normalized, indicating that oxidative stress had greatly declined (Figure 13). Pyroglutamate was well within normal limits and sulfate levels also normalized, indicating improved glutathione availability. L-lactate was still high-normal (Figure 14), although there was close to a 50% reduction. The citric acid cycle intermediates (not shown), L-lactate, 8-OHdG, and glutathione status had all improved, suggesting overall improved mitochondrial health. Oral $B_{12}$ supplementation was not adequate to address TL's deficiency, as shown by the rising follow-up methylmalonate (Figure 15). Autistic children with GI lymphoid nodular hyperplasia, a condition associated with the MMR vaccination, had concurrent elevation of urinary methylmalonic acid.[32]

At TL's 10-month visit, he was reported as being in mainstream nursery school, and was indistinguishable from the "normal" children. His parents took before and after videos. They were very pleased with TL's success, as TL's father notes in Figure 16.

# CONCLUSION

ASD is currently the most commonly diagnosed pediatric neurodevelopmental condition. Since the 1980s, the incidence has increased an alarming 20-fold, from 5 in 10,000 to about 1 in 100 today with a higher rate in boys since the M:F ratio is about 4:1. Recent studies have suggested that there have been real increases and that at least 50% of the increases cannot be explained away by increased awareness, changed diagnostic criteria or diagnostic substitution (e.g. children formerly labeled mentally retarded now diagnosed with ASD).[64,65]

Genetics and environment are both recognized as playing causal roles in ASD. Genetic lesions have been found in methylation, sulfuration, glutathione conjugation, the immune system, and the mitochondrial electron transport chain.[58,59] Genetic or epigenetic alteration to enzymatic function can increase cofactor nutrient demand.[60] Nutrient deficiencies due to poor diet or gastrointestinal malabsorption conditions, infections, food reactions, and toxic exposures are also potential triggers or disease mediators.[7,9,11,16,28]

Although TL's recovery from ASD was dramatic, it is not considered rare among clinicians using a biomedical approach.

An association between ASD and vaccines, including the MMR, has been suggested, although the validity of this claim has been challenged.[20,32] Indeed, a great deal of recent controversy surrounds the formal retraction of the 1998 Wakefield article that suggested a link between MMR and ASD.[31] At the same time, however, the argument for environmental impact on ASD precipitation (and many other diseases) is gaining support.[61,66-68] In this case, it appears that both toxic exposures and the MMR vaccine may have had roles in the development of ASD.

Although TL's recovery from ASD was dramatic, it is not considered rare among clinicians using a biomedical approach. Such an approach addresses the interplay of environment and genetics on central nervous system dysregulation, nutrient imbalances, oxidative stress, inflammation, and gastrointestinal pathology.[7,9,10] Because the metabolic lesions in ASD vary widely, laboratory evaluations are used to identify each individual's specific imbalances, allowing for individualized treatment.

Despite the successes, the greater medical community has struggled with fully recognizing the need for this whole-systems approach to treating ASD and often dismisses it by associating it only with extreme or risky practices without understanding the underlying principles or great range of low risk interventions. There is a need for more detailed case reports to be published in the peer-reviewed literature both to document efficacy and to detail practices to conventional medical practitioners who do not have training in the types of assessments and treatments that appear to be most medically effective for ASD. There is also a need to document the impact of functional medicine treatment regimens on neuropsychological and brain function. Such evidence would challenge the conventional framework that autism is purely a fixed genetically caused brain lesion.[69]

Given the surprisingly high and growing incidence of this disorder, well-designed trials are strongly needed to validate the efficacy of the biomedical approach to treating ASD. A functional medicine approach (see appendix A) is well suited to designing a research methodology that, by honoring autism's daunting heterogeneity and complexity, has the best chance of succeeding in validating efficacy of this approach.

---

**Authors: Kara Fitzgerald, ND; Mark Hyman, MD**

**Case Clinicians: Mark Hyman, MD, Chairman, Institute for Functional Medicine; Kathie Swift, MS, RD**

## References


1. CDC. Autism Spectrum Disorders. http://www.cdc.gov/ncbddd/autism/data.html. Accessed 5/15/2010, 2010.
2. CDC. Prevalence of Autism Spectrum Disorders --- Autism and Developmental Disabilities Monitoring Network, 14 Sites, United States, 2002. *MMWR* [http://www.cdc.gov/mmwr/preview/mmwrhtml/ss5601a2.htm. Accessed 07/17/07.
3. Newschaffer CJ, Croen LA, Daniels J, et al. The epidemiology of autism spectrum disorders. *Annu Rev Public Health. 2007;28:235-258.*
4. Rimland B, Baker SM. Brief report: alternative approaches to the development of effective treatments for autism. *J Autism Dev Disord. Apr 1996;26(2):237-241.*
5. O'Hara NH, Szakacs GM. The recovery of a child with autism spectrum disorder through biomedical interventions. *Altern Ther Health Med. Nov-Dec 2008;14(6):42-44.*
6. Baker SM. Sidney MacDonald Baker, MD: taking a biomedical approach to autism treatment. Interview by Frank Lampe and Suzanne Snyder. *Altern Ther Health Med. Nov-Dec 2008;14(6):60-69.*
7. Deth R, Muratore C, Benzecry J, Power-Charnitsky VA, Waly M. How environmental and genetic factors combine to cause autism: A redox/methylation hypothesis. *Neurotoxicology. Jan 2008;29(1):190-201.*
8. Vojdani A, O'Bryan T, Green JA, et al. Immune response to dietary proteins, gliadin and cerebellar peptides in children with autism. *Nutr Neurosci. Jun 2004;7(3):151-161.*
9. James SJ, Cutler P, Melnyk S, et al. Metabolic biomarkers of increased oxidative stress and impaired methylation capacity in children with autism. *Am J Clin Nutr. Dec 2004;80(6):1611-1617.*
10. Poling JS, Frye RE, Shoffner J, Zimmerman AW. Developmental regression and mitochondrial dysfunction in a child with autism. *J Child Neurol. Feb 2006;21(2):170-172.*
11. Kidd PM. Autism, an extreme challenge to integrative medicine. Part 2: medical management. *Altern Med Rev. Dec 2002;7(6):472-499.*
12. Bischoff SC, Grabowsky J, Manns MP. Quantification of inflammatory mediators in stool samples of patients with inflammatory bowel disorders and controls. *Dig Dis Sci. Feb 1997;42(2):394-403.*
13. Jyonouchi H, Geng L, Ruby A, Reddy C, Zimmerman-Bier B. Evaluation of an association between gastrointestinal symptoms and cytokine production against common dietary proteins in children with autism spectrum disorders. *J Pediatr. May 2005;146(5):605-610.*
14. Liu Z, Li N, Neu J. Tight junctions, leaky intestines, and pediatric diseases. *Acta Paediatr. Apr 2005;94(4):386-393.*
15. Margutti P, Delunardo F, Ortona E. Autoantibodies associated with psychiatric disorders. *Curr Neurovasc Res. May 2006;3(2):149-157.*
16. James SJ, Melnyk S, Jernigan S, et al. Metabolic endophenotype and related genotypes are associated with oxidative stress in children with autism. *Am J Med Genet B Neuropsychiatr Genet. Dec 5 2006;141(8):947-956.*
17. Williams MT, Simonet L. In vivo suppression of stearyl CoA desaturase activity by griseofulvin: evidence against the involvement of lipid peroxidation. *Toxicol Appl Pharmacol. Dec 1988;96(3):541-549.*
18. Williams TA, Mars AE, Buyske SG, et al. Risk of autistic disorder in affected offspring of mothers with a glutathione S-transferase P1 haplotype. *Arch Pediatr Adolesc Med. Apr 2007;161(4):356-361.*
19. Wakefield AJ, Puleston JM, Montgomery SM, Anthony A, O'Leary JJ, Murch SH. Review article: the concept of entero-colonic encephalopathy, autism and opioid receptor ligands. *Aliment Pharmacol Ther. Apr 2002;16(4):663-674.*
20. Blaylock RL. A possible central mechanism in autism spectrum disorders, part 1. *Altern Ther Health Med. Nov-Dec 2008;14(6):46-53.*
21. Megson MN. Is autism a G-alpha protein defect reversible with natural vitamin A? *Med Hypotheses. Jun 2000;54(6):979-983.*
22. Frissora CL, Cash BD. Review article: the role of antibiotics vs. conventional pharmacotherapy in treating symptoms of irritable bowel syndrome. *Aliment Pharmacol Ther. Jun 1 2007;25(11):1271-1281.*
23. Fumi AL, Trexler K. Rifaximin treatment for symptoms of irritable bowel syndrome. *Ann Pharmacother. Mar 2008;42(3):408-412.*

24. Majewski M, Reddymasu SC, Sostarich S, Foran P, McCallum RW. Efficacy of rifaximin, a nonabsorbed oral antibiotic, in the treatment of small intestinal bacterial overgrowth. *Am J Med Sci. May 2007;333(5):266-270.*

25. Jawhara S, Poulain D. Saccharomyces boulardii decreases inflammation and intestinal colonization by *Candida albicans* in a mouse model of chemically-induced colitis. *Med Mycol. Dec 2007;45(8):691-700.*

26. Pham M, Lemberg DA, Day AS. Probiotics: sorting the evidence from the myths. *Med J Aust. Mar 3 2008;188(5):304-308.*

27. Haas RH. Autism and mitochondrial disease. *Dev Disabil Res Rev. Jun;16(2):144-153.*

28. Kidd PM. Autism, an extreme challenge to integrative medicine. Part: 1: The knowledge base. *Altern Med Rev. Aug 2002;7(4):292-316.*

29. Kidd PM. Bipolar disorder and cell membrane dysfunction. Progress toward integrative management. *Altern Med Rev. Jun 2004;9(2):107-135.*

30. Wakefield AJ, Murch SH, Anthony A, et al. Ileal-lymphoid-nodular hyperplasia, non-specific colitis, and pervasive developmental disorder in children [see comments]. *Lancet. 1998;351(9103):637-641.*

31. Retraction--Ileal-lymphoid-nodular hyperplasia, non-specific colitis, and pervasive developmental disorder in children. *Lancet. Feb 6;375(9713):445.*

32. Wakefield AJ, Murch SH, Anthony A, et al. Ileal-lymphoid-nodular hyperplasia, non-specific colitis, and pervasive developmental disorder in children. *Lancet. Feb 28 1998;351(9103):637-641.*

33. Uribarri J, Oh MS, Carroll HJ. D-lactic acidosis. A review of clinical presentation, biochemical features, and pathophysiologic mechanisms. *Medicine (Baltimore). Mar 1998;77(2):73-82.*

34. Vernia P, Latella G, Magliocca FM, Caprilli R. Fecal organic anions in diarrhoeal diseases. *Scand J Gastroenterol Suppl. 1987;129:105-109.*

35. Goodwin BL, Ruthven CR, Sandler M. Gut flora and the origin of some urinary aromatic phenolic compounds. *Biochem Pharmacol. Jun 15 1994;47(12):2294-2297.*

36. Tischendorf FW, Brattig NW, Lintzel M, et al. Eosinophil granule proteins in serum and urine of patients with helminth infections and atopic dermatitis. *Trop Med Int Health. Dec 2000;5(12):898-905.*

37. Arvola T, Moilanen E, Vuento R, Isolauri E. Weaning to hypoallergenic formula improves gut barrier function in breast-fed infants with atopic eczema. *J Pediatr Gastroenterol Nutr. Jan 2004;38(1):92-96.*

38. Berni Canani R, Rapacciuolo L, Romano MT, et al. Diagnostic value of faecal calprotectin in paediatric gastroenterology clinical practice. *Dig Liver Dis. Jul 2004;36(7):467-470.*

39. Caldarini MI, Pons S, D'Agostino D, et al. Abnormal fecal flora in a patient with short bowel syndrome. An in vitro study on effect of pH on D-lactic acid production. *Dig Dis Sci. Aug 1996;41(8):1649-1652.*

40. Bull G, Shattock P, Whiteley P, et al. Indolyl-3-acryloylglycine (IAG) is a putative diagnostic urinary marker for autism spectrum disorders. *Med Sci Monit. Oct 2003;9(10):CR422-425.*

41. Wright B, Brzozowski AM, Calvert E, et al. Is the presence of urinary indolyl-3-acryloylglycine associated with autism spectrum disorder? *Dev Med Child Neurol. Mar 2005;47(3):190-192.*

42. Ashwood P, Anthony A, Torrente F, Wakefield AJ. Spontaneous mucosal lymphocyte cytokine profiles in children with autism and gastrointestinal symptoms: mucosal immune activation and reduced counter regulatory interleukin-10. *J Clin Immunol. Nov 2004;24(6):664-673.*

43. Pavone L, Fiumara A, Bottaro G, Mazzone D, Coleman M. Autism and celiac disease: failure to validate the hypothesis that a link might exist. *Biol Psychiatry. Jul 1 1997;42(1):72-75.*

44. Villalta D, Alessio MG, Tampoia M, et al. Diagnostic accuracy of IgA anti-tissue transglutaminase antibody assays in celiac disease patients with selective IgA deficiency. *Ann N Y Acad Sci. Aug 2007;1109:212-220.*

45. Atkinson W, Sheldon TA, Shaath N, Whorwell PJ. Food elimination based on IgG antibodies in irritable bowel syndrome: a randomised controlled trial. *Gut. Oct 2004;53(10):1459-1464.*

46. Macdonald TT, Monteleone G. Immunity, inflammation, and allergy in the gut. *Science. Mar 25 2005;307(5717):1920-1925.*

47. Amminger GP, Berger GE, Schafer MR, Klier C, Friedrich MH, Feucht M. Omega-3 fatty acids supplementation in children with autism: a double-blind randomized, placebo-controlled pilot study. *Biol Psychiatry. Feb 15 2007;61(4):551-553.*

48. Johnson SM, Hollander E. Evidence that eicosapentaenoic acid is effective in treating autism. *J Clin Psychiatry. Jul 2003;64(7):848-849.*

**49.** Deth R, Muratore C, Benzecry J, Power-Charnitsky VA, Waly M. How environmental and genetic factors combine to cause autism: A redox/methylation hypothesis. *Neurotoxicology. Oct 13 2007.*

**50.** Jackson AA, Badaloo AV, Forrester T, Hibbert JM, Persaud C. Urinary excretion of 5-oxoproline (pyroglutamic aciduria) as an index of glycine insufficiency in normal man. *Br J Nutr. Sep 1987;58(2):207-214.*

**51.** Yu YM, Ryan CM, Fei ZW, et al. Plasma L-5-oxoproline kinetics and whole blood glutathione synthesis rates in severely burned adult humans. *Am J Physiol Endocrinol Metab. Feb 2002;282(2):E247-258.*

**52.** Gregus Z, White C, Howell S, Klaassen CD. Effect of glutathione depletion on sulfate activation and sulfate ester formation in rats. *Biochem Pharmacol. Nov 15 1988;37(22):4307-4312.*

**53.** Correia C, Coutinho AM, Diogo L, et al. Brief report: High frequency of biochemical markers for mitochondrial dysfunction in autism: no association with the mitochondrial aspartate/glutamate carrier SLC25A12 gene. *J Autism Dev Disord. Nov 2006;36(8):1137-1140.*

**54.** Bressler JP, Olivi L, Cheong JH, Kim Y, Bannona D. Divalent metal transporter 1 in lead and cadmium transport. *Ann N Y Acad Sci. Mar 2004;1012:142-152.*

**55.** Chauhan A, Chauhan V, Brown WT, Cohen I. Oxidative stress in autism: increased lipid peroxidation and reduced serum levels of ceruloplasmin and transferrin--the antioxidant proteins. *Life Sci. Oct 8 2004;75(21):2539-2549.*

**56.** Mousain-Bosc M, Roche M, Polge A, Pradal-Prat D, Rapin J, Bali JP. Improvement of neurobehavioral disorders in children supplemented with magnesium-vitamin $B_6$. I. Attention deficit hyperactivity disorders. *Magnes Res. Mar 2006;19(1):46-52.*

**57.** Gupta S, Rossignol DA. Autism spectrum disorders: rising prevalence drives research on causes and cures. *Ann Clin Psychiatry. Oct-Dec 2009;21(4):193.*

**58.** Herbert MR. Autism: A Brain Disorder, or a Disorder that Affects the Brain. *Clinical Neuropsychiatry. 2005;2(6):354-379.*

**59.** Ames BN. A role for supplements in optimizing health: the metabolic tune-up. *Arch Biochem Biophys. Mar 1 2004;423(1):227-234.*

**60.** Curtis LT, Patel K. Nutritional and environmental approaches to preventing and treating autism and attention deficit hyperactivity disorder (ADHD): a review. *J Altern Complement Med. Jan-Feb 2008;14(1):79-85.*

**61.** Burrows CJ, Muller JG, Kornyushyna O, et al. Structure and potential mutagenicity of new hydantoin products from guanosine and 8-oxo-7,8-dihydroguanine oxidation by transition metals. *Environmental health perspectives.* Oct 2002;110 Suppl 5:713-717.

**62.** Whiteley P, Haracopos D, Knivsberg AM, et al. The ScanBrit randomised, controlled, single-blind study of a gluten- and casein-free dietary intervention for children with autism spectrum disorders. *Nutr Neurosci.* Apr 2010;13(2):87-100.

**63.** Rossignol DA, Frye RE. Mitochondrial dysfunction in autism spectrum disorders: a systematic review and meta-analysis. *Mol Psychiatry.* Jan 25 2011.

**64.** McDonald ME, Paul JF. Timing of increased autistic disorder cumulative incidence. *Environ Sci Technol.* Mar 15 2010;44(6):2112-2118.

**65.** Hertz-Picciotto I, Delwiche L. The rise in autism and the role of age at diagnosis. *Epidemiology (Cambridge, Mass.* Jan 2009;20(1):84-90.

**66.** Herbert MR. Contributions of the environment and environmentally vulnerable physiology to autism spectrum disorders. *Current opinion in neurology.* Apr 2010;23(2):103-110.

**67.** Herbert MR. Autism: The Centrality of Active Pathophysiology and the Shift from Static to Chronic Dynamic Encephalopathy. In: Chauhan A, Chauhan V, Brown T, eds. *Autism : oxidative stress, inflammation, and immune abnormalities.* Boca Raton, FL: Taylor & Francis; 2009: 427 p.

**68.** Chauhan A, Chauhan V, Brown WT, Cohen I. Oxidative stress in autism: increased lipid peroxidation and reduced serum levels of ceruloplasmin and transferrin--the antioxidant proteins. *Life Sci.* Oct 8 2004;75(21):2539-2549.

**69.** Herbert MR. Learning from the autism catastrophe: key leverage points. *Alternative therapies in health and medicine.* Nov-Dec 2008;14(6):28-30.

# Attention Deficit Hyperactivity Disorder

*Attention Deficit Hyperactivity Disorder (ADHD) is considered a neurobehavioral developmental disorder involving attention regulation and hyperactivity. ADHD is the most prevalent behavioral disorder in children.[1, 2] It occurs at a rate of up to 18% in school-age children, and the incidence might be even higher: in privately insured children, it was, at 28%, the number-one pediatric diagnosis. Symptoms of childhood ADHD persist into adulthood at a rate of up to 66%.[3-5] Stimulant medications, including methylphenidate[6] and amphetamines[7]—the most common drug classes used in treating ADHD—carry significant risks that include, in particular, growth retardation, seizures and cardiovascular events. Not surprisingly, ADHD is a serious public health concern that results in an annual cost to society (as estimated in 2005) of 52 billion U.S. dollars.[8]*

## 12-Year-Old Male with Attention Deficit Hyperactivity Disorder*

| | |
|---|---|
| **Symptoms and Conditions** | Muscle spasms, audio sensitivity, hyperkeratosis pilaris, asthma, allergies, headache, hives, sinusitis, atopic dermatitis, aphthous stomatitis, GERD, nausea, IBS, pruritus ani, anxiety, insomnia |
| **Medications** | Cetirizine (Zyrtec®), albuterol, levalbuterol inhaler (Xopenex®), flunisolide (Nasarel or AeroBid®), cimetidine (Tagamet®), acetaminophen, and ibuprofen |
| **Tests Used** | Multiprofile panel assessing nutrients, fatty acids, amino acids, organic acids, essential elements, oxidative stress and inflammation markers, and whole blood toxic metals; food-specific IgG antibodies, celiac panel; urine toxic elements test; complete blood count; comprehensive metabolic panel |
| **Imbalances Identified** | Essential element and vitamin deficiencies; elevated saturated and trans fatty acids; elevated arachidonic acid/eicosapentaenoic acid ratio (AA/EPA); multiple food sensitivities; antigliadin antibodies; elevated urine lead and low neurotransmitter metabolites; GI fungal overgrowth |
| **Treatments** | Zinc, magnesium, multivitamin and mineral, vitamin D, pyridoxal 5′ phosphate ($B_6$), EPA and docosahexaenoic acid (DHA), 5-HTP, fluconazole, probiotics. Diet: Modified elimination diet: no dairy, peanuts, gluten, sugar, or trans fatty acids. Reduce saturated fat intake. Whole foods, minimally processed; organic diet. DMSA chelation therapy to start in 2 months. |
| **Outcome** | Symptom-free for the first time in his life; dysgraphia improved (see Figure 6 ); eliminated all medications; mood and behavior stabilized; insomnia resolved; improved in school, academically and socially |
| **Discussion/ Significance** | Etiologically, ADHD is considered to be a neurodevelopmental disorder; medications are designed to increase prefrontal cortex catecholamine production. This case, however, suggested that ADHD may be a condition involving multiple system imbalances, with co-morbidities such as dysgraphia, IBS, reflux, atopy, and environmental allergies sharing similar pathophysiology. A systems approach, including an extensive history with comprehensive laboratory assessment, allowed the causal factors to be identified and treated, resulting in a remarkable resolution of all of the patient's complaints. ADHD is the most prevalent behavioral disorder in children, and is a very costly health issue.[1, 2] Medication therapy comes with significant risks. The treatment approach employed in this case, with the demonstrated success, deserves a serious, second look. |

* This case was modified with permission by Kara Fitzgerald, ND, and Mark Hyman, MD, and published by The Institute for Functional Medicine in its *Textbook of Functional Medicine,* 2010.

# CASE HISTORY

PJ presented at age 12 with significant attention deficit hyperactivity disorder (ADHD), dysgraphia, environmental allergies, asthma, insomnia, eczema, canker sores, migraine headaches, muscle cramps, stomach pain, nausea, and diarrhea. He was first diagnosed with ADHD at age 5. He repeated kindergarten because of attention and behavioral difficulties. He began methylphenidate (Ritalin®) in first grade and continued to take it through fourth grade, although it did not change his behavior significantly. The drug was discontinued in fourth grade because of growth retardation. Once off the medication, he gained weight while also increasing his intake of junk food and deli meats.

**ADHD is diagnosed in up to 28% of the pediatric population.**

PJ had never received a positive teacher's report. No longer taking methylphenidate, he continued to be disruptive and unfocused. He excelled in math but had severe dysgraphia (Figure 6). (Dysgraphia, an ADHD comorbidity,[3] is defined as illegible handwriting and spelling errors.)

PJ's environmental allergies included reactions to tree pollen and mold with symptoms of sinus congestion, postnasal drip, sore throats, and hives, for which he took cetirizine (Zyrtec®). Although his mother had removed his bedroom carpet and installed hardwood floors, he showed minimal improvement in his symptoms. His mother noted that dairy worsened his sinus congestion and postnasal drip. PJ usually developed full-blown sinusitis about twice a year, for which he was prescribed antibiotics. PJ's house had an unaddressed mold infestation of an unknown type. Although he had numerous environmental allergies, PJ had shown no drug allergies.

As a toddler, he had developed asthma, hyperkeratosis pilaris, and eczema. For the asthma, PJ was maintained on albuterol, levalbuterol (Xopenex®) and flunisolide (AeroBid®). Since the asthma caused difficulty with breathing at night, he did not sleep well. PJ also suffered from cold-induced asthma attacks. His skin and anus were frequently itchy, and he frequently got canker sores in his mouth.

**Etiologically, ADHD is considered to be a neurodevelopmental disorder; medications are designed to increase prefrontal cortex catecholamine production. This case, however, suggested that ADHD may be a condition involving multiple system imbalances, with co-morbidities such as dysgraphia, IBS, reflux, atopy, and environmental allergies sharing similar pathophysiology.**

PJ suffered from migraine headaches with hypersensitivity to light and sound and had muscle cramps and spasms. For these complaints, he was given acetaminophen and ibuprofen. His stomach pain was treated with cimetidine. He also complained of nausea and had frequent bouts of diarrhea.

Although he was a healthy baby, weighing 7 lb, 10 oz, his vaginal delivery had been difficult. He was treated for hyperbilirubinemia. PJ had been breastfed for 10 months and then given soy formula to treat a "sensitive stomach." Gluten-containing grains were introduced before he turned one year of age. He was prone to diaper rash, had sensitive skin, and received frequent antibiotics for otitis media as a toddler. He received a full vaccine schedule, including annual influenza shots. Although PJ sustained a concussion at age 5, his subsequent CAT scan was normal.

His mother had migraine headaches, sinusitis and food allergies. His sister had environmental allergies. PJ's father was in good health.

His usual dietary intake included eggs, bacon and cereal for breakfast; sandwiches, cookies, peanut butter and crackers for lunch; pizza, chicken, pork, broccoli, green beans, and rice, pasta, or potatoes for dinner. He had strong cravings for sugar and pasta and consumed sugary foods daily. He felt better when he avoided dairy products.

# Initial Laboratory Results

**Laboratory tests ordered and rationale:**

1. **Multiprofile panel**: A comprehensive assessment of fatty acids, amino acids, organic acids, essential elements, oxidative stress and inflammation markers and whole blood toxic metals. The profile assists in finding individual etiopathogenic factors and in consideration of subsequent individualized treatment options. (Not all findings are discussed below. Panel results not grouped together)
2. **Food-specific IgG antibodies and celiac panel**: Food reactions, including gluten sensitivity, may be found at higher rates in atopy and ADHD.
3. **Urine toxic elements**: Toxic metals, particularly lead, have been associated with ADHD.
4. **CBC and comprehensive metabolic panel**: Standard general health assessments.

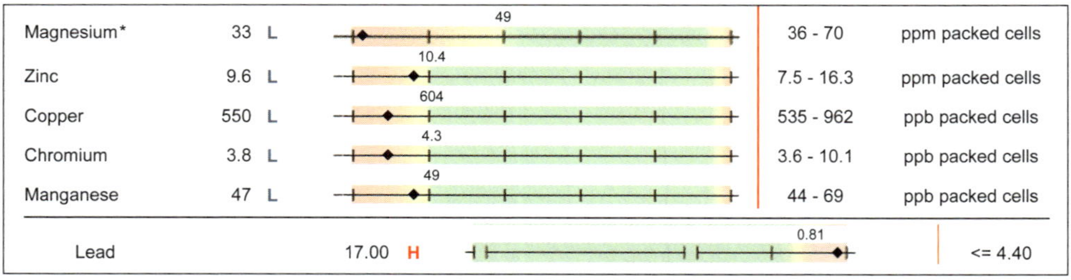


**Figure 1. Red blood cell minerals and urine toxic metals.** Red blood cell essential element levels were low and low-normal in PJ. Six-hour urine toxic elements test with oral DMPS (2,3-dimercapto-1-propanesulfonic acid) challenge showed elevated lead. (Urine toxic units µg/g creatinine)

NOTES

| | Result | Flag | Chart markers | Reference range | Units |
|---|---|---|---|---|---|
| **Vitamin A** | | | | | |
| Retinol | 0.33 | L | 0.36 – 0.74 | 0.29 - 1.05 | mg/L |
| β-Carotene | <0.01 | L | 0.15 – 1.70 | 0.10 - 2.71 | mg/L |
| **Vitamin E** | | | | | |
| alpha-Tocopherol | 8.0 | L | 9.8 – 25.1 | 6.8 - 31.7 | mg/L |
| gamma-Tocopherol | 0.15 | L | 0.26 – 2.06 | 0.06 - 2.99 | mg/L |
| **Vitamin D** | | | | | |
| 25-Hydroxyvitamin D | 12 | L | 16 – 32 | 10 - 64 | ng/mL |
| Xanthurenate | 0.65 | H | 0.47 | <= 0.74 | |
| Kynurenate | 2.0 | H | 1.9 | <= 2.7 | |

**Figure 2. Serum vitamins and urinary organic acids.** Direct and functional assessment of vitamin levels demonstrated multiple deficiencies. The urinary organic acids kynurenate (KYNA) and xanthurenate may rise with $B_6$ deficiency.[9] (Organic acid units: µg/mg creatinine)

| | Results uM | Flag | Chart markers | Reference range |
|---|---|---|---|---|
| ***Saturated*** | | | | |
| Palmitic (16:0) | 2,450 | H | 792 – 1,794 | 667 - 2,526 |
| Stearic (18:0) | 600 | H | 294 – 511 | 250 - 629 |
| Arachidic (20:0) | 6.0 | H | 1.5 – 3.2 | 1.3 - 4.7 |
| Behenic (22:0) | 4.0 | H | 0.8 – 2.0 | 0.6 - 2.9 |
| Lignoceric (24:0) | 3.00 | H | 0.84 – 1.66 | 0.63 - 2.45 |
| ***Trans*** | | | | |
| Palmitelaidic (16:1n7t) | 1.2 | H | 0.4 | <= 1.8 |
| Total C:18 Trans | 45 | H | 42 | <= 59 |
| ***Polyunsaturated Omega-3*** | | | | |
| Alpha Linolenic (18:3n3) | 30 | | 20 | 13 - 80 |
| Eicosapentaenoic (20:5n3) | 45 | | 17 | 5 - 210 |
| Docosahexaenoic (22:6n3) | 80 | | 59 | 31 - 213 |
| ***Polyunsaturated Omega-6*** | | | | |
| Arachidonic (20:4n6) | 785 | H | 201 – 451 | 158 - 521 |

**Figure 3. Serum fatty acids.** Elevated saturated fatty acids, trans fatty acids, and arachidonic acid (AA). Omega 3 fatty acids were within normal limits. (Units: µM)

**IgG (TOTAL) Reactive Foods (BLOOD)**

| | | | |
|---|---|---|---|
| Bean, Kidney (+1) | Milk, Cow's (+3) | Peanut (+2) | Walnut (+1) |
| Cheese (+1) | Mustard (+1) | R. Seed (Canola) (+1) | Yeast, Brewer's (+2) |

| | Results | Reference Limits |
|---|---|---|
| IgG anti-gliadin | HN 17 | normal 0–19 units |

**Figure 4. Food-specific IgG antibodies.** Multiple IgG food sensitivities were found in PJ, including a high-normal production of antigliadin antibodies. Together, these findings suggested intestinal hyperpermeability.

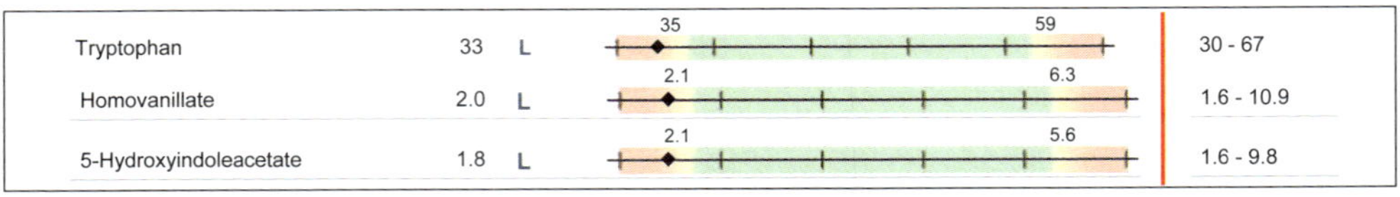


**Figure 5. Tryptophan and urinary neurotransmitter metabolites.** First quintile levels of tryptophan, homovanillate (HVA), and 5-Hydroxyindoleacetate (5-HIAA) were found. HVA and 5-HIAA are metabolites of dopamine and serotonin, respectively. (Tryptophan units: µmol/L; neurotransmitter metabolite units: µg/mg creatinine)

### Other Laboratory Results

Although PJ's serum chemistries and complete blood count were within normal limits, his lymphocyte count was higher than his neutrophil count. Clinical experience suggests that this finding, when combined with his history of antibiotic use and complaint of anal itching, indicates a fungal presence.

## Initial Assessment

- ADHD
- Muscle spasms
- Audio sensitivity
- Hyperkeratosis pilaris
- Asthma
- Allergies
- Headache
- Hives
- Sinusitis
- Atopic dermatitis
- Aphthous stomatitis
- GERD
- Nausea

- IBS
- Pruritus ani
- Anxiety
- Multiple nutrient deficiencies
- Hypovitaminosis D
- Fatty acid imbalance
- Multiple IgG food sensitivities
- Gluten sensitivity
- Intestinal hyperpermeability
- Yeast overgrowth
- Lead toxicity
- Neurotransmitter insufficiency
- PMH: diaper rash, otitis media
- FMH: food and environmental allergies, migraine headaches, sinusitis

## Initial Plan

- Diet:
  - Modified elimination diet based on test results. No dairy, peanuts, gluten, sugar, or trans fatty acids. Reduce saturated fat intake. Whole foods, minimally processed; organic diet. Organic dark chocolate is fine.
- Zinc citrate 20 mg, 1 tab QD
- Magnesium glycinate 120 mg, 2 caps QHS
- Multivitamin/mineral (MVM), 2 tabs QD
- Vitamin $D_3$ 1000 IU, 1 cap QD
- Pyridoxal 5' phosphate (activated $B_6$) 50 mg, 1 cap QD
- EPA/DHA 6:1, 1 cap BID
- 5-HTP 50–100 mg QHS as needed for sleep
- Broad spectrum probiotics, 2 caps QAM
- Fluconazole 100 mg, 1 tab QD × 30 days
- After 2 months on the treatment protocol:
  - Start DMSA (dimercaptosuccinic acid) 100 mg, one twice a day for 3 days every other week (such as MTW)—in effect, the schedule provides for 3 consecutive days on the DMSA followed by 11 days off. Continue that schedule for 6 months and then repeat the DMPS challenge and RBC essential elements tests.

**Treatment plan rationale:** Dietary changes were determined by PJ's clinical history, IgG food sensitivities, antigliadin antibodies, intestinal hyperpermeability, fatty acid deficiency and suspected fungal overgrowth.[10-12] Processed foods containing preservatives and dyes were removed. Fluconazole was prescribed, given the clinical and laboratory evidence for *Candida* overgrowth. Clinical experience suggests that long-term fluconazole with dietary changes will produce the best outcome. Probiotic therapy—considered to be beneficial for treatment of intestinal hyperpermeability, immune hypersensitivity, food sensitivities and IBS—was used to support microbiota.

Nutrient interventions were based on both laboratory and clinical findings: a multivitamin and mineral formula for general nutrient needs with extra zinc for immune dysfunction, diarrhea and allergies;[13-15] magnesium for muscle cramps, insomnia, anxiety and autosensitivity.[16] Additional $B_6$ and vitamin D were given as indicated by the research associated with PJ's condition.[17,18] The vitamin D dosage was based on an attempt to achieve a level of serum vitamin D between 40 and 70 ng/mL.[19] Anti-inflammatory omega-3 fatty acids were used to minimize the pro-inflammatory arachidonic acid cascade, offsetting the elevated AA/EPA ratio.[20-23] 5-HTP was prescribed to provide substrate for serotonin production while preserving tryptophan. Since CNS serotonin is methylated to produce melatonin, an increase in serotonin was expected to help with insomnia.[24]

Since oral chelation with DMSA is one of the main treatments for lead toxicity, it was prescribed for PJ. Pulse dosing DMSA and concurrent detoxification and essential minerals supplementation were prescribed to minimize adverse reactions.[25] Prior to the initiation of DMSA, it was determined that his kidney function and bowel movements were good; in addition, his nutritional deficiencies (particularly those of essential minerals and amino acids), were remediated and impaired methylation was improved. Follow-up testing was ordered to monitor treatment efficacy.

## Two-Month Follow-up

After he began his treatment, which included removing yeast and antigenic foods and adding the needed micronutrients and probiotics, PJ's mother noted that he was much less disruptive in the classroom. He was sleeping though the night and his headaches and runny nose improved. He hadn't required cetirizine or flunisolide for some time. His asthma symptoms improved and were no longer triggered by cold. Light, sound, and smell sensitivities were reduced considerably. PJ tolerated supplements and diet changes well because he felt so much better when he followed the plan. No changes were made to PJ's treatment plan at his two-month visit.

## Six-Month Follow-up

PJ's mother reported that he was free from his chronic symptoms for the first time in his life. His dysgraphia improved considerably (see Figure 6). He no longer required his medications, including antihistamines (cetirizine and cimetidine), bronchodilators, steroid inhaler, acetaminophen, and ibuprofen. His mood and behavior had stabilized, and his ability to focus improved greatly. His hyperactivity symptoms, including disruptiveness, irritability, and anxiety, were gone. His hives, asthma, runny nose and post nasal drip, anal itching, stomachaches, nausea, diarrhea, headaches, muscle cramps, and sensitivity to loud noises were all completely resolved. He slept soundly at night and was doing well in school, academically and socially.

Just after his 6-month follow-up, PJ's mother wrote the following:

> *"We had a meeting this morning at PJ's school, where the teachers, school counselor, parents, and principal all got together to review "the plan" for kids with special educational needs (in PJ's case prompted by the ADHD diagnosis). This was the first time in his entire schooling history that everything seems to be going well. The input from his teachers was that he is "a different kid" from the boy they saw in the first half of the year and that they're amazed by the difference. The school nurse hasn't seen him in months (he used to be in her office several times a week). The school psychologist said that his social skills are very good as well as age appropriate, and that she sees no problems at all. She also noted that PJ seems very proud of himself and his new health, and that he's taking good "ownership" of all the changes in his diet. He even seems to be "shrugging it off" when the other kids at school call him an "alien" because he doesn't drink soda.*
>
> *This was just such a fantastic meeting and I wanted to pass along the good news and say Thank You!"*
>
> **~ PJ's mother**

## Follow-up Laboratory Results

Follow-up testing revealed normalization of the lymphocyte/neutrophil ratio and improvement in his nutritional status, including normalized levels of vitamin E and beta carotene, RBC minerals, and tryptophan. His saturated fatty acids and trans fatty acids were all within their normal ranges, reducing the concern about dysinsulinemia and confirming PJ's commitment to following dietary changes. He still required vitamins A and D. The dietary changes and supplement interventions not only eliminated his presenting complaints, but radically improved his prognosis for developing conditions such as diabetes or cardiovascular disease.

# DISCUSSION

Individuals with ADHD focus excessively on specific stimuli without the ability to discriminate between the relevant and the non-relevant. Hyperactivity and impulsivity are also components of the condition. Executive function and, therefore, attention and behavioral inhibition are primary activities of the frontal lobes. MRIs of individuals diagnosed with ADHD demonstrate decreased activation of the frontal cortex, including lower levels of neurotransmitters. Neurotransmitters in the frontal lobe are primarily the catecholamines, dopamine and norepinephrine. ADHD medications target these neurotransmitters, increasing their availability. Serotonergic receptors, which have been linked to attention capability, may also play a role in ADHD pathophysiology.

ADHD is thought to result from a complex interplay between genes and environment. Variants of the gene that codes for dopamine-related proteins, including transport, receptor and enzyme proteins, have been implicated in ADHD.[5,26] Recognized environmental contributors to ADHD include head injuries, food preservatives and dyes, toxins, infectious exposure, food allergens, and nutrient insufficiencies.[27-30] A full understanding of the genetics of ADHD may depend upon understanding multiple gene-environment interactions.[31]

At 12 years of age, PJ was on an overwhelming pharmacopoeia, including cetirizine, albuterol, levalbuterol inhaler, flunisolide, cimetidine, acetaminophen and ibuprofen without good result. While methylphenidate, specifically designed to address low prefrontal cortex catecholamine status, did not improve his school performance in any measurable way, it did cause growth retardation and was therefore discontinued. Side effects of his medications may also have contributed to the pathogenesis of his numerous complaints. For example, cimetidine has been associated with nutritional deficiencies and gastrointestinal bacterial overgrowth from gastric acid inhibition.[32] Glutathione depletion results from acetaminophen use,[33] and intestinal permeability increases with use of nonsteroidal anti-inflammatory medications such as ibuprofen.[34] Flunisolide has also been shown to inhibit growth in children.[35]

Recognized environmental contributors to ADHD include head injuries, food preservatives and dyes, toxins, infectious exposure, food allergens, and nutrient insufficiencies.

Very low levels of zinc and magnesium and low-normal levels of other minerals were found. These findings were not surprising given PJ's poor diet, GI inflammation and cimetidine use. Zinc deficiency is implicated in asthma, atopic dermatitis, allergies and ADHD.[13-15] Magnesium deficiency is also implicated in headaches, insomnia, muscle cramps and spasms.[16] Copper and manganese are important cofactors in the antioxidant enzyme superoxide dismutase. Chromium as chromodulin may increase cellular glucose uptake by potentiating insulin receptor activity.[36]

DMPS (2,3-dimercapto-1-propanesulfonic acid) provocation challenge demonstrated an elevated urine lead level (Figure 1). Although whole blood assay is considered the gold standard for identifying lead toxicity, urinary lead concentration has also been shown to increase with toxicity.[36] On account of the fact that exposure to lead may result in cognitive deficits at levels commonly encountered in blood, numerous recommendations have been made to reduce it to safer threshold levels.[36] Lead toxicity and environmental toxins such as household mold have been linked to cognitive and behavioral problems, including ADHD, in children.[29,37-39] Sources of lead include toys, paint, contaminated soil, lead plumbing, and glazed pottery.[36] Essential mineral deficiencies may allow for increased uptake of toxic metals.[25] Thus, the patient must be tested for and treated with essential minerals during chelation therapy.

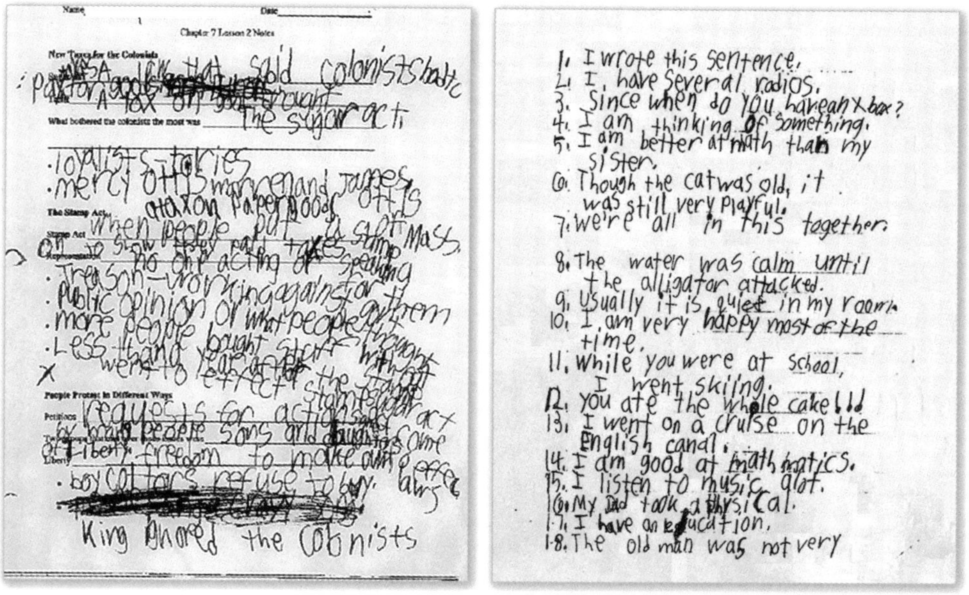


**Figure 6. PJ's pre- and post-treatment writing samples.** PJ was described by his teachers as "a different kid" from the boy they saw in the first half of the year. They were amazed by the difference.

Figure 2 demonstrated that levels of the fat-soluble vitamins in PJ's serum were low (for E, A, and D) or undetectable (for beta carotene). Such a pattern can indicate fat malabsorption, but in PJ's case the cause was thought to be poor dietary habits. The low level of vitamin D probably played a role in PJ's imbalanced immune response, contributing to both his chronic infections and hypersensitivities. Hypovitaminosis D has been implicated in asthma, general development problems, and mood disorders.[17] The optimal level of serum vitamin D is now thought to lie between 40 to 70 ng/mL; individuals with serious diseases should maintain levels between 55 to 70 ng/mL.[19]

Figure 2 also revealed a functional need for $B_6$. Elevations of the organic acids xanthurenate and kynurenate demonstrated a $B_6$ insufficiency, because the enzymes required to metabolize them further are $B_6$ dependent.[40] A number of PJ's symptoms may have been attributable to insufficient $B_6$, including ADHD, mood disturbances, and insomnia.[18]

Plasma free fatty acid levels (primarily that of palmitic acid) roughly approximate plasma triglyceride levels.[36] The numerous high-normal saturated fatty acids shown in Figure 3 indicated that, at age 12, PJ probably had higher than optimal triglyceride levels most likely caused by insulin-stimulated up-regulation of liver fatty acid synthesis. Given PJ's high-sugar diet, early onset of dysinsulinemia was not surprising, although mild chromium deficiency could be another underlying factor contributing to dysinsulinemia. The elevated levels of trans fatty acids (TFAs) shown in Figure 3 were further evidence of PJ's poor food choices. TFAs are strongly implicated in metabolic syndrome and cardiovascular disease.[41]

Of the polyunsaturated omega fatty acids, the pro-inflammatory eicosanoid precursor arachidonic acid (AA) was very elevated (Figure 3) and was found in much greater quantity than the anti-inflammatory omega-3 fatty acid eicosapentaenoic acid (EPA), creating a relative deficiency of EPA. AA is implicated in the pathogenesis of allergies and asthma,[21,23] while EPA insufficiency and a low EPA/AA ratio are implicated in ADHD.[20, 22]

The plasma fatty acid analysis revealed that, had PJ continued with his present diet and lifestyle, he would have incurred, as an adult, an increased risk of continued inflammatory conditions including heart disease, diabetes, and cancer. Addressing these findings early not only treated his initial complaints, but significantly reduced his future risk of ill health.

ELISA testing for IgG response to 90 different foods demonstrated a strong positive reaction to dairy (+3), a reaction to peanuts (+2), and mild positive reactions (+1 or +2) to seven other foods, indicating intestinal hyperpermeability and GI inflammation (Figure 4).[10-12] These sensitivities are associated with the pathogenesis of atopic dermatitis, asthma and ADHD.[42-44] Additionally, PJ's IgG antigliadin antibodies were trending high at 17 units. Clinical experience warranted minimizing gluten intake.

When introduced into the diet prior to age 1, as in the case of PJ, gluten-containing grains are associated with a statistically significant increase in the incidence of celiac disease in susceptible patients.[45] Furthermore, the use of soy formula in infants with a first-degree relative with allergies (as in the case of PJ) is associated with increased incidence of allergies, food intolerances, and eczema.[46] Early antibiotic use is also associated with an increased incidence of atopic conditions, including asthma.[47-50]

The urinary neurotransmitter metabolites for dopamine and serotonin, homovanillate (HVA) and 5-hydroxyindoleacetate (5-HIAA), were low normal in PJ, suggesting lower total body neurotransmitter turnover (Figure 5). Corroborative evidence of the risk of serotonin insufficiency was found in the low-normal plasma tryptophan, the amino acid precursor to serotonin. Furthermore, two important nutrients involved in dopamine and serotonin synthesis, $B_6$ and magnesium, were both reported as insufficient in PJ. Genetic and metabolic research has linked imbalances, with regard to uptake, synthesis, and breakdown of CNS dopamine and serotonin, to ADHD, although no consistent pattern has been noted.[51, 52] Serotonin imbalance has also been implicated in insomnia[24] and IBS.[53]

---

NOTES

# CONCLUSION

ADHD is thought to be an issue of insufficient prefrontal cortex catecholamine production caused by a complex interplay between gene predisposition and environment exposures. The standard therapeutic goal is therefore designed to increase prefrontal cortex catecholamine production. The case of PJ, however, suggested that ADHD may be a condition involving multiple system imbalances, with comorbidities such as dysgraphia, IBS, reflux, atopy, and environmental allergies sharing similar etiologic factors. Environmental causes of ADHD in PJ's case appeared to be gluten sensitivity, lead exposure, and poor diet, which in turn contributed to intestinal hyperpermeability, IgG food sensitivities, and significant nutrient deficiencies. Interestingly, while neurotransmitter imbalances were identified on laboratory testing, their involvement in the etiology of his condition appeared secondary to other issues. Treating multiple system dysfunctions led to remarkable resolution of PJ's ADHD, his dysgraphia, and all of his other complaints. Use of a systems approach, including an extensive history with comprehensive laboratory assessment, allowed the causal factors to be identified and treated. While ADHD is the most prevalent behavioral disorder in children and a very costly health condition,[1,2] medication therapy comes with significant risks and often very limited success. Therefore, clinicians must become skilled in the use of other approaches, such as the comprehensive assessment, dietary modifications, and nutritional therapies exemplified by this case.

**Treating multiple system dysfunctions led to remarkable resolution of PJ's ADHD, his dysgraphia, and all of his other complaints.**

**Authors: Kara Fitzgerald, ND; Mark Hyman, MD**

**Case Clinicians: Mark Hyman, MD, Chairman, Institute for Functional Medicine; Kathie Swift, MS, RD**

## References

1. Jensen PS, Garcia JA, Glied S, et al. Cost-effectiveness of ADHD treatments: findings from the multimodal treatment study of children with ADHD. *Am J Psychiatry.* Sep 2005;162(9):1628-1636.
2. Richters JE, Arnold LE, Jensen PS, et al. NIMH collaborative multisite multimodal treatment study of children with ADHD: I. Background and rationale. *J Am Acad Child Adolesc Psychiatry.* Aug 1995;34(8):987-1000.
3. Adi-Japha E, Landau YE, Frenkel L, Teicher M, Gross-Tsur V, Shalev RS. ADHD and dysgraphia: underlying mechanisms. *Cortex.* Aug 2007;43(6):700-709.
4. CDC. Public Health Issues in ADHD: Individual, System, and Cost Burden of the Disorder Workshop. http://www.cdc.gov/ncbddd/adhd/workshops/publichealth.html. Accessed 6/12/2010, 2010.
5. Madras BK, Miller GM, Fischman AJ. The dopamine transporter and attention-deficit/hyperactivity disorder. *Biol Psychiatry.* Jun 1 2005;57(11):1397-1409.
6. RxList. Methylphenidate. http://www.rxlist.com/script/main/srchcont_rxlist.asp?src=methylphenidate. Accessed 6/21/2010.
7. RxList. Amphetamines and ADHD. http://www.rxlist.com/script/main/srchcont_rxlist.asp?src=amphetamines+adhd. Accessed 6-21-2010, 2010.
8. CDC. Attention-Deficit / Hyperactivity Disorder (ADHD). http://www.cdc.gov/ncbddd/adhd/data.html. Accessed 6/10/2010, 2010.
9. Lord RS BJ, ed. *Laboratory Evaluations for Integrative and Functional Medicine.* Atlanta: Metametrix Institute; 2008:31.

10. Atkinson W, Sheldon TA, Shaath N, Whorwell PJ. Food elimination based on IgG antibodies in irritable bowel syndrome: a randomised controlled trial. *Gut.* Oct 2004;53(10):1459-1464.

11. DeMeo MT, Mutlu EA, Keshavarzian A, Tobin MC. Intestinal permeation and gastrointestinal disease. *J Clin Gastroenterol.* Apr 2002;34(4):385-396.

12. Macdonald TT, Monteleone G. Immunity, inflammation, and allergy in the gut. *Science.* Mar 25 2005;307(5717):1920-1925.

13. Wintergerst ES, Maggini S, Hornig DH. Contribution of selected vitamins and trace elements to immune function. *Ann Nutr Metab.* 2007;51(4):301-323.

14. Arnold LE, DiSilvestro RA. Zinc in attention-deficit/hyperactivity disorder. *J Child Adolesc Psychopharmacol.* Aug 2005;15(4):619-627.

15. Yorbik O, Ozdag MF, Olgun A, Senol MG, Bek S, Akman S. Potential effects of zinc on information processing in boys with attention deficit hyperactivity disorder. *Prog Neuropsychopharmacol Biol Psychiatry.* Apr 1 2008;32(3):662-667.

16. Altura BM, Altura BT. Tension headaches and muscle tension: is there a role for magnesium? *Med Hypotheses.* Dec 2001;57(6):705-713.

17. Holick MF. Vitamin D deficiency. *N Engl J Med.* Jul 19 2007;357(3):266-281.

18. Mousain-Bosc M, Roche M, Polge A, Pradal-Prat D, Rapin J, Bali JP. Improvement of neurobehavioral disorders in children supplemented with magnesium-vitamin B6. II. Pervasive developmental disorder-autism. *Magnes Res.* Mar 2006;19(1):53-62.

19. Cannell JJ, Hollis BW. Use of vitamin D in clinical practice. *Altern Med Rev.* Mar 2008;13(1):6-20.

20. Matsudaira T. Attention deficit disorders—drugs or nutrition? *Nutr Health.* 2007;19(1-2):57-60.

21. Serrano-Mollar A, Closa D. Arachidonic acid signaling in pathogenesis of allergy: therapeutic implications. *Curr Drug Targets Inflamm Allergy.* Apr 2005;4(2):151-155.

22. Sorgi PJ, Hallowell EM, Hutchins HL, Sears B. Effects of an open-label pilot study with high-dose EPA/DHA concentrates on plasma phospholipids and behavior in children with attention deficit hyperactivity disorder. *Nutr* J. Jul 13 2007;6(1):16.

23. Wenzel SE. Arachidonic acid metabolites: mediators of inflammation in asthma. *Pharmacotherapy.* Jan-Feb 1997;17(1 Pt 2):3S-12S.

24. Bucci L. Migraine, insomnia, reactive depression due to brain serotonin deficiency. *Br J Psychiatry.* Jun 1988;152:867-868.

25. Bressler JP, Olivi L, Cheong JH, Kim Y, Maerten A, Bannon D. Metal transporters in intestine and brain: their involvement in metal-associated neurotoxicities. *Hum Exp Toxicol.* Mar 2007;26(3):221-229.

26. Madras BK, Miller GM, Fischman AJ. The dopamine transporter: relevance to attention deficit hyperactivity disorder (ADHD). *Behav Brain Res.* Mar 10 2002;130(1-2):57-63.

27. Willmott C, Ponsford J, Hocking C, Schonberger M. Factors contributing to attentional impairments after traumatic brain injury. *Neuropsychology.* Jul 2009;23(4):424-432.

28. Sinn N. Nutritional and dietary influences on attention deficit hyperactivity disorder. *Nutr Rev.* Oct 2008;66(10):558-568.

29. Curtis LT, Patel K. Nutritional and environmental approaches to preventing and treating autism and attention deficit hyperactivity disorder (ADHD): a review. *J Altern Complement Med.* Jan-Feb 2008;14(1):79-85.

30. Froehlich TE, Lanphear BP, Auinger P, et al. Association of tobacco and lead exposures with attention-deficit/hyperactivity disorder. *Pediatrics.* Dec 2009;124(6):e1054-1063.

31. Coghill D, Banaschewski T. The genetics of attention-deficit/hyperactivity disorder. *Expert Rev Neurother.* Oct 2009;9(10):1547-1565.

32. Evenepoel P. Alteration in digestion and absorption of nutrients during profound acid suppression. *Best Pract Res Clin Gastroenterol.* Jun 2001;15(3):539-551.

33. Kon K, Ikejima K, Okumura K, et al. Role of apoptosis in acetaminophen hepatotoxicity. *J Gastroenterol Hepatol.* Jun 2007;22 Suppl 1:S49-52.

34. Mielants H, Goemaere S, De Vos M, et al. Intestinal mucosal permeability in inflammatory rheumatic diseases. I. Role of antiinflammatory drugs. *J Rheumatol.* Mar 1991;18(3):389-393.

35. Sharek PJ, Bergman DA. Beclomethasone for asthma in children: effects on linear growth. *Cochrane Database Syst Rev.* 2000(2):CD001282.

36. Lord RS, Bralley JA, eds. *Laboratory Evaluations for Integrative and Functional Medicine.* 2nd ed. Duluth, GA: Metametrix Institute; 2008.

37. Banerjee TD, Middleton F, Faraone SV. Environmental risk factors for attention-deficit hyperactivity disorder. *Acta Paediatr.* Sep 2007;96(9):1269-1274.

38. Braun JM, Kahn RS, Froehlich T, Auinger P, Lanphear BP. Exposures to environmental toxicants and attention deficit hyperactivity disorder in U.S. children. *Environ Health Perspect.* Dec 2006;114(12):1904-1909.

39. Kidd PM. Attention deficit/hyperactivity disorder (ADHD) in children: rationale for its integrative management. *Altern Med Rev.* Oct 2000;5(5):402-428.

40. Council NRCUSCoDAFaNBNR. *Human vitamin B6 requirements: proceedings of a workshop: Letterman Army.* Washington, DC: National Academy of Sciences; 1976.

41. Mozaffarian D. Trans fatty acids - Effects on systemic inflammation and endothelial function. *Atheroscler Suppl.* May 2006;7(2):29-32.

42. Del Giudice MM, Rocco A, Capristo C. Probiotics in the atopic march: highlights and new insights. *Dig Liver Dis.* Dec 2006;38 Suppl 2:S288-290.

43. Newmark SC. ADHD and food sensitivity. *Altern Ther Health Med.* May-Jun 2002;8(3):18; author reply 18.

44. Schnoll R, Burshteyn D, Cea-Aravena J. Nutrition in the treatment of attention-deficit hyperactivity disorder: a neglected but important aspect. *Appl Psychophysiol Biofeedback.* Mar 2003;28(1):63-75.

45. Norris JM, Barriga K, Hoffenberg EJ, et al. Risk of celiac disease autoimmunity and timing of gluten introduction in the diet of infants at increased risk of disease. *Jama.* May 18 2005;293(19):2343-2351.

46. Osborn DA, Sinn J. Soy formula for prevention of allergy and food intolerance in infants. *Cochrane Database Syst Rev.* 2004(3):CD003741.

47. Kozyrskyj AL, Ernst P, Becker AB. Increased risk of childhood asthma from antibiotic use in early life. *Chest.* Jun 2007;131(6):1753-1759.

48. Farooqi IS, Hopkin JM. Early childhood infection and atopic disorder. *Thorax.* Nov 1998;53(11):927-932.

49. Shreiner A, Huffnagle GB, Noverr MC. The "Microflora Hypothesis" of allergic disease. *Adv Exp Med Biol.* 2008;635:113-134.

50. Wickens K, Pearce N, Crane J, Beasley R. Antibiotic use in early childhood and the development of asthma. *Clin Exp Allergy.* Jun 1999;29(6):766-771.

51. Oades RD. Dopamine-serotonin interactions in attention-deficit hyperactivity disorder (ADHD). *Prog Brain Res.* 2008;172:543-565.

52. Oades RD. Dopamine may be 'hyper' with respect to noradrenaline metabolism, but 'hypo' with respect to serotonin metabolism in children with attention-deficit hyperactivity disorder. *Behav Brain Res.* Mar 10 2002;130(1-2):97-102.

53. Sikander A, Rana SV, Prasad KK. Role of serotonin in gastrointestinal motility and irritable bowel syndrome. *Clin Chim Acta.* May 2009;403(1-2):47-55.

# 4 Cardiovascular and Related Conditions

## Hypertension

*Hypertension is responsible for roughly one-in-six adult deaths annually in the United States and is associated with five of the top nine causes of death.[1] Ten trillion dollars is the estimated annual cost worldwide of the direct and indirect effects of hypertension.[2, 3] In the U.S. alone, costs estimated at almost $74 billion in 2009 placed a huge economic burden on the health care system.[4] The prevalence of hypertension increases with advancing age to the point where more than half of people 60 to 69 years of age and at least three-fourths of those 70 years of age and older are affected.[5] Most individuals with hypertension do not have it adequately controlled.[1, 6] Medication noncompliance due to avoidance of side effects is suggested to be a primary factor.[6] The epidemic incidence of hypertension and its significant cost to society indicate that a well-tolerated, cost-effective approach to treatment is urgently needed.*

### 48-Year-Old Male with Resistant Hypertension on Triple Therapy

| | |
|---|---|
| **Symptoms and Conditions** | Recent past history of hypertensive crisis, complicated by diastolic dysfunction and congestive heart failure; significant medication side effects, including weakness, fatigue, erectile dysfunction and dizziness |
| **Medications** | Amlodipine and olmesartan (Azor®); carvedilol (Coreg CR®) |
| **Tests Used** | Asymmetric dimethylarginine (ADMA), high sensitivity C-reactive protein (hsCRP), 8-hydroxy-2-deoxyguanosine (8-OHdG), quinolinate, red blood cell magnesium, vitamin D |
| **Imbalances Identified** | Elevated ADMA, hsCRP, 8-OHdG, and quinolinate; low red blood cell magnesium; low serum vitamin D |
| **Treatments** | Arginine, ascorbic acid, magnesium, and vitamin D; dietary and exercise modifications |
| **Outcome** | Decreased mean systolic and diastolic blood pressure from 162/104 to 130/85 over four months, allowing for a reduction in his antihypertensive medications to tolerable dosages that did not invoke side effects; 25 pound weight loss. |
| **Discussion and Significance** | Evidence suggests, and this case demonstrates, that effective, well-tolerated, non-pharmacological approaches to hypertension are available.[4,7] In this case, laboratory analysis was used to identify the underlying metabolic imbalances contributing to the patient's hypertension. The findings enabled the development of a personalized treatment protocol that was effective in reducing the patient's blood pressure to safer levels. The treatment allowed for a medication reduction that was sufficient to eliminate the side effects the patient had been experiencing. Because of the potential for significant improvements in morbidity, mortality and cost savings with the approach employed in this case, further research is warranted. |

# CASE HISTORY

JF was 48 when he presented with a history of pharmaceutically managed hypertension. His goal was to decrease his medications, as he felt they were adversely affecting his quality of life. He experienced erectile dysfunction (ED), which he felt was exacerbated by the medication. He also complained of other medication-related side effects, including dizziness, fatigue, and general weakness. A little over ten years earlier, during a routine office visit, JF's physician discovered a blood pressure of 147/95 mmHg; the patient chose not to be concerned about blood pressure at that time, as he felt fine. However, ten years later, JF was not feeling well and was under a great deal of stress. He was also taking a number of "herbal stimulants," which he later discontinued. He visited his doctor, who found his blood pressure to be 250/160 mmHg. JF was immediately hospitalized for hypertensive crisis, complicated by diastolic dysfunction and congestive heart failure. The initial hospital treatment included diuresis with furosemide. His doctor then initiated triple antihypertensive therapy including a combination calcium channel blocker/angiotensin receptor blocker (amlodipine and olmesartan medoxomil 20 mg/40 mg) and 40 mg of extended release carvedilol, a non-selective beta blocker. Since a follow-up echocardiogram demonstrated improvement in diastolic dysfunction and hypertension, JF and his physician discontinued furosemide treatment. However, he remained on the three other blood pressure medications. It was at this time that JF sought the care of an integrative physician to support him in finding alternative options for controlling his hypertension.

Additional history revealed that the patient had all but four of his dental amalgam fillings removed just prior to the hypertensive crisis. JF also had a history of multiple root canals for abscesses that resulted from dental caries. He was 35 pounds overweight. Though yoga was his main form of exercise, he did it intermittently. He reported his stress level to be 3 out of 10 (0 as lowest stress level possible, 10 as highest stress level possible) at the time of his visit. He took a variety of supplements; including vitamin E, fish oil, CoQ10, and magnesium citrate. His diet included a good deal of simple carbohydrate foods, such as white rice, potato and pasta, with some sweets.

**Ten trillion dollars is the estimated annual cost world wide of the direct and indirect effects of hypertension. In the United States, more than half of people 60 to 69 years of age and at least three-fourths of those 70 years of age have hypertension.**

JF's family history included a father who was a heavy smoker, deceased at age 50 from myocardial infarction, and a 76-year-old mother who had hypertension. He had two healthy sisters and one 53-year-old brother with hypertension (medicated) and coronary artery disease, status post stent placement.

JF's blood pressure was 162/104.

---

NOTES

# Initial Laboratory Results

**Laboratory tests ordered and rationale:**

1. **ADMA and arginine**: Evaluation of nitric oxide inhibition (ADMA) and nitric oxide substrate availability (arginine) Imbalances of both have been associated with hypertension.
2. **Urinary organic acids**: In this case, the organic acid profile was used to evaluate oxidative stress and inflammation.
3. **Lipid panel with fasting insulin and hsCRP**: Evaluation of metabolic imbalances and inflammation associated with cardiovascular disease
4. **Fat-soluble vitamins E and D, and CoQ10**: Nutrients required for cardiovascular function

| Test | Result | Marker | Reference range |
|---|---|---|---|
| Asymmetric Dimethylarginine (ADMA) | 0.62 H | 0.54 | 0.26 - 0.67 |
| Arginine | 109 H | 54 | 37 - 101 |

**Figure 1. ADMA and arginine.** Result showed a fifth quintile elevation of both plasma ADMA and arginine. (Units: µmol/L)

| Test | Result | Reference range | Units |
|---|---|---|---|
| c-Reactive Protein (HS) | 10.3 H | <= 3.0 | mg/L |
| Quinolinate | 5.7 H | <= 5.8 | |

**Figure 2. Inflammation markers.** Results showed a significant elevation of hsCRP. The urinary organic acid quinolinate was high-normal in the fifth quintile. (Quinolinate units: µg/mg creatinine)

| Test | Result | Marker | Reference range |
|---|---|---|---|
| 8-Hydroxy-2-deoxyguanosine ** | 9.4 H | 5.3 | <= 7.6 |

** Units for 8-Hydroxy-2-deoxyguanosine are ng/mg creatinine

**Figure 3. Oxidative stress.** The urinary organic acid 8-OHdG was significantly elevated. (Units: ng/mg creatinine)

| Test | Result | Marker | Reference range | Units |
|---|---|---|---|---|
| RBC Magnesium | 40 L | 49 | 36 - 70 | ppm packed cells |

**Figure 4. Red blood cell magnesium.** The magnesium level was suboptimal.

| | | | |
|---|---|---|---|
| Triglycerides | 209 H | 35 - 160 | mg/dL |
| Insulin | 2.2 | 2.0 - 12.0 | uIU/mL |
| Total Cholesterol | 189 | <= 200 | mg/dL |
| HDL Cholesterol | 25 L | 30 - 85 | mg/dL |

**Figure 5. Cardiovascular markers.** Findings indicated hypertriglyceridemia with low HDL; insulin and total cholesterol were within normal limits.

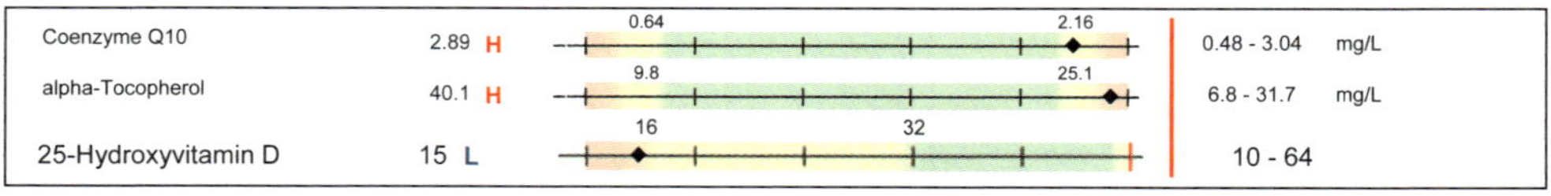


**Figure 6. Fat-soluble nutrients.** Elevated serum CoQ10, elevated vitamin E, and low vitamin D. (CoQ10 and vitamin E units: mg/L; vitamin D units: ng/mL)

# Initial Assessment

- Hypertension (elevated ADMA and arginine)
- Congestive heart failure
- Hypertriglyceridemia
- Erectile dysfunction
- High triglyceride/HDL ratio suggests insulin resistance
- Hypomagnesemia
- Hypovitaminosis D
- Oxidative stress (elevated 8OHdG)
- Systemic inflammation (elevated hs-CRP and quinolinate)
- Periodontal disease

# Initial Plan

- Titrate magnesium citrate up slowly to bowel tolerance
- Sustained release arginine: begin with 500 mg a day, and gradually increase to 3000 mg a day, in divided doses; begin after magnesium dosage stabilization
- Calcium ascorbate with bioflavonoids, 2000 mg a day for oxidative stress
- Vitamin $D_3$, 4000 IU per day for 3 months
- Oral irrigation daily (for periodontal disease)
- ½ tsp of cinnamon powder daily
- Low glycemic-index DASH diet (Dietary Approaches to Stop Hypertension)
- Decrease supplemental vitamin E
- Continue fish oil (essential fatty acids)
- Exercise program
- Recheck hsCRP and 8OHdG in 8 weeks
- Recheck vitamin $D_3$ in 3 months; goal > 55 ng/mL

**Treatment plan rationale:** The high ADMA level may have contributed to a relative arginine deficiency (despite an elevated plasma arginine finding) resulting in reduced nitric oxide availability that contributed to hypertension. Therefore, arginine supplementation was initiated. Magnesium was also needed, as indicated by the low RBC finding, which has specifically been associated with hypertension.[8] Ascorbate and bioflavonoids were introduced for their cardiovascular-protective, antioxidant and anti-inflammatory potential.[9,10]

Vitamin D was initiated based on the laboratory finding. Hypovitaminosis D is associated with hypertension, inflammation and increased oxidative stress.[11] JF was advised to begin oral irrigation, given his history of periodontal disease. Cinnamon was recommended because it has been shown to help diminish insulin sensitivity and to have antimicrobial properties that would further support the treatment of periodontal disease.[12] A sugar-free, low glycemic-index (DASH-type) diet with exercise was also prescribed for insulin resistance. Despite elevated serum levels, CoQ10 was continued because it is nontoxic at higher levels and may be beneficial.[13] However, since vitamin E supplementation has mixed safety reviews in the literature, his self-prescribed dosage was reduced based on the elevated finding.[14,15] It was recommended he continue fish oil for vascular disease risk reduction.[16]

**The high ADMA level may have contributed to a relative arginine deficiency (despite an elevated plasma arginine finding) resulting in reduced nitric oxide availability that contributed to hypertension.**

## One-Month Follow-up

JF's average blood pressure was 141/93. He was following the dietary suggestions, taking supplements as directed and had initiated exercise. He was pleased to report a five pound weight loss. It was suggested he reduce the amlodipine/olmesartan combination to 10 mg/20 mg per day and the carvedilol from 50 mg twice per day to 25 mg in the morning and 12.5 mg in evening. He was otherwise advised to continue the plan as directed.

## Four-Month Follow-up

JF's average blood pressure was 130/85. He was following all aspects of his plan as prescribed. He stated that he felt calmer, and was now walking daily and biking 3 to 4 days a week. His weight loss was at 25 pounds. He noted improvement with ED. He was very pleased with his progress, and was motivated to continue to improve. He was advised to remain on the amlodipine/olmesartan dose of 10 mg/20 mg and reduce the carvedilol to 12.5 mg once in the morning (at which dose he had no side effects). No other changes were made to his plan.

## Four-Month Follow-up Laboratory Results

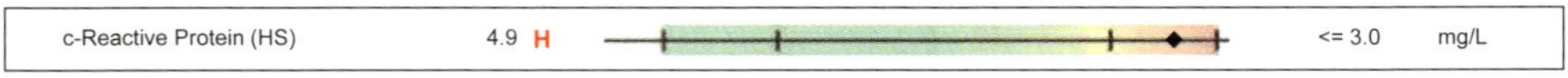


**Figure 7. Follow-up hsCRP.** Follow-up hsCRP demonstrated significant improvement (baseline level was 10.3).

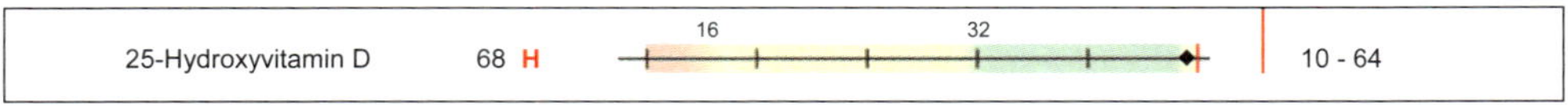


**Figure 8. Follow-up vitamin D.** Target level of > 55 ng/mL had been achieved.

# DISCUSSION

Hypertension is directly or indirectly associated with five of the top nine causes of death in the U.S., including heart disease, cerebrovascular disease, diabetes, renal disease, and essential hypertension.[1] Lifestyle risk factors play a significant role in hypertension etiology, including poor diet and nutrition, imbalanced salt and potassium intake, inactivity, and smoking. There is also a recognized genetic component.[1] Essential element deficiency, in particular that of magnesium, is strongly implicated as a contributing factor (Table 1).[17, 18]

| Cause of Death* | Year of Publication: Number of Subjects | | | | | | |
|---|---|---|---|---|---|---|---|
| | Calcium | Magnesium | Zinc | Selenium | Potassium | Chromium | Copper |
| Heart disease | 2006: 110,792[36] | 2006: 4,035[37]<br>2003: 7,172[38]<br>1999: 2,316[39, 40]<br>1992: 930[41] | 2006: 4,035[37]<br>2005: 70[42] | 2005: 70[42]<br>1996: 3[43] | 1979: 21[44] | 1992: 76[45]<br>1991: 63[46] | 2001: 80[47] |
| Malignant neoplasms | 2007: 2,110[48]<br>2006: 45,306[49] | 2005: 61,433[50] | 2006: 857[51] | 2006: 218[52, 53]<br>1998: 974[54] | | | 2006: 3,352[55] |
| Cerebrovascular diseases | 2006: 110,792[36]<br>1999: 85,764[56] | 1998: 13,922[57]<br>1998: 43,738[58] | | 2004: 1103[59] | 2002: 5,600[60]<br>2001: 9,805[61] | | 1995: 149[62] |
| Chronic respiratory diseases | | 1997: 20[63] | | 1995: 79[64]<br>1983: 81[65] | | | |
| Diabetes mellitus | 2006: 83,779[66] | 2004: 39,345[67]<br>1994: 20[68]<br>1992: 37[69] | 2004: 39,345[67]<br>1994: 20[68] | 2005: 1,247[70]<br>2005: 92[71]<br>2005: 194[72] | | 2006: 36[73]<br>1997: 180[74] | |
| Alzheimer's disease | | 2005: 6[75] | | 1986: 25[76] | | | 2005: 32[77] |
| Nephritis, nephritic syndrome | | | 2005: 72[72] | 1985: 78[78] | | | |
| Liver disease | | | 1995: 253[79] | 1992: 188[80] | | | |
| Essential hypertension | 1991: 1,928[81]<br>1985: 80[82]<br>1982: 90[83] | 2005: 12,344[12]<br>1999: 7,731[84]<br>1998: 60[85]<br>1992: 30,681[86] | 1995: 62[87] | 1998: 57[88]<br>1992: 3,016[89] | 2001: 17,030[90] | 1991: 63[46] | 1995: 62[87] |

**Table 1. Reports Showing Associations of Essential Element Insufficiency with the Top Causes of Death in the United States (2005*).** Conditions associated with hypertension include heart disease, cerebrovascular disease, diabetes mellitus, nephritis and nephritic syndrome, and essential hypertension.[31] NOTE: References in this table are to Lord RS, Bralley JA, eds. *Laboratory Evaluations for Integrative and Functional Medicine.* 2nd ed. Duluth, GA: Metametrix Institute; 2008: 152-154.

The patient had multiple imbalances that can contribute to hypertension, including an elevated ADMA (Figure 1). ADMA has been shown to impair nitric oxide function, and therefore has adverse effects on blood pressure, erectile function, and other nitric oxide-dependent activities.[19,20] Treatment with arginine and N-acetylcysteine has been shown to reduce both systolic and diastolic mean arterial blood pressure, total cholesterol, oxidized LDL, and high-sensitivity C-reactive protein.[21] ADMA synthesis, clearance, and regulation of nitric oxide synthase are illustrated in Figure 9. Arginine, the substrate for nitric oxide, was high-normal in JF. Any elevation of ADMA may cause a relative L-arginine deficiency resulting in lowered nitric oxide production. Thus, supplementation with arginine, even in states of apparent sufficiency, may be indicated.[22] In this case, treatment included sustained-release arginine to address both the high blood pressure and erectile dysfunction.[23]

**The patient was able to lower the dosages of his medications to tolerable, side-effect-free levels. In so doing, he improved his health and well-being, while significantly reducing the risk of recurrence of a hypertensive crisis, congestive heart failure and other associated diseases.**

Laboratory assessment also revealed elevated quinolinate and hs-CRP (Figure 2), both of which are associated with systemic inflammation, possibly from insulin resistance and/or an occult infection (e.g., periodontal disease).[17,24,25] Anti-inflammatory treatment approaches were used, including ascorbic acid and magnesium supplementation. JF was also put on an oral hygiene regimen using an oral irrigation system, and was instructed to avoid sugars and processed carbohydrates. Cinnamon was prescribed because of its apparent favorable effect on insulin sensitivity and its antimicrobial properties.[12]

An elevation of 8-OHdG was discovered (Figure 3). This elevation correlates with DNA oxidative damage. In association with hypertension, nitric oxide is thought to lose its beneficial physiological effects in the presence of oxygen radicals.[21] Therefore, additional vitamin C was given as an antioxidant to address oxidative stress; on follow-up testing, the hsCRP was significantly reduced (Figure 7).

Despite supplementation with magnesium, JF's RBC magnesium level was low (Figure 4). RBC magnesium concentrations significantly lower in hypertensive patients than in controls have been reported.[8] Additionally, magnesium deficiency has been associated with multiple hypertension-related causes of death (Table 1).[26,27]

Elevated triglycerides and low HDL are indicative of probable insulin resistance despite the normal fasting insulin (Figure 5). The TG/HDL ratio has a high predictive value of a first coronary event regardless of BMI.[28] The DASH diet, exercise and cinnamon were started to improve insulin sensitivity.

JF's elevated coenzyme Q10 and alpha-tocopherol levels (Figure 6) were likely from supplementation, so his vitamin E dosage was decreased. His elevated serum CoQ10 was determined to be advantageous for him. CoQ10 is nontoxic at higher levels, and is beneficial for patients with high 8-OHdG and cardiovascular risks.[13] Since vitamin E supplementation has had mixed reviews in the literature, it was considered wise to keep that level within normal limits.[14,15] Figure 6 also shows that his vitamin D level was low.

Vitamin D insufficiency has been associated with hypertension, inflammation and oxidative stress.[11] Persons with chronic disease are recommended to maintain levels between 55 and 70 ng/mL, as was the goal in this case.[29] The four-month follow-up vitamin D level was 68 ng/mL (Figure 8), right in the target range.

JF initially presented with an elevated blood pressure of 162/104, despite three different antihypertensive medications. He was 30 pounds overweight, under much stress, and he consumed a poor diet. His history included a hypertensive crisis resulting in diastolic dysfunction and congestive heart failure. After four months of treatment using nutrients and diet and lifestyle intervention, his average blood pressure was 135/85. He lost 25 pounds. His medications were reduced: amlodipine and olmesartan medoxomil 20 mg/40 mg to 10 mg/20 mg and carvedilol 40 mg to 12.5 mg. At these amounts, he reported resolution or improvement in all side effects, including ED. It was anticipated that continued adherence to supplement protocol, with adjustments of dosages as needed, and an increasingly vigorous exercise program would further reduce his blood pressure over time.

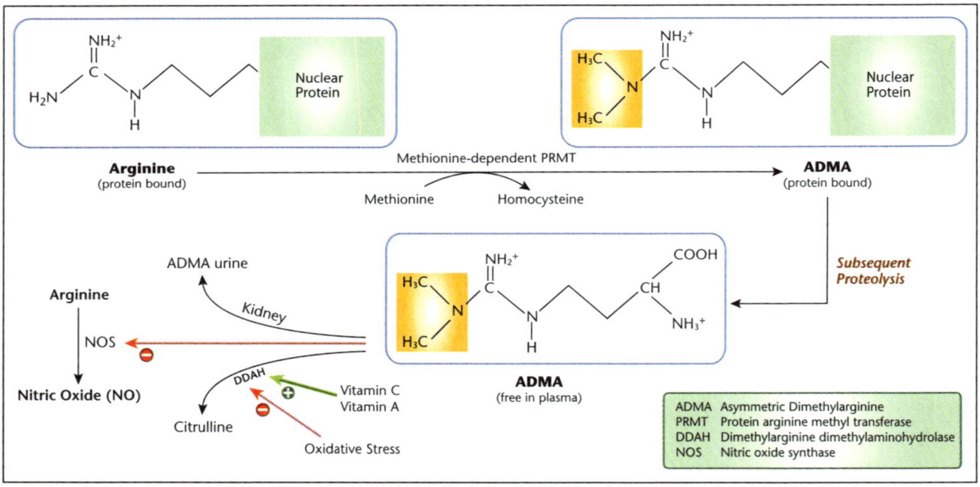


**Figure 9. ADMA Synthesis, Clearance, & Regulation of NOS.** Methylation of the terminal nitrogen atom of the arginine side chain in nuclear proteins produces protein-bound ADMA that is released on proteolysis. The released ADMA binds to NOS, slowing its activity in NO formation, thus regulating the rate of NO synthesis. The half-life of ADMA is governed partly by DDAH activity that causes degradation to citrulline. Because DDAH is susceptible to damage by cellular oxidants, its protection by vitamin C and vitamin A allows normal ADMA removal and, thus, normal NO formation.

NOTES

# CONCLUSION

Hypertension is a worldwide epidemic.[30] The morbidity, mortality and financial cost to society of untreated or undertreated hypertension are remarkably high. Despite this fact, a 2010 report from the Institute of Medicine noted that hypertension is a neglected disease. It is suggested that medication-related side effects are partly responsible.

As demonstrated in this case study, however, resistant hypertension was modified using a combination of lifestyle changes and nutrients. Using advanced laboratory analysis to identify the specific factors associated with the patient's hypertension, an effective, individualized plan was designed. The patient was able to lower the dosages of his medications to tolerable, side-effect-free levels. In so doing, he improved his health and well-being, while significantly reducing the risk of recurrence of a hypertensive crisis, congestive heart failure and other associated diseases.

**Evidence suggests, and this case demonstrates, that effective, well-tolerated, non-pharmacological approaches to hypertension are available.**

Given the dire consequences of hypertension on health, investigation into the efficacy of this safe and effective individualized-plan approach to treatment is warranted.

---

**Author: Kara Fitzgerald, ND**

**Case Clinician: Todd LePine, MD**

## References

1. NHLBI National Heart Lung and Blood Institute. The Seventh Report of the Joint National Committee on Prevention, Detection, Evaluation, and Treatment of High Blood Pressure (JNC 7) http://www.nhlbi.nih.gov/guidelines/hypertension/jnc7full.htm
2. Gaziano TA, Bitton A, Anand S, Weinstein MC. The global cost of nonoptimal blood pressure. *J Hypertens.* Jul 2009;27(7):1472-1477.
3. Lawes CM, Vander Hoorn S, Rodgers A. Global burden of blood-pressure-related disease, 2001. *Lancet.* May 3 2008;371(9623):1513-1518.
4. Lloyd-Jones D, Adams RJ, Brown TM, et al. Heart Disease and Stroke Statistics--2010 Update: A Report From the American Heart Association. *Circulation.* Feb 23;121(7):e46-e215.
5. Burt VL, Whelton P, Roccella EJ, et al. Prevalence of hypertension in the US adult population. Results from the Third National Health and Nutrition Examination Survey, 1988-1991. *Hypertension.* Mar 1995;25(3):305-313.
6. Thrall G, Lip GY, Lane D. Compliance with pharmacological therapy in hypertension: can we do better, and how? *J Hum Hypertens.* Sep 2004;18(9):595-597.
7. Padiyar A. Nonpharmacologic management of hypertension in the elderly. *Clin Geriatr Med.* May 2009;25(2):213-219.
8. Li Y, Ma A, Sun Y, et al. Magnesium status and dietary intake of mid-old people in a rural area of China. *Magnes Res.* Jun 2009;22(2):66-71.
9. Nijveldt RJ, van Nood E, van Hoorn DE, Boelens PG, van Norren K, van Leeuwen PA. Flavonoids: a review of probable mechanisms of action and potential applications. *Am J Clin Nutr.* Oct 2001;74(4):418-425.

10. Wannamethee SG, Lowe GD, Rumley A, Bruckdorfer KR, Whincup PH. Associations of vitamin C status, fruit and vegetable intakes, and markers of inflammation and hemostasis. *Am J Clin Nutr.* Mar 2006;83(3):567-574; quiz 726-567.

11. Gouni-Berthold I, Krone W, Berthold HK. Vitamin D and cardiovascular disease. *Curr Vasc Pharmacol.* Jul 2009;7(3):414-422.

12. Solomon TP, Blannin AK. Changes in glucose tolerance and insulin sensitivity following 2 weeks of daily cinnamon ingestion in healthy humans. *Eur J Appl Physiol.* Apr 2009;105(6):969-976.

13. Eriksson JG, Forsen TJ, Mortensen SA, Rohde M. The effect of coenzyme Q10 administration on metabolic control in patients with type 2 diabetes mellitus. *Biofactors.* 1999;9(2-4):315-318.

14. Gutierrez AD, de Serna DG, Robinson I, Schade DS. The response of gamma vitamin E to varying dosages of alpha vitamin E plus vitamin C. *Metabolism.* Apr 2009;58(4):469-478.

15. Riccioni G, D'Orazio N, Palumbo N, et al. Relationship between plasma antioxidant concentrations and carotid intima-media thickness: the Asymptomatic Carotid Atherosclerotic Disease In Manfredonia Study. *Eur J Cardiovasc Prev Rehabil.* Jun 2009;16(3):351-357.

16. Harris WS. The omega-3 index: from biomarker to risk marker to risk factor. *Curr Atheroscler Rep.* Nov 2009;11(6):411-417.

17. Lord RS, Bralley JA, eds. *Laboratory Evaluations for Integrative and Functional Medicine.* 2nd ed. Duluth, GA: Metametrix Institute; 2008.

18. Hatzistavri LS, Sarafidis PA, Georgianos PI, et al. Oral magnesium supplementation reduces ambulatory blood pressure in patients with mild hypertension. *Am J Hypertens.* Oct 2009;22(10):1070-1075.

19. Boger RH. Asymmetric dimethylarginine, an endogenous inhibitor of nitric oxide synthase, explains the "L-arginine paradox" and acts as a novel cardiovascular risk factor. *J Nutr.* Oct 2004;134(10 Suppl):2842S-2847S; discussion 2853S.

20. Selcuk MT, Selcuk H, Temizhan A, et al. Asymmetric dimethylarginine plasma concentrations and L-arginine/asymmetric dimethylarginine ratio in patients with slow coronary flow. *Coron Artery Dis.* Nov 2007;18(7):545-551.

21. Martina V, Masha A, Gigliardi VR, et al. Long-term N-acetylcysteine and L-arginine administration reduces endothelial activation and systolic blood pressure in hypertensive patients with type 2 diabetes. *Diabetes Care.* May 2008;31(5):940-944.

22. Vladimirova-Kitova LG. Asymmetric dimethylarginine--mechanisms and targets for therapeutic management. *Folia Med (Plovdiv).* 2008;50(1):12-21.

23. Miller AL. The effects of sustained-release-L-arginine formulation on blood pressure and vascular compliance in 29 healthy individuals. *Altern Med Rev.* Mar 2006;11(1):23-29.

24. Sabatine MS, Morrow DA, Jablonski KA, et al. Prognostic significance of the Centers for Disease Control/American Heart Association high-sensitivity C-reactive protein cut points for cardiovascular and other outcomes in patients with stable coronary artery disease. *Circulation.* Mar 27 2007;115(12):1528-1536.

25. Yan E, Chen S, Hong K, et al. Insulin, hs-CRP, leptin, and adiponectin. An analysis of their relationship to the metabolic syndrome in an obese population with an elevated waist circumference. *Metab Syndr Relat Disord.* Spring 2008;6(1):64-73.

26. Townsend MS, Fulgoni VL, 3rd, Stern JS, Adu-Afarwuah S, McCarron DA. Low mineral intake is associated with high systolic blood pressure in the Third and Fourth National Health and Nutrition Examination Surveys: could we all be right? *Am J Hypertens.* Feb 2005;18(2 Pt 1):261-269.

27. Woods KL, Fletcher S. Magnesium and myocardial infarction. *Lancet.* Jun 18 1994;343(8912):1565-1566.

28. Cordero A, Andres E, Ordonez B, et al. Usefulness of triglycerides-to-high-density lipoprotein cholesterol ratio for predicting the first coronary event in men. *Am J Cardiol.* Nov 15 2009;104(10):1393-1397.

29. Cannell JJ, Hollis BW. Use of vitamin D in clinical practice. *Altern Med Rev.* Mar 2008;13(1):6-20.

30. Chockalingam A, Campbell NR, Fodor JG. Worldwide epidemic of hypertension. *Can J Cardiol.* May 15 2006;22(7):553-555.

31. Lord RS, Bralley JA. *Laboratory Evaluations for Integrative and Functional Medicine.* 2nd ed. Duluth: Metametrix Institute; 2008:71.

# Statin-Induced Myopathy

*Heart disease (HD) is the number one killer in the United States.[1] In 2006, the direct and indirect costs associated with cardiovascular disease in the United States were estimated at 400 billion dollars.[2] Statin therapy for cholesterol reduction is a mainstay intervention for cardiovascular disease (CVD) as reflected in atorvastatin's status as the number one prescribed medication in the United States.[3] Statin therapy, however, is also associated with side effects that signal mitochondrial distress. A commonly reported statin-induced symptom is myaglia, which is defined as muscle pain without an associated elevation of serum creatine kinase (CK). In clinical trials, the reports of myalgia vary from less than 1% to 25% of patients.[4] Myopathy is a general term defined as an abnormal condition or disease of muscle tissue. Myopathy includes myalgia, myositis (inflammation of muscle tissue associated with elevated CK) and the very serious condition rhabdomyolysis (extreme myositis). Histological findings in statin-induced myopathy demonstrate electron chain dysfunction making "mitochondrial myopathy" the more precise term.[5] Mitochondrial myopathy has been associated with statin-induced CoQ10 depletion.[5] Given the density of mitochondria in cardiomyocytes, and CoQ10's role in mitochondrial energy production, depletion has long been associated with increased risk for heart disease.[6-7] In the case below, mitochondrial-specific organic acids, serum CoQ10, vitamin D and clinical history all suggest statin-induced mitochondrial myopathy, despite normal serum CK.*

## 57-Year-Old Male with Statin-Induced Myopathy

| | |
|---|---|
| **Additional Symptoms and Conditions** | Myalgia, hyperlipidemia, depression, fatigue |
| **Medication** | Atorvastatin (Lipitor®) |
| **Tests Used** | CoQ10; vitamin D; organic acids; serum creatine kinase |
| **Imbalances Identified** | Low serum CoQ10 and vitamin D with elevated citric acid cycle intermediates |
| **Treatments** | CoQ10; vitamin $D_3$; reduce simple carbohydrates; consume a whole-foods based, high-fiber diet; exercise program; discontinue atorvastatin |
| **Outcome** | Resolution of symptoms; maintenance of healthy cholesterol levels without medication |
| **Discussion/ Significance** | In this case, the side effects of fatigue, myalgia, exercise intolerance and depression required cessation of statin therapy. Laboratory evaluation of nutrients and mitochondrial function guided appropriate nutrient interventions. Assessment of mitochondrial health and the nutrients involved in mitochondrial function may be pivotal in determining who is most vulnerable to statin-induced side effects. |

# CASE HISTORY

BT, a 57-year-old male, presented with fatigue, severe depression and myalgia. His fatigue and myalgia became worse with exercise. He was taking 40 mg of the cholesterol-lowering medication atorvastatin for many months. The onset of fatigue, myalgia and exercise intolerance occurred after the introduction of the statin.

# Initial Laboratory Results

**Laboratory tests ordered and rationale:**

1. **Urinary organic acids**: Provides a functional assessment of mitochondrial activity
2. **CoQ10**: Deficiency may occur with statin therapy and may be associated with statin-induced side effects.
3. **Vitamin D**: Deficiency is associated with depression and statin-induced myalgia.
4. **Serum creatine kinase**: Elevation indicates muscle injury. In cases of elevation, isozymes may be obtained to determine involved organ system.

| | | | | |
|---|---|---|---|---|
| **Carbohydrate Metabolism** *(B1, B3, Cr, Lipoic Acid, CoQ10)* | | | | |
| Pyruvate | 2.1 | | 3.9 | <= 6.4 |
| L-Lactate | 23 | H | 14 | 3 - 46 |
| β-Hydroxybutyrate | <DL* | | 2.1 | <= 9.9 |
| **Energy Production (Citric Acid Cycle)** *(B comp., CoQ10, Amino acids, Mg)* | | | | |
| Citrate | 610 | H | 601 | 56 - 987 |
| Cis-Aconitate | 42 | | 51 | 18 - 78 |
| Isocitrate | 79 | | 98 | 39 - 143 |
| a-Ketoglutarate | 13.9 | | 19.0 | <= 35.0 |
| Succinate | 49.9 | H | 11.6 | <= 20.9 |
| Fumarate | 0.55 | | 0.59 | <= 1.35 |
| Malate | 6.0 | H | 1.4 | <= 3.1 |
| Hydroxymethylglutarate | 6.9 | H | 3.6 | <= 5.1 |

**Figure 1. Urinary organic acids.** Elevations in lactic acid and citric acid cycle intermediates suggested a functional need for CoQ10. The cholesterol synthetic pathway was also inhibited, as shown by the elevation of hydroxymethylglutarate. (Units: μg/mg creatinine)

| | | | | | |
|---|---|---|---|---|---|
| **Vitamin D** | | | | | |
| 25-Hydroxyvitamin D | 15 | L | 16 / 32 | 10 - 64 | ng/mL |
| **Coenzyme Q10** | 0.60 | L | 0.64 / 2.16 | 0.48 - 3.04 | mg/L |

**Figure 2. Serum vitamin D and CoQ10.** Both levels were in the low range.

**Pertinent Negative Results:**

- Serum creatine kinase was within normal limits.

## Initial Assessment

Statin-induced mitochodropathy presenting with:

- Myalgia
- Depression
- Fatigue
- Exercise intolerance

**Mitochondrial myopathy has been associated with statin-induced CoQ10 depletion.**

## Initial Plan

- Discontinue atorvastatin
- CoQ10 300 mg, 1 cap PO QD
- Vitamin $D_3$ 2000 IU, 1 cap PO QD
- Reduce simple carbohydrates; eat a whole-foods, high-fiber diet
- Cardiovascular exercise program

**Treatment rationale:** BT's treatment was straightforward: Discontinue the most likely cause of the myalgia, which was atorvastatin; begin CoQ10 and vitamin D as laboratory findings demonstrated low normal levels; institute dietary changes and an exercise program for long-term cholesterol control.

## Four-Month Follow-up

The patient responded well to the interventions. The myalgia, fatigue and depression resolved with the cessation of atorvastatin and the introduction of nutrients. Exercise tolerance improved and healthy cholesterol levels were maintained through diet and exercise.

# DISCUSSION

Statin therapy has been associated with side effects that suggest mitochondrial distress, such as fatigue and myalgia, symptoms experienced by BT.[8] Individuals with comorbidities such as diabetes, or genetic variants in CYP450 enzymes or mitochondrial proteins may be at particular risk of statin-related side effects.[8-11] Exercise has been shown to precipitate statin myopathy and the potentially life-threatening but rare rhabdomyolysis.[12] Nutrient deficiencies generated by statin use may be associated with increased side effects, and may be particularly pronounced if coupled with genetic vulnerability.[11]

In Figure 1, BT's urinary organic acid results showed an accumulation of hydroxymethylglutarate (HMG), demonstrating the chief mechanism of statin drugs: inhibition of HMG-CoA reductase (Figure 3). Inhibition of HMG-CoA reductase decreases endogenous cholesterol production, thereby potentially reducing cholesterol-based compounds such as CoQ10, sex hormones, bile acid, and cholecalciferol.[8] When HMG-CoA reductase is chronically inhibited, the aforementioned compounds may become depleted. Depletion of CoQ10 in particular may result in a mitochondropathy, as evidenced in this case by imbalanced mitochondrial markers, including the elevated lactate and citric acid cycle intermediates (Figure 1). These data corroborated the findings in Figure 2, which showed low-normal serum CoQ10. HMG-CoA reductase inhibition may therefore have ultimately resulted in lowered energy (ATP) production via CoQ10 depletion (Figure 3). Since the mitochondria reside most densely in tissue with high energy demands, heart muscle is among the first to be affected. CoQ10 deficiency has been associated with mitochondrial myopathy, fatigue, heart disease and Parkinson disease.[5-7]

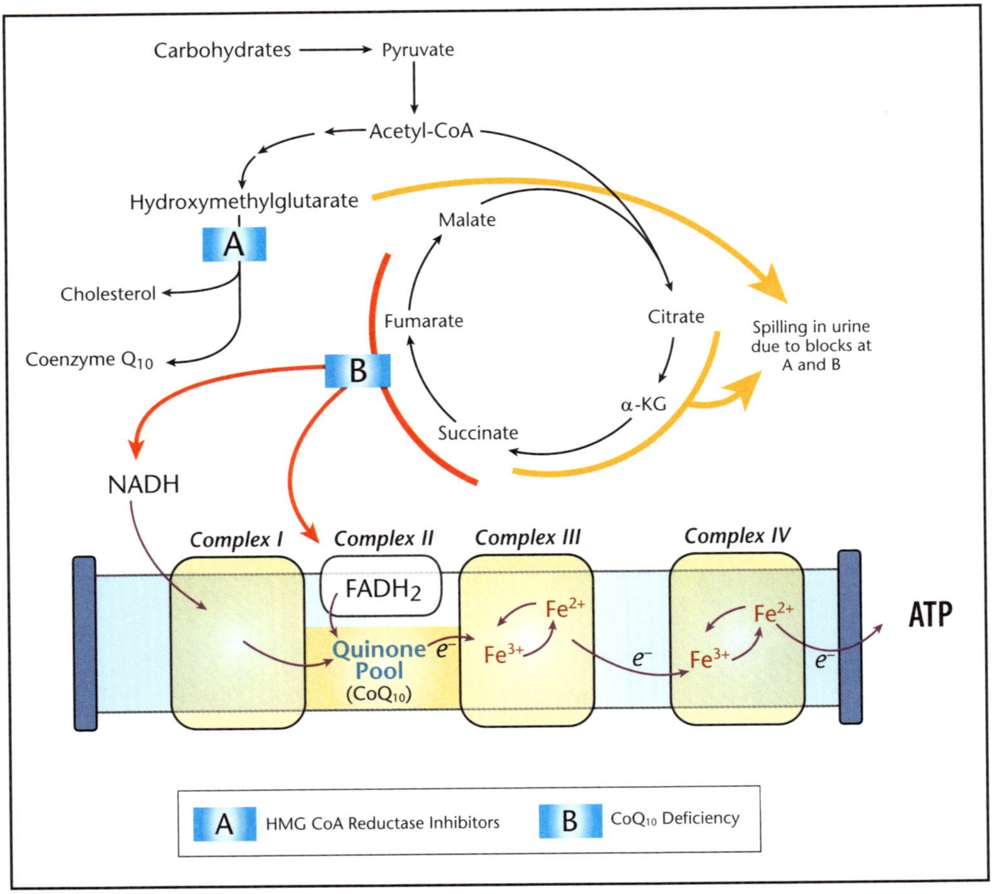


**Figure 3. Markers of Coenzyme Q10 Synthesis and Function.** Elevation of organic acids in urine can reveal inhibition of the coenzyme Q10 biosynthetic pathway (A) or interruptions of the electron transport system (B) from inability to sustain adequate CoQ10 levels in the inner mitochondrial membrane. Both endogenous regulators, such as glucagon and statin drugs, act at the HMG-CoA reductase enzyme gateway to inhibit two-carbon unit entry into the pathway that leads to synthesis of cholesterol and CoQ10. Accumulation of intermediates of the citric acid cycle, on the other hand, signals a functional insufficiency of inner mitochondrial membrane CoQ10 to sustain the flow of electrons.

While it has been understood for more than 20 years that statin drugs reduce CoQ10 levels and that CoQ10 depletion can induce mitochondrial myopathy, current standard guidelines don't recommend routine use of CoQ10 in people taking statins.[5] Atorvastatin in particular has been shown to significantly reduce CoQ10 very quickly—in as little as two weeks—and by more than 50% after 30 days of therapy.[13] As discussed, it is speculated that the deficiency of CoQ10 is the cause of statin myopathy, exercise intolerance, and myoglobinuria.[14] Research on the resolution of fatigue and myalgia with CoQ10 supplementation has been mixed when patients continue on statin therapy.[15] However, significant improvement of symptoms such as myalgia, fatigue, dyspnea, memory loss, and peripheral neuropathy was demonstrated with 240 mg/day CoQ10 supplementation when the statin was discontinued.[14]

**Depression has been linked to statin therapy and may be associated with lower brain cholesterol levels.**

Since myalgia could signal rhabdomyolysis, a serum creatine kinase (CK) level should be obtained in anyone reporting muscle pain while on statin therapy.

BT's vitamin D was shown to be low in Figure 2. While vitamin D depletion has not been directly associated with statin therapy, a recent study demonstrated that supplementation of high-dose vitamin $D_2$ led to a resolution of statin-induced myalgia in 92% of the study population. This finding suggests a link between statin-induced myalgia and vitamin D deficiency or insufficiency.[16]

Depression—also experienced by BT—has been linked to statin therapy and may be associated with lower brain cholesterol levels.[17] Vitamin D deficiency has been linked to depression.[18] It may be that CoQ10 and vitamin D assessment should take place prior to and during statin therapy, with treatment initiated as indicated. Cholesterol levels should also be periodically monitored and when warranted, prompt medication adjustment if found to be low or low-normal. Indeed, in one study, an increased incidence of death occurred after six years of 5 mg simvastatin therapy when LDL levels fell below 80 mg/dL.[5,19]

In this case, BT responded very favorably to treatment that included cessation of atorvastatin, introduction of CoQ10, vitamin D, dietary changes and exercise. His program was successful in resolving his myalgia, fatigue, and depression. His exercise tolerance was improved, and he was able to maintain healthy cholesterol levels, thereby significantly reducing his risk for CVD.

# CONCLUSION

Statin-related side effects, including fatigue, exercise intolerance and myalgia suggest mitochondrial vulnerability associated with CoQ10 depletion. Depression has also been associated with statin use. Vitamin D appears to be associated with statin myalgia, although the mechanism has yet to be elucidated. Mitochondrial vulnerability may be increased in persons with certain genetic variants in mitochondrial and P450 proteins and comorbid conditions such as diabetes.[8] Functional assessment of mitochondrial health using organic acids, as well as direct assessment of nutrients including serum CoQ10 and vitamin D, may be key in determining who is at risk for statin-induced side effects. In this case, side effects required cessation of medication. However, identification and treatment of nutrient deficiencies, along with appropriate diet and exercise, successfully resolved side effects while keeping lipids at an acceptable level and significantly reducing risk for CVD. This type of program may be utilized in lieu of, or in conjunction with, statin therapy.

**Authors: Kara Fitzgerald, ND; Elizabeth Redmond, PhD**
**Case Clinician: Cathryn Harbor, MD**

## References

1. Leading Causes of Death. Centers for Disease Control and Prevention Web Site. National Center for Health Statistics. FastStats. http://www.cdc.gov/nchs/FASTATS/lcod.htm. Accessed March 1, 2010.
2. Gaziano TA. Reducing the growing burden of cardiovascular disease in the developing world. *Health affairs (Project Hope).* Jan-Feb 2007;26(1):13-24.
3. Top 15 U.S Pharmaceutical Products by Sales. IMS Health. http://www.imshealth.com/deployedfiles/imshealth/Global/Content/StaticFile/Top_Line_Data/2008_Top_15_Products_by_U.S._Sales.pdf. Accessed March 1, 2010.
4. Thompson PD, Clarkson P, Karas RH. Statin-associated myopathy. *JAMA.* Apr 2 2003;289(13):1681-1690.
5. Lehmann J, Kauffman J. Statins Including Baycol: Questionable Cholesterol Control. In: O'Donnell J, ed. *Drug Injury: Liability, Analysis and Prevention.* 2nd ed: Lawyers & Judges Publishing; 2005:469-478.
6. Littarru GP, Ho L, Folkers K. Deficiency of coenzyme Q10 in human heart disease. II. *Int J Vitam Nutr Res.* 1972;42(3):413-434.
7. Littarru GP, Ho L, Folkers K. Deficiency of coenzyme Q10 in human heart disease. I. *Int J Vitam Nutr Res.* 1972;42(2):291-305.
8. Golomb BA, Evans MA. Statin adverse effects : a review of the literature and evidence for a mitochondrial mechanism. *Am J Cardiovasc Drugs.* 2008;8(6):373-418.
9. Eckel RH. Approach to the patient who is intolerant of statin therapy. *J Clin Endocrinol Metab.* May 2010;95(5):2015-2022.
10. Ghatak A, Faheem O, Thompson PD. The genetics of statin-induced myopathy. *Atherosclerosis.* Jun 2010;210(2):337-343.
11. Christopher-Stine L. Statin myopathy: an update. *Curr Opin Rheumatol.* Nov 2006;18(6):647-653.
12. Unnikrishnan D, Satish B. Exertion-induced rhabdomyolysis in a patient on statin therapy. *Nephrol Dial Transplant.* Jan 2005;20(1):244.
13. Rundek T, Naini A, Sacco R, Coates K, DiMauro S. Atorvastatin decreases the coenzyme Q10 level in the blood of patients at risk for cardiovascular disease and stroke. *Archives of neurology.* Jun 2004;61(6):889-892.
14. Langsjoen PH, Langsjoen JO, Langsjoen AM, Lucas LA. Treatment of statin adverse effects with supplemental Coenzyme Q10 and statin drug discontinuation. *BioFactors (Oxford, England).* 2005;25(1-4):147-152.
15. Marcoff L, Thompson PD. The role of coenzyme Q10 in statin-associated myopathy: a systematic review. *Journal of the American College of Cardiology.* Jun 12 2007;49(23):2231-2237.
16. Ahmed W, Khan N, Glueck CJ, et al. Low serum 25 (OH) vitamin D levels (<32 ng/mL) are associated with reversible myositis-myalgia in statin-treated patients. *Transl Res.* Jan 2009;153(1):11-16.
17. Morales K, Wittink M, Datto C, et al. Simvastatin causes changes in affective processes in elderly volunteers. *Journal of the American Geriatrics Society.* Jan 2006;54(1):70-76.
18. Check your vitamin D intake to avoid multiple health consequences. Three 2008 studies link low vitamin D levels to depression, hip fractures, and increased risk of death. *DukeMedicine healthnews.* Nov 2008;14(11):9-10.
19. Matsuzaki M, Kita T, Mabuchi H, et al. Large scale cohort study of the relationship between serum cholesterol concentration and coronary events with low-dose simvastatin therapy in Japanese patients with hypercholesterolemia. *Circ J.* Dec 2002;66(12):1087-1095.

# Supraventricular Tachycardia

*Supraventricular tachycardia (SVT) refers to a group of tachyarrhythmias originating in the atrial or atrioventricular (AV) nodal tissue. Paroxysmal supraventricular tachycardia (PSVT) is episodic, with abrupt onset and termination. PSVTs are a common clinical condition and unlike ventricular tachycardia, they are generally not life-threatening; however, heart failure, myocardial ischemia or infarction and pulmonary edema can result from increased heart rate. SVTs should therefore be monitored and treated. Heart palpitations, dizziness, anxiety and shortness of breath are the most common SVT symptoms. Because of the alarming nature of these symptoms, SVT is a frequent cause of emergency room(ER) and physician visits. Indeed, about 50,000 ER visits per year are due to SVT episodes.[1] SVTs are more common in women, the elderly, and those with comorbid heart conditions, although all ages are affected.[2-7] Smoking, caffeine, alcohol and certain medications may increase risk of PSVT. While treatment can be challenging, beta blockers, digoxin or calcium channel blockers are first-line long-term therapies. Less commonly recognized, but likely significant, is the role of nutritional deficiencies in causing or contributing to PSVT.[8-12]*

## 56-Year-Old Female with Paroxysmal Supraventricular Tachycardia

| | |
|---|---|
| **Symptoms and Conditions** | Dizziness, heart palpitations |
| **Medications** | Propranolol (Inderal®) |
| **Tests Used** | Plasma amino acids, erythrocyte essential elements |
| **Imbalances Identified** | Very low taurine and magnesium |
| **Treatments** | Taurine, magnesium, arginine |
| **Outcome** | Reduced incidence of tachycardic episodes; medication reduced 50% |
| **Discussion/Significance** | In this case, laboratory analysis uncovered pronounced taurine and magnesium deficiencies in a long-time vegetarian with PSVT. Laboratory assessment of nutrient status, which can help identify a deficiency before pathological changes occur, may be of particular importance for those consuming a nutrient-restricted diet. The degree of deficiency identified can inform dosage decisions, thus helping to improve outcomes. Treating this patient's nutrient deficiencies resulted in sufficient improvement of PSVT to allow a 50% reduction in medication. Laboratory assessment of nutrients required for normal cardiac conduction function may be of benefit in individuals with PSVT. |

# CASE HISTORY

LK was 56 years old when she presented with paroxysmal supraventricular tachycardia (PSVT), for which she took 120 mg of the beta-adrenergic receptor blocker propranolol. The PSVT caused heart palpitations and dizziness. LK was a strict vegetarian for years and reported taking many supplements. She reported no other complaints. Being very health conscious, LK did not anticipate that her PSVT could be associated with nutrient deficiencies.

# Initial Laboratory Results

**Laboratory tests ordered and rationale:**

1. **Plasma amino acids**: Insufficiency of taurine and other amino acids may be associated with increased risk of cardiac disease, including arrhythmias.[10,13]
2. **Erythrocyte essential elements**: Insufficient magnesium and other essential elements may be associated with cardiac disease, including arrhythmias.[9,11]

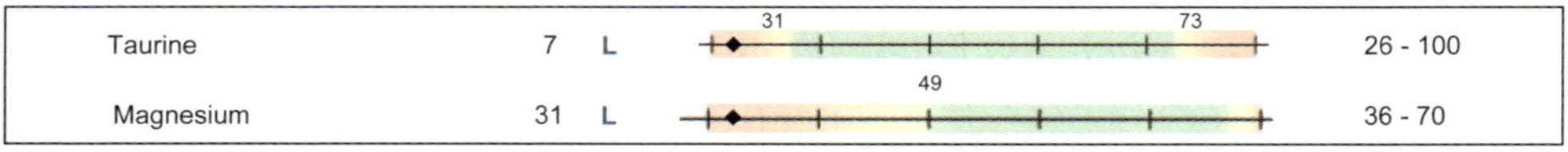


**Figure 1. Taurine and magnesium.** Very low levels of plasma taurine and erythrocyte magnesium were found in this patient. (Taurine units: µmol/L; magnesium units: ppm packed cells)

# Initial Assessment

- Paroxysmal supraventricular tachycardia
- Taurine deficiency
- Magnesium deficiency

# Initial Plan

- Taurine 500 mg, 1 cap PO QD
- Magnesium 500 mg, 1 tab PO BID
- Arginine 500 mg, 1 cap PO BID

**Treatment plan rationale:** Taurine and magnesium were initiated based on the laboratory findings of deficiency. Insufficient levels of taurine, magnesium and arginine have been associated with cardiac arrhythmia.[8-12] The research findings prompted the addition of arginine to the treatment protocol, although levels were tested and found to be normal.[8,9]

# Six-Month Follow-up

LK reported a reduction in PSVT episodes. Propranolol was reduced by 50%.

# DISCUSSION

LK presented with a history of PSVT, for which she took 120 mg per day of propranolol. She was otherwise a health-conscious, years-long vegetarian who reported taking a number of supplements. She had no other significant medical concerns. Probably because of her healthy habits, she did not believe the PSVT was associated with nutrient deficiencies. Her tests (Figure 1), however, showed significantly low taurine and magnesium. Taurine comes primarily from foods of animal origin; thus, taurine is usually low in vegans[14] and vegetarians.[15] Because taurine deficiency is a common occurrence in vegetarians, it is suggested that vegetarian diets be supplemented with taurine to maintain optimal levels.[15,16]

Deficiencies of both nutrients have been associated with cardiac dysfunction, including arrhythmia.[8-12] It has been hypothesized that cardiac arrhythmias of unknown origin in healthy individuals may be symptoms of taurine and arginine deficiency.[8,9]

The prescribed treatment involved ingestion of one gram each of magnesium, taurine, and arginine per day. Six-month follow-up revealed improvement in PSVT episodes and a subsequent 50% reduction in medication use. At one gram per day, the taurine dose prescribed was moderate. Perhaps a higher taurine dose would have provided a better outcome, particularly given the patient's low dietary intake of the amino acid. Taurine is largely non-toxic, and doses up to 12 grams per day have been used in research trials.[17] A follow-up plasma taurine level would have assisted in assessing the success of the intervention.

**There are many roles for taurine in cardiovascular function: protection against ischemia-reperfusion injury, modulation of intracellular calcium concentration, and antioxidant and blood pressure-lowering effects.**

There are many roles for taurine in cardiovascular function:[18] protection against ischemia-reperfusion injury, modulation of intracellular calcium concentration, and antioxidant and blood pressure-lowering effects,[19] for example. Supplementation with taurine is useful in preventing arrhythmias, regulating excitability of the myocardium, and protecting against free radical damage.[20] It has also been shown to lower homocysteine levels.[21] People who eat little or no meat or seafood have been shown to have greater platelet aggregation; taurine can prevent this phenomenon.[8]

Taurine is distinctive as an amino acid in that it does not become incorporated into proteins, as other amino acids do. It is a sulfur-containing amino acid considered to be conditionally essential; many individuals do not synthesize sufficient taurine. It is found abundantly in cardiac muscle, retina, brain, and liver.

Magnesium is well known for its cardio-modulation effects and deficiencies may be associated with congestive heart failure, PVST, and hypertension.[22-24] Studies have shown magnesium to be an effective treatment for supraventricular arrhythmias, with no side effects; other therapies, such as those involving calcium channel blockers, produced side effects of hypotension and cardiac failure.[25] Insufficient intake of magnesium is generally found in those consuming a Western diet.[12,26]

# CONCLUSION

For those who suffer from it, PSVT is a frightening occurrence that prompts a high number of ER visits each year. While its course is generally not life-threatening, there are occasions where prolonged rapid heart rate can result in serious complications including heart failure and pulmonary edema. As such, PSVT must be monitored and treated. Long-term medication management of PSVT primarily relies on antihypertensives that have potentially significant side effects.

In this case, the patient lived a healthy lifestyle and consumed a healthy, vegetarian diet. She also took a number of supplements. Despite her efforts, however, she experienced PSVT that required daily treatment with propranolol. Closer inspection of nutritional status using laboratory testing revealed significant deficiencies of two key nutrients required for cardiac function. Deficiencies of magnesium and taurine have both been associated with cardiac arrhythmias. Because taurine is a conditionally essential amino acid found in animal protein, deficiency is common in vegetarians. Magnesium is a common deficiency in those eating a Western diet.

**PSVT is a frightening occurrence that prompts a high number of ER visits each year. While its course is generally not life-threatening, there are occasions where prolonged rapid heart rate can result in serious complications including heart failure and pulmonary edema.**

When supplementation of these nutrients was undertaken, the patient experienced a reduction in the PSVT episodes and was able to reduce her medication use by 50%. It is possible with increased dosing of the nutrients, particularly taurine, that further abatement of PSVT would have been achieved. Moreover, follow-up laboratory evaluation to ensure repletion may have also been beneficial.

The effects of nutrient deficiencies can be far-reaching and serious. Testing for status, however, has yet to become routine clinical practice. Nutrient supplementation is well-tolerated and safe; it addresses the cause of an illness rather than just focusing on symptom abatement. In this case, supplementation led to improvement in symptoms and quality of life and to reduced reliance on medication.

---

**Authors: Kara Fitzgerald, ND; Terry Pollock, MS; Christie Egeston, MS**
**Case Clinician: Kathleen Power, DC**

## References


1. Murman DH, McDonald AJ, Pelletier AJ, Camargo CA, Jr. U.S. emergency department visits for supraventricular tachycardia, 1993-2003. *Acad Emerg Med.* Jun 2007;14(6):578-581.
2. Baine WB, Yu W, Weis KA. Trends and outcomes in the hospitalization of older Americans for cardiac conduction disorders or arrhythmias, 1991-1998. *J Am Geriatr Soc.* Jun 2001;49(6):763-770.
3. Cairns CB, Niemann JT. Intravenous adenosine in the emergency department management of paroxysmal supraventricular tachycardia. *Ann Emerg Med.* Jul 1991;20(7):717-721.
4. Campbell RW. Supraventricular tachycardia. Occasional nuisance or frequent threat? *Eur Heart J.* Jul 1996;17 Suppl C:21-25.
5. Connors S, Dorian P. Management of supraventricular tachycardia in the emergency department. *Can J Cardiol.* Mar 1997;13 Suppl A:19A-24A.
6. Harrison TR, Fauci AS. Harrison's principles of internal medicine. 17th ed. New York: McGraw-Hill, Health Professions Division; 2008:p . 1426
7. Luderitz B, Manz M. Pharmacologic treatment of supraventricular tachycardia: the German experience. *Am J Cardiol.* Aug 20 1992;70(5):66A-73A; discussion 73A-74A.
8. Eby G, Halcomb WW. Elimination of cardiac arrhythmias using oral taurine with l-arginine with case histories: Hypothesis for nitric oxide stabilization of the sinus node. *Med Hypotheses.* 2006;67(5):1200-1204.
9. Nielsen FH, Milne DB, Klevay LM, Gallagher S, Johnson L. Dietary magnesium deficiency induces heart rhythm changes, impairs glucose tolerance, and decreases serum cholesterol in post menopausal women. *J Am Coll Nutr.* Apr 2007;26(2):121-132.
10. Azuma J, Hasegawa H, Sawamura A, et al. Taurine for treatment of congestive heart failure. *Int J Cardiol.* 1982;2(2):303-304.
11. Palatnik A. And the beat goes on. *Nursing.* 2008;38(2):56cc51-56cc53.
12. Lord RS, Bralley JA, eds. *Laboratory Evaluations for Integrative and Functional Medicine.* Duluth: Metametrix Institute; 2008:84, 229.
13. Lord RS, Bralley JA, eds. *Laboratory Evaluations for Integrative and Functional Medicine.* Atlanta: Metametrix Institute; 2008:229.
14. Laidlaw SA, Shultz TD, Cecchino JT, Kopple JD. Plasma and urine taurine levels in vegans. *Am J Clin Nutr.* 1988;47(4):660-663.
15. McCarty MF. Sub-optimal taurine status may promote platelet hyperaggregability in vegetarians. *Med Hypotheses.* 2004;63(3):426-433.
16. Rana SK, Sanders TA. Taurine concentrations in the diet, plasma, urine and breast milk of vegans compared with omnivores. *Br J Nutr.* 1986;56(1):17-27.
17. Revised Codex Standard for Canned Pears. *Codex Stan.* 2001(61):3.
18. Wojcik OP, Koenig KL, Zeleniuch-Jacquotte A, Costa M, Chen Y. The potential protective effects of taurine on coronary heart disease. *Atherosclerosis.* Jan;208(1):19-25.
19. Xu YJ, Arneja AS, Tappia PS, Dhalla NS. The potential health benefits of taurine in cardiovascular disease. *Exp Clin Cardiol.* Summer 2008;13(2):57-65.
20. Sanderson SL, Gross KL, Ogburn PN, et al. Effects of dietary fat and L-carnitine on plasma and whole blood taurine concentrations and cardiac function in healthy dogs fed protein-restricted diets. *Am J Vet Res.* Oct 2001;62(10):1616-1623.
21. Ahn CS. Effect of taurine supplementation on plasma homocysteine levels of the middle-aged Korean women. *Adv Exp Med Biol.* 2009;643:415-422.
22. Durham D, Worthley LI. Cardiac arrhythmias: diagnosis and management. The tachycardias. *Crit Care Resusc.* Mar 2002;4(1):35-53.
23. Iezhitsa IN. Potassium and magnesium depletions in congestive heart failure--pathophysiology, consequences and replenishment. *Clin Calcium.* Nov 2005;15(11):123-133.

24. Iezhitsa IN, Onishchenko NV, Churbakova NV, Parshev VV, Petrov VI, Spasov AA. Effect of magnesium supplementation containing mineral bishofit ($MgCl_2 \times 6H_2O$) solution and pyridoxine hydrochloride on erythrocyte magnesium depletion and behaviour of rats after three-month alcoholization. *Magnes Res.* Dec 2002;15(3-4):179-189.

25. Gullestad L, Birkeland K, Molstad P, Hoyer MM, Vanberg P, Kjekshus J. The effect of magnesium versus verapamil on supraventricular arrhythmias. *Clin Cardiol.* 1993;16(5):429-434.

26. Vormann J. Magnesium: nutrition and metabolism. *Mol Aspects Med.* Feb-Jun 2003;24(1-3):27-37.

# 5 Endocrine and Metabolic Disorders

## Adrenal Fatigue

*In primary care, fatigue is a complaint in more than 20% of all patient contacts, and accounts for more than 18 million physician visits in the United States annually.[1, 2] In unpublished data from the US General Social Survey, at least one fatigue-associated symptom was found in 78% of all women and in 73% of all men.[2] Many cases elude diagnosis, and patients frequently do not pursue follow-up care, although at least half of all cases demonstrate unfavorable outcomes.[3] Adrenal fatigue (stress-induced subclinical adrenal insufficiency) is a well-recognized cause of fatigue in integrative medicine,[4-6] but its diagnostic validity is challenged by the conventional medical community,[7] who consider frank adrenal insufficiency (the most common cause being exogenous steroid withdrawal) to be the recognized clinical entity. Research, however, supports the occurrence of chronic stress-induced hypocortisolemic states.[8-10] Furthermore, a remarkable 75% to 90% of all primary care visits are reported to be related to stress.[11] Taken together, these facts suggest that adrenal fatigue may be a common cause of idiopathic fatigue.*

### 29-Year-Old Female with Adrenal Fatigue

| | |
|---|---|
| **Symptoms and Conditions** | Weight gain, salt craving, severe constipation, mild hypotension |
| **Tests Used** | Four-point salivary cortisol assay, thyroid panel, fasting insulin and blood sugar, iron panel, blood chemistries |
| **Imbalances Identified** | Very low salivary cortisol (adrenal fatigue), high-normal thyroid stimulating hormone (subclinical hypothyroidism), high-normal insulin (subclinical dysinsulinemia) |
| **Treatments** | Adrenal gland concentratrate with B vitamins, adrenal botanical formula, vitamin C, multivitamin mineral formula, fiber, dietary changes with elimination of dairy and reduction in simple carbohydrates, stress reduction techniques |
| **Outcome** | Improved energy, weight loss |
| **Discussion/ Significance** | While there are numerous etiologies of fatigue that must be ruled out, adrenal fatigue is a likely finding in many individuals, particularly if prolonged stress is a significant historical component. Hypothyroidism and dysinsulinemia may accompany adrenal fatigue. Using multi-specimen salivary cortisol testing with quintile data ranking, the sensitivity to identify subtle perturbations in circadian release is possible. Formal, well-designed trials evaluating adrenal fatigue may allow for broader recognition of this condition within the healthcare community. |

# CASE HISTORY

TJ was 29 years old when she presented with longstanding fatigue. She stated that the fatigue she had felt throughout college had recently worsened. The increased fatigue correlated with the completion of graduate school, which was followed by a move to a new city and the start of a new job. She described her fatigue as being worse in the evening, rating her energy level at 3 out of 10 (0 as lowest energy possible, 10 as highest energy possible). She tended to avoid late night parties, and rested most weekends. She slept well and awoke rested. TJ felt her best in the morning and used this time to maintain a regular exercise schedule of aerobic and anaerobic activities. She used some caffeine as a stimulant but tried to avoid excessive intake. She gained weight easily in her thighs, buttocks, and abdomen. Although she tended to gain it when she was feeling very stressed, she was not a binge eater. She craved salt. She occasionally had severe constipation. In spite of the fact that an elimination diet undertaken while in college revealed dairy, eggs, and soy as constipation triggers, she continued to consume forms of dairy. Her menstrual cycle was regular, with minimal PMS. She denied having had fever or myalgia. Her physical exam was unremarkable, with no fever or lymphadenopathy. Her blood pressure was low normal at 100/60 LAS.

Adrenal fatigue is a well-recognized cause of fatigue in integrative medicine, but its diagnostic validity is challenged by the conventional medical community, who consider frank adrenal insufficiency to be the recognized clinical entity. Research, however, supports the occurrence of chronic stress-induced hypocortisolemic states.

**Laboratory tests ordered and rationale:**

1. **Four point-measurement of salivary cortisol**: Evaluate etiology of stress-induced fatigue
2. **Thyroid panel**: Rule out hypothyroidism, a common cause of fatigue
3. **Fasting insulin and blood sugar**: Rule out dysinsulinemia, a common imbalance with fatigue and weight gain
4. **Iron panel**: Rule out iron deficiency, a common cause of fatigue
5. **Blood chemistries**: Rule out general metabolic dysfunctions, infection, macro- or microcytic anemia. All may be a cause of or associated with fatigue.

NOTES

## Initial Laboratory Results

| Cortisol - Saliva | Results | | Percentile Ranking by Quintile (1st, 2nd, 3rd, 4th, 5th; 20%, 40%, 60%, 80%) | | 95% Reference Interval | |
|---|---|---|---|---|---|---|
| Cortisol - AM | 1.8 | L | 4.3 | 20.7 | 2.4 - 33.7 | nM |
| Cortisol - Noon | 0.5 | L | 1.9 | 8.7 | 1.2 - 17.8 | nM |
| Cortisol - PM | 0.3 | L | 0.9 | 5.5 | 0.5 - 12.1 | nM |
| Cortisol - MN | <0.33 | L | 0.4 | 3.6 | 0.3 - 11.0 | nM |
| Total Cortisol | UC* | | 11.0 | 34.8 | 8.2 - 50.9 | nM |

*Unable to Calculate

**Figure 1. Baseline salivary cortisol.** All measurements were low.

| DHEA - Saliva | | | | | |
|---|---|---|---|---|---|
| DHEA (Noon - PM Average) | 2.8 | 1.2 | 4.6 | 0.8 - 7.5 | ng/mL |

**Figure 2. Dehydroepiandrosterone sulfate (DHEA-S).** Within normal limits.

| | Results | Reference Limits |
|---|---|---|
| Thyroid Stimulating Hormone (TSH) | 2.7 | 0.5–5.0 mIU/L |
| Fasting Insulin | 7.0 | 2.0–12.0 µIU/mL |

**Figure 3. Baseline TSH and fasting insulin.** Levels reported were higher than optimal.[8,12]

### Pertinent negative laboratory results:

- Complete blood count and serum blood chemistries were within normal limits.
- Iron panel was within normal limits.

## Initial Assessment

- Adrenal fatigue
- Subclinical hypothyroidism
- Constipation
- Food sensitivities
- Mild insulin resistance

## Initial Plan

- Adrenal glandular formula (with B vitamins)
- Adrenal botanical formula (Cordyceps mycelium, *Panax ginseng, and Rhodiola rosea)*
- Vitamin C, 1–3 grams/day
- Multivitamin mineral formula
- Re-evaluate adrenal and thyroid function in four months
- Stress-reduction techniques discussed
- Recommend continued exercise to tolerance
- Recommend complete dairy elimination with reduction in simple carbohydrates including grains, starchy vegetables, and high-sugar fruits
- Recommend minimize or discontinue coffee
- Recommend fiber formula with added prune extract

**Treatment plan rationale:** Nutrient and botanical preparations associated with adrenal function were initiated. Adrenal gland extract void of active hormone has a long been used as a supportive intervention for hypoadrenalism. Cordyceps mycelium, *Panax ginseng,* and *Rhodiola rosea* have demonstrated favorable modulation of adrenal function, stress and fatigue.[5, 13] Vitamins C and B complex have also been shown to be helpful in normalizing adrenal function.[5] Stress reduction techniques were taught and exercise was encouraged. It was recommended that the coffee be discontinued, because of its well-recognized potentiation of the stress response.[14] A low glycemic, low simple carbohydrate diet was started to assist in improving insulin sensitivity. For constipation, fiber with prune extract was started and complete dietary elimination of dairy products was suggested.[15]

In primary care, fatigue is a complaint in more than 20% of all visits, and stress is a factor in 75% to 90% of all visits.

## Four-Month Follow-up

TJ reported that the supplements improved her energy and constipation was much better when she eliminated dairy altogether and used the fiber. She also noticed her clothes fit better. She was pleased with her progress. She noticed that one day, after having two cups of coffee, she became very tired. TJ therefore decided to eliminate coffee and switch to green tea, which did not have the same effect on her.

## Four-Month Follow-up Laboratory Results

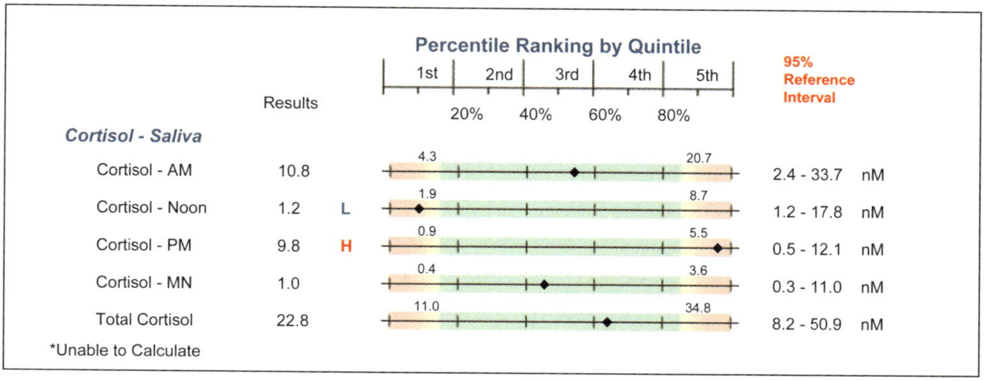


**Figure 4. Four-month follow-up salivary cortisol.** Some improvements noted in all measurements. DHEA-S (not shown) was within normal limits.

| | | Results | Reference Limits |
|---|---|---|---|
| Thyroid Stimulating Hormone (TSH) | | 1.8 | 0.5–5.0 mIU/L |
| Free T4 | | 1.3 | 0.8–1.5 ng/dl |
| T3 total | | 124 | 87–180 ng/dl |
| Fasting Insulin | HN | 5.7 | 2.0–12.0 µIU/mL |
| Fasting blood sugar | | 85 | 70–99 mg/dl |

**Figure 5. Follow-up thyroid study and fasting insulin.** Improvements noted, although fasting insulin still slightly higher than optimal.[8, 12]

# Four-Month Follow-up Plan

- Reduce adrenal formulas
- Continue other nutrients and lifestyle suggestions as directed
- Re-evaluate adrenal function in six months

# Ten-Month Follow-up

TJ was happy to report that she could finally be adventurous in her life, that she had enough energy to step out and explore her new city and meet new people. Her endurance and coping ability improved. Her stress response improved. She lost 13 pounds, requiring her to buy a smaller pant size. Her GI function was good as long as she avoided her trigger foods, particularly dairy. TJ was very pleased with her progress, but noted that her fatigue would return if she didn't supplement regularly with the adrenal support products.

## Ten-Month Follow-up Laboratory Results

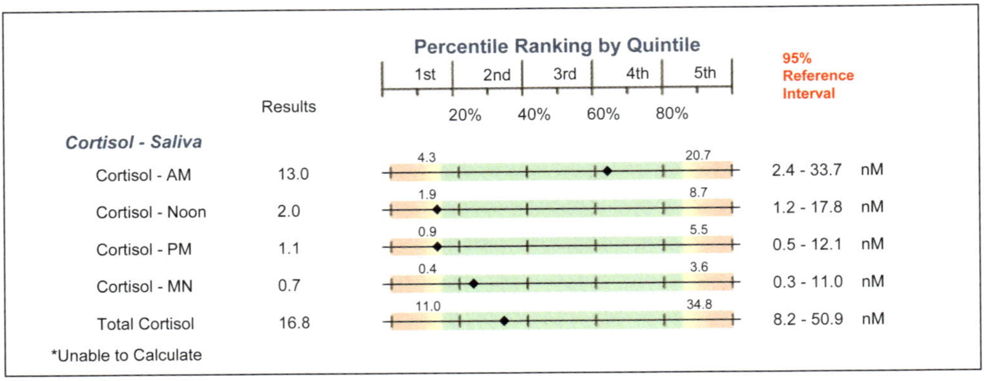


**Figure 6. Ten-month follow-up salivary cortisol.** Although improvements were noted in all areas, all measurements (with the exception of AM) were at low-normal levels. DHEA S (not shown) was within normal limits.

## Ten-Month Follow-up Plan

- Continue plan
- Re-evaluate thyroid and adrenal function, fasting blood sugar, and insulin in six months

# DISCUSSION

TJ presented as a typical adrenal fatigue patient, in that the onset of her fatigue was preceded by long-term stress. TJ also complained of salt craving and constipation and exhibited low-normal blood pressure; these signs and symptoms are associated with low cortisol (Table 1). Laboratory analysis confirmed TJ's clinical picture—very low or undetectable baseline salivary cortisol (Figure 1) on all measurements. DHEA-S was normal and remained normal in all laboratory evaluations, which may be somewhat unusual. The levels of DHEA are generally believed to drop first on account of its significantly higher quantitative demands.[16] Figure 3 indicated subclinical hypothyroidism, based on a TSH greater than 2.0.[12] TJ also had an insulin level of 7.0, which may be considered suboptimal.[8] The serum chemistry was normal, ruling out other common findings associated with low cortisol, including sodium and potassium imbalance; this result was somewhat surprising, given TJ's reported salt craving. Her complete blood count and iron studies results were also within normal limits, ruling out infection, metabolic dysfunction and anemia as potential causes of fatigue.

**Hypothyroidism and dysinsulinemia may accompany adrenal fatigue and should be evaluated and treated if warranted.**

Treatment included botanicals and nutrients designed to improve the stress response,[5] as well as stress-reduction techniques and dietary changes to reduce dysinsulinemia. TJ was also advised to begin a fiber supplement and to completely eliminate from her diet the foods she previously identified as contributing to constipation. While constipation was most likely a function of food sensitivities, bowel flora imbalance secondary to stress may have been a complicating factor.[17,18] At her ten-month follow-up, TJ was pleased to report on how much her life had improved with ongoing treatment. She also reported a 13-pound weight loss. Figure 6 showed normalization of all salivary cortisol measurements. However, results remained in the low-normal range. TJ also indicated that she required ongoing adrenal support to maintain energy. The treatment plan was continued, with further follow-up laboratory testing ordered at six months.

Elevated TSH frequently accompanies adrenal hypofunction. In frank adrenal insufficiency with hypothyroidism, treatment of the thyroid alone may result in an adrenal crisis.[20] Thus, evaluation of thyroid function is indicated in the adrenal fatigue patient (as is the evaluation of adrenal function in the hypothyroid patient.) Dysinsulinemia is also seen in adrenal insufficiency,[18] which suggests that dysinsulinemia may also be present in adrenal fatigue.[4] These latter two findings may have been associated with TJ's tendency to gain, rather than lose, weight, which is a more common sign of frank cortisol deficiency.

**Table 1. Signs and Symptoms of Cortisol Deficiency and Excess.[16]**

| Deficiency | Excess |
|---|---|
| ♦ Chronic weakness | ♦ Sugar craving |
| ♦ Weight loss | ♦ Central obesity |
| ♦ Fatigue | ♦ Insulin resistance |
| ♦ Decreased stress tolerance | ♦ Weakness |
| ♦ Anorexia | ♦ Shakiness between meals |
| ♦ Alternating diarrhea and constipation | ♦ Irritability |
| ♦ Salt craving | ♦ Hypertension |
| ♦ Postural dizziness | ♦ Easy bruising |
| ♦ Muscle or joint pain | ♦ Amenorrhea |
| ♦ Hyperpigmentation | ♦ Impotence |
| ♦ Hypotension | ♦ Oily skin |
| ♦ Anemia | ♦ Sleep disturbances |
| | ♦ Headache |

There are a number of possible reasons for the difficulty in accepting adrenal fatigue as a valid, measurable condition. First, the multiplicity of potential symptoms (Table 1), can make the diagnosis difficult.[4-6] Also, objective diagnosis requires multiple measurements to capture perturbations in circadian cortisol.[21] Since blood remains the gold-standard specimen, divided specimen collection is less likely to occur in routine clinical practice.[21] Furthermore, since ranges set for blood cortisol are designed to capture frank deficiency and excess states, subclinical deficiency may be missed. Saliva, while long-used in integrative circles, is a relative newcomer among specimen types. Although not frequently tested by conventional doctors, salivary cortisol is easily collected over time, at multiple points, allowing the results of its assay to capture subtle perturbations in circadian cortisol dysregulation.[21] It has been reported that circadian assessments of cortisol using saliva and serum were shown to be correlated. In our experience, salivary cortisol reference ranges that include quintile rankings (a frequent tool used in research to sort data) have more subtle interpretive power. With greater acceptance of salivary cortisol testing, formal recognition of adrenal fatigue as a clinical entity may develop.

# CONCLUSION

Fatigue and stress are common complaints, and they play a role in the majority of primary care visits. Far too often, however, the cause of the fatigue is never found. Perhaps as a result, more than half of all fatigue patients fail to return for follow-up visits, which may contribute to the high incidence of unfavorable outcomes found in this population.

The cluster of symptoms experienced by TJ is a common finding in any clinical practice. Without recognition of adrenal fatigue as a legitimate clinical complaint, TJ would have been one of the patients for whom no diagnosis was found. Fortunately, her clinician recognized her presentation as chronic stress-induced adrenal fatigue, and she performed the appropriate evaluations. TJ responded very favorably to a treatment program directed at supporting adrenal function and stress reduction; it was safe, straightforward and relatively easy to implement.

**The cluster of symptoms experienced by TJ is a common finding in any clinical practice. Without recognition of adrenal fatigue as a legitimate clinical complaint, TJ would have been one of the patients for whom no diagnosis was found.**

With the advent of salivary cortisol testing with quintile ranges, the ease of multiple collections with the sensitivity to identify subtle perturbations in circadian release is possible. Formal, well-designed trials that evaluate adrenal fatigue may allow for broader recognition of this condition among healthcare practitioners.

---

**Author: Kara Fitzgerald, ND**
**Case Clinician: Kara Fitzgerald, ND**

## References


1. CDC. Ambulatory Care Use and Physician Visits. http://www.cdc.gov/nchs/fastats/docvisit.htm. Accessed 6/28/2010, 2010.
2. Lewis G, Wessely S. The epidemiology of fatigue: more questions than answers. *J Epidemiol Community Health.* Apr 1992;46(2):92-97.
3. Nijrolder I, van der Windt D, van der Horst H. Prediction of outcome in patients presenting with fatigue in primary care. *Br J Gen Pract.* Apr 2009;59(561):e101-109.
4. Wilson JL. *Adrenal Fatigue: The 21st Century Stress Syndrome.* 1st ed: Smart Books; 2002.
5. Head KA, Kelly GS. Nutrients and botanicals for treatment of stress: adrenal fatigue, neurotransmitter imbalance, anxiety, and restless sleep. *Altern Med Rev.* Jun 2009;14(2):114-140.
6. Selye H. *The Stress of Life.* New York: McGraw-Hill; 1956.
7. Nippoldt T. Is there such a thing as adrenal fatigue? http://www.mayoclinic.com/health/adrenal-fatigue/AN01583.
8. Hanley AJ, Williams K, Stern MP, Haffner SM. Homeostasis model assessment of insulin resistance in relation to the incidence of cardiovascular disease: the San Antonio Heart Study. *Diabetes Care.* Jul 2002;25(7):1177-1184.
9. Vythilingam M, Gill JM, Luckenbaugh DA, et al. Low early morning plasma cortisol in posttraumatic stress disorder is associated with co-morbid depression but not with enhanced glucocorticoid feedback inhibition. *Psychoneuroendocrinology.* Sep 17 2009.
10. Maldonado EF, Fernandez FJ, Trianes MV, et al. Cognitive performance and morning levels of salivary cortisol and alpha-amylase in children reporting high vs. low daily stress perception. *Span J Psychol.* May 2008;11(1):3-15.
11. AIS. America's Number One Health Problem. http://www.stress.org/americas.htm. Accessed 6/28/2010, 2010.
12. Wartofsky L, Dickey RA. The evidence for a narrower thyrotropin reference range is compelling. *J Clin Endocrinol Metab.* Sep 2005;90(9):5483-5488.
13. Koh JH, Kim KM, Kim JM, Song JC, Suh HJ. Antifatigue and antistress effect of the hot-water fraction from mycelia of Cordyceps sinensis. *Biol Pharm Bull.* May 2003;26(5):691-694.
14. Lane JD, Pieper CF, Phillips-Bute BG, Bryant JE, Kuhn CM. Caffeine affects cardiovascular and neuroendocrine activation at work and home. *Psychosom Med.* Jul-Aug 2002;64(4):595-603.
15. WebMD. The Basics of Constipation. http://www.webmd.com/digestive-disorders/digestive-diseases-constipation. Accessed 6/28/2010, 2010.
16. Lord RS, Bralley JA, eds. *Laboratory Evaluations for Integrative and Functional Medicine.* 2nd ed. Duluth, GA: Metametrix Institute; 2008.
17. Higashikawa F, Noda M, Awaya T, Nomura K, Oku H, Sugiyama M. Improvement of constipation and liver function by plant-derived lactic acid bacteria: A double-blind, randomized trial. *Nutrition.* Jul 21 2009.
18. Kearney DJ, Brown-Chang J. Complementary and alternative medicine for IBS in adults: mind-body interventions. *Nat Clin Pract Gastroenterol Hepatol.* Nov 2008;5(11):624-636.
19. Abdullatif HD, Ashraf AP. Reversible subclinical hypothyroidism in the presence of adrenal insufficiency. *Endocr Pract.* Sep-Oct 2006;12(5):572.
20. Shulman DI, Palmert MR, Kemp SF. Adrenal insufficiency: still a cause of morbidity and death in childhood. *Pediatrics.* Feb 2007;119(2):e484-494.
21. Dorn LD, Lucke JF, Loucks TL, Berga SL. Salivary cortisol reflects serum cortisol: analysis of circadian profiles. *Ann Clin Biochem.* May 2007;44(Pt 3):281-284.

# Type 2 Diabetes Mellitus

*A diabetic is diagnosed in the United States every 20 seconds.[1] Diabetes mellitus (DM) is the seventh leading cause of death in the United States, with type 2 diabetes mellitus (DMII) accounting for 90 to 95% of all diabetes. Significant comorbidities include heart disease, hypertension, respiratory infection, kidney disease, stroke, retinopathy, neuropathy, and dementia, of which all except the last three are among the top ten causes of death in the U.S. These comorbidities are all linked by common underlying mechanisms. Treating the underlying causes and mechanisms can prevent or reverse most of these comorbidities. Pre-diabetes was found in more than 40% of the population between 1988 and 1994, and 7% of all adolescents have been diagnosed with impaired fasting glucose. The estimated annual cost to society of diabetes-related concerns in the U.S. is $218 billion. Hypoglycemic medications, while very important in minimizing diabetic-associated sequelae, have long carried risks. Most recently rosiglitazone (Avandia®) was shown to increase risk of myocardial infarction by 43%,[2] which is a concern in any population, but particularly so in a group already vulnerable to cardiovascular (CV) events.*

A diabetic is diagnosed in the U.S. every 20 seconds… Significant comorbidities include heart disease, hypertension, respiratory infection, kidney disease, stroke, retinopathy, neuropathy, and dementia, of which all except the last three are among the top ten causes of death in the U.S.

*Lifestyle intervention has been shown to reduce the incidence of diabetes by 71% in those 60 years of age and older, and by 58% in all adults. Such findings strongly suggest that diabetes, while subject to genetic influence, is primarily a disease of lifestyle choice and increasingly environmental toxicity.[3, 4]*

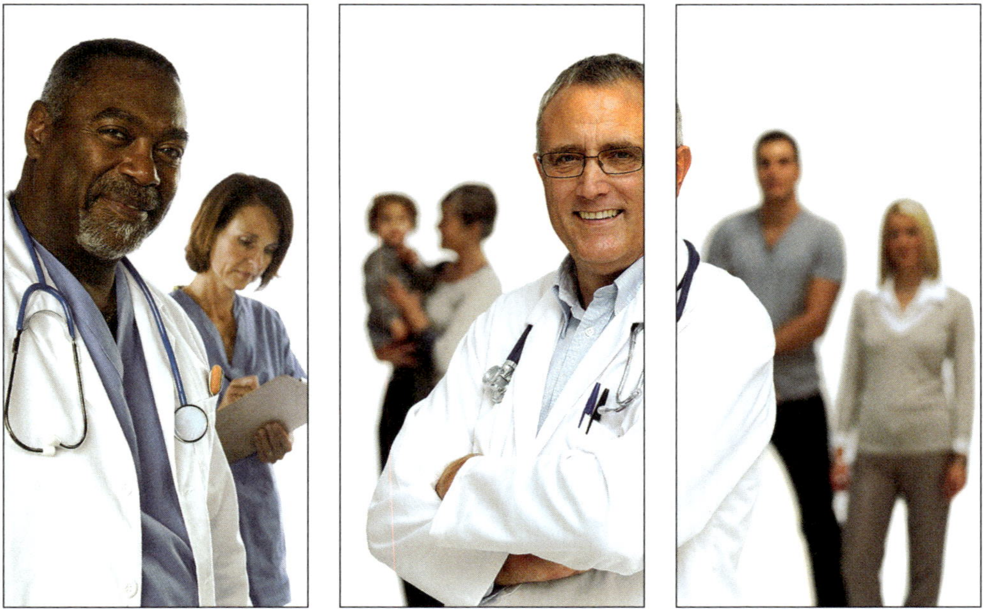

## 56-Year-Old Female with Type 2 Diabetes Mellitus

| | |
|---|---|
| **Additional Symptoms and Conditions** | Obesity, hypertension, elevated cholesterol and sleep apnea |
| **Medications** | Atorvastatin (Lipitor®), glyburide (Micronase®) metformin (Glucophage®) metoprolol, amlodipine and benazepril (Lotrel®), aspirin, One-a-Day multivitamin and mineral |
| **Tests Used** | Fasting insulin, hemoglobin A1C, urinalysis, metabolic panel, thyroid panel, hs-CRP and fibrinogen, lipids, lipoprotein subclasses with lipoprotein (a), vitamin D, multi-profile metabolic panel (organic acids, fatty acids, amino acids, fat soluble vitamins, essential elements and oxidative stress markers) |
| **Imbalances Identified** | Elevated A1C, elevated fasting blood sugar, presence of urinary glucose, elevated liver enzymes; subclinical hypothyroidism; lipid particle and Lp (a) abnormalities, hypovitaminosis D; biotin and B-complex deficiency; subclinical mitochondropathy; elevated arachidonic acid; low-normal essential elements; lipid peroxidation |
| **Treatments** | Nutrients for glucose regulation, antioxidants, essential elements, mitochondrial nutrients, protein-based medicinal food, fiber, essential fatty acids, niacin, vitamin D, biotin; low carbohydrate/low glycemic diet; exercise |
| **Outcome** | 30-pound weight loss, blood pressure improved, sleep apnea resolved, fasting blood sugar average 91 to 111; A1C normalized; liver enzymes normalized; lipids, D and B vitamins, and mitochondrial markers improved; reduction in metformin usage; elimination of glyburide and metoprolol; began regular exercise |
| **Discussion/ Significance** | Despite polypharmacy, the patient presented with very poorly controlled type 2 diabetes and typical comorbidities, including hypertension, hyperlipidemia, obesity and sleep apnea. Her risk was high for experiencing serious diabetic-related complications, including kidney, cardiovascular and/or cerebrovascular diseases. Furthermore, pharmacologic interventions, while important in reducing glucose and improving insulin response, have significant risks associated with usage. Laboratory evaluation of metabolic and nutrient imbalances guided the development of a safe, individualized program that was rapidly effective. |

# CASE HISTORY

CK, a 56-year-old female presented to the clinic with type 2 diabetes (DMII), obesity, high blood pressure, elevated cholesterol and sleep apnea. CK was diagnosed with diabetes in 1999 and was prescribed glyburide and metformin. She did not regularly test her blood sugar, although she did attempt to adhere to a healthy diet, including oatmeal for breakfast, chicken and other lean protein with salads for lunch and dinner. However, she craved sugary foods and consumed much candy and ice cream at night. She generally felt ravenous before lunch and dinner, and experienced nausea and mood swings when she waited too long to eat. She also had wine with dinner most nights. These habits provided palliation for her high-stress job as a university professor and researcher.

CK was diagnosed with hypertension in 1997, for which she took metoprolol and amlodipine/benazepril. She did not monitor her blood pressure levels regularly. She was diagnosed with hyperlipidemia in 2003 for which she took atorvastatin. CK had sleep apnea for years, but did not use a CPAP machine. She experienced occasional constipation. She felt well in the mornings, and meditated daily for 15 minutes, but was frequently sleepy after lunch and dinner.

CK's past medical history was unremarkable, with the exception of mononucleosis at age 16.

CK's father died at 55 years of age from a cerebrovascular accident. He also had coronary artery disease. CK's father was adopted, and therefore extended paternal family history was unknown. CK's mother died at 70 years of age. She was diagnosed with type 2 diabetes and heart disease. CK has no siblings. CK's maternal aunts have type 2 diabetes.

Despite polypharmacy, the patient presented with very poorly controlled type 2 diabetes and typical comorbidities, including hypertension, hyperlipidemia, obesity, and sleep apnea.

CK did not smoke. She meditated for 15 minutes each morning. She took a one-per-day multivitamin and mineral supplement. She traveled a great deal for work and went out 1 to 2 nights per week. CK generally did not exercise, but did some limited walking during vacations.

CK's significant physical exam findings included a blood pressure of 160/104 (left arm seated) and a heart rate of 94 beats per minute. She weighed 190 pounds and was 5'2" tall. Her body mass index (BMI) was 34.7, considered obese, and her waist-to-hip ratio (WHR) was slightly above optimal at 0.89.

**Laboratory tests ordered and rationale:**

1. **Fasting insulin, hemoglobin A1C, urinalysis*, metabolic panel*, thyroid panel, hs-CRP and fibrinogen**: Comprehensive, standard laboratory assessments for DMII and associated inflammation.
2. **Lipids, lipoprotein subclasses with lipoprotein (a)**: Lipid subclass assessment may be a more sensitive predictor of cardiovascular risk in metabolic syndrome than a standard lipid assay. Lp(a) is an independent risk marker for cardiovascular disease that is not responsive to statin therapy.[5-7]
3. **Vitamin D**: Low levels are associated with increased inflammation and increased incidence of numerous diseases.[8]
4. **Multi-profile metabolic panel***: A comprehensive assessment including organic acids, fatty acids, amino acids, fat soluble vitamins, essential elements and oxidative stress markers; assists in detecting individual etiopathogenic factors and in individualizing treatment plans.
5. **Stool test**: Assessment of GI microbial status and GI function. Imbalances may be associated with glycemic regulation and obesity.[9]

**Only significant findings are discussed below.*

# Initial Laboratory Results

| | | Results | Reference Limits |
|---|---|---|---|
| Fasting Insulin | HN | 9.0 | 2–12 uIU/mL |
| A1C | H | 9.9% | 0.0–5.9% non-diabetic range |
| Fasting blood glucose | H | 312 | 65–99 mg/dL |
| Urinary glucose | H | 3+ | Negative |
| hs-CRP | | 0.7 (low risk) | < 1.0 mg/L |
| Alanine aminotransferase (ALT) | H | 56 | 6–40 U/L |
| Aspartate aminotransferase (AST) | | 20 | 10–35 U/L |
| Thyroid Peroxidase Antibodies | | < 10 | 0–34 IU/mL |
| Thyroglobulin Antibodies | | < 10 | 0–20 IU/mL |
| Thyroid Stimulating Hormone (TSH) | HN | 2.6 | 0.3–5.5 μIU/mL |
| Free T4 | | 1.1 | 0.8–1.8 ng/dl |
| T3 total | | 286 | 230–420 pg/dL |

**FIGURE 1. Standard laboratory assessments.** Numerous high markers of insulin resistance despite hypoglycemic therapies. Liver enzyme ALT elevation suggested early non-alcoholic fatty liver disease. Thyroid panel result was within normal limits, although the TSH was suboptimal. Fibrinogen, microalbumin and kidney function test results were within normal limits.

| | | Results | Reference Limits |
|---|---|---|---|
| LDL | | 100 | < 100 mg/dL |
| HDL | | 64 | > 40 mg/dL |
| Triglycerides | | 101 | < 150 |
| LDL particles | H | 1608 | OR < 1000 nmol/L |
| Small LDL particles | H | 1320 | OR < 850 nmol/L |
| LDL size | L | 20.3 | 20.6–23.0 nm |
| Small HDL particles | L | 6.9 | > 9.0 μmol/L |
| Lipoprotein(a) | H | 423 | 0–74 nmol/L |

**Figure 2. Lipid panel with lipoprotein subclasses with Lp(a).** Despite a normal lipid panel (on statin), the elevated Lp(a), small particle size of HDL and LDL and increased quantity of LDL particles suggested metabolic syndrome.

| | Results ng/mL | Quintile Ranking | 95% Reference Interval |
|---|---|---|---|
| 25-Hydroxyvitamin D | 17 L | 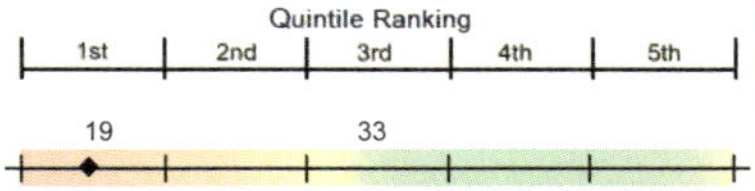 | 12 - 83 |



**Figure 3. Serum vitamin D.** Results demonstrated insufficiency

| | | | | |
|---|---|---|---|---|
| a-Ketoisocaproate | 1.01 | H | 0.34 | <= 0.52 |
| a-Keto-β-Methylvalerate | 2.91 | H | 0.38 | <= 1.10 |
| β-Hydroxyisovalerate | 12.6 | H | 7.6 | <= 11.5 |
| Methylmalonate | 1.1 | | 1.7 | <= 2.3 |

**Figure 4. Urinary organic acid B vitamin markers.** Beta-Hydroxyiosvalerate is a sensitive and specific biomarker for biotin insufficiency.[10] The two alpha-keto acid elevations have been associated with increased need for thiamin and may also suggest a need for niacin, pantothenic acid, riboflavin and alpha-lipoic acid. Methylmalonate, a biomarker for intracellular $B_{12}$ status, was shown to be within normal limits. (Units: µg/mg creatinine)

| | | | | |
|---|---|---|---|---|
| Pyruvate | 1.3 | | 3.9 | <= 6.4 |
| L-Lactate | 51 | H | 14 | 3 - 46 |
| β-Hydroxybutyrate | 16.1 | H | 2.1 | <= 9.9 |
| Hydroxymethylglutarate | 4.1 | H | 3.6 | <= 5.1 |

**Figure 5. Urinary organic acid mitochondrial markers.** Elevated lactate, B-hydroxybutyrate, hydroxymethylglutarate and normal pyruvate were found. Together, they suggest mitochondropathy. (Units: µg/mg creatinine)

| | | | | |
|---|---|---|---|---|
| Eicosapentaenoic (20:5n3) | 130 | | 17 | 5 - 210 |
| Docosahexaenoic (22:6n3) | 111 | | 59 | 31 - 213 |
| Arachidonic (20:4n6) | 500 | H | 201 / 451 | 158 - 521 |

**Figure 6. Omega-3 and -6 fatty acids.** Normal omega-3 fatty acids EPA and DHA with high-normal omega-6 fatty acid AA were found. (Units: µM)

| | | | | | |
|---|---|---|---|---|---|
| Magnesium* | 36 | L | 49 | 36 - 70 | ppm packed cells |
| Selenium | 0.14 | L | 0.19 | 0.14 - 0.47 | ppm whole blood |
| Chromium | 3.6 | L | 4.3 | 3.6 - 10.1 | ppb packed cells |
| **Vanadium** | **0.01** | LN | | **0.10 – 0.28** | **ppm packed cells** |

**Figure 7. Red blood cell essential elements.** All found at low-normal levels.

| | | | | |
|---|---|---|---|---|
| Lipid Peroxides | 2.65 | H | 1.72 | <= 2.60 |

**Figure 8. Serum lipid peroxides.** Elevated level demonstrated increased oxidative stress. (Units: nmol/mL)

## Initial Assessment

- Type 2 diabetes
- Obesity
- Hypertension
- Hyperlipidemia
- Sleep apnea
- Subclinical fatty liver disease
- Subclinical hypothyroidism
- Hypovitaminosis D
- Mitochondropathy
- Oxidative stress

## Initial Plan

- Dietary Intervention
  - Begin low carbohydrate/low glycemic diet; have protein with each meal. Chew food adequately, eat slowly and allow digestion time. Protein-based snacks in afternoon
- Lifestyle Intervention
  - Increase exercise—begin interval training.
  - Monitor fasting blood sugar and 2 hour post prandial blood sugar QD.
  - Sleep apnea: Recommend mandibular repositioning appliance and home sleep study
- Nutrient Support
  - Nutrients for glucose metabolism (chromium, vanadium, alpha-lipoic acid (ALA), n-acetyl cysteine (NAC), biotin, banaba leaf extract, *Gymnema sylvestre*), 1 packet PO BID
  - Fiber complex (konjac mannan, sodium alginate, xanthan gum), 4 capsules before meals with water
  - Medicinal food containing rice protein powder, medium chain triglycerides, vitamins and minerals specific for hepatic function, 2 scoops QAM (mix/blend with ice, unsweetened soy milk and berries; add 2 TBSP ground flax.)
  - Nutrients for mitochondrial support (including: magnesium, CoQ10, creatine, acetyl-carnitine), 1 tab PO BID
  - EPA/DHA 720 mg, 2 Gelcaps PO BID
  - CoQ10 100 mg, 1 tab PO BID
  - R-alpha-lipoic acid (R-ALA) 100 mg, 1 cap PO QD

- Cinnamon (Cinnamomum burmannii) extract, 2 caps PO BID
- Biotin 8 mg, 1 capsule QD
- Vitamin $D_3$ 10,000 IU, daily

- Discontinue:
  - Multivitamin mineral formula
- Medication
  - Niacin sustained release 500 mg, 1 tablet QHS
- Continue:
  - Atorvastatin 10 mg, 1 tab QHS
  - Glyburide 5 mg, 1 tab QD
  - Metformin 500 mg, 1 tab TID
  - Metoprolol 25 mg 1 tab QD
  - Lotrel 10 mg–20 mg, 1 cap QD
  - Aspirin 81 mg, 1 tab QD
- Follow-up Laboratory Tests Ordered:
  - Hemoglobin AIC
  - Fasting blood glucose
  - Urinary microalbumin

**Treatment plan rationale:** Intensive dietary intervention was recommended to reduce glycemic load and increase phytonutrient density, in combination with addressing meal timing and frequency. A regular exercise program was initiated to improve insulin sensitivity and increase VO2max and mitochondrial number and efficiency. Supplementation of glucose metabolism-supportive nutrients was initiated, including a specifically-designed product with chromium, vanadium, alpha-lipoic acid (ALA), NAC, biotin, and botanicals banaba leaf and *Gymnema sylvestre*. Extra biotin was also given, based on research using higher doses in insulin resistance (IR), and the significant biotin deficiency identified (Figure 4).[11] All nutrients prescribed have shown efficacy in improving insulin sensitivity in human trials.[1, 11-16] Additional lipoic acid was also given in the form of R-ALA, which may be more potent than ALA,[17] and may therefore be more effective for IR. A fiber complex including Konjac-mannan (KJM) was initiated. KJM has been shown to improve insulin sensitivity.[18] Fiber is also a demonstrated hypolipidemic agent.[19] KJM may have similar promise. A proprietary rice protein and nutrient-based medicinal food was given. Research suggests this medicinal food benefits hepatic function, and was therefore prescribed for the suspected subclinical fatty liver.[20] The medicinal food contains B vitamins and essential elements, both found to be insufficient in this patient (Figures 4 and 7). The

**After making dietary changes and taking supplements, CK reported improvement in energy, particularly in the mid-afternoon and evening.**

anti-inflammatory fatty acids EPA and DHA have been shown to reduce the pro-inflammatory fatty acid arachidonic acid, which was found to be elevated (Figure 6). Both fatty acids also have demonstrated benefit in hypertriglyceridemia.[21] Mitochondrial supportive nutrients, including CoQ10, creatine, carnitine, and magnesium were started based on the organic acid findings (Figure 5) and high lipid peroxide level (Figure 8), which suggested an oxidative stress picture and mitochondropathy. Niacin has been shown to effectively reduce lipids, including Lp(a), which was found to be very high. Atorvastatin, which CK was taking, has not been shown effective at lowering Lp(a).[22] Vitamin D was given for the identified deficiency (Figure 3). The multivitamin and mineral formula was stopped because it didn't supply enough of the specific nutrients required.

## Four-Month Follow-up

After making dietary changes and taking supplements, CK reported improvement in energy, particularly in the mid-afternoon and evening. Her morning blood sugar average was 90. She noted that her skin was clearer. Protein-based afternoon snacks were very helpful in improving mood and energy, and reducing cravings. Fiber was helping with bowel movements. She was exercising on treadmill 30 minutes per day on most days. Her weight loss was at 20 lbs. Her sleep apnea resolved without any interventions. She was very pleased with her progress.

CK admitted that she followed the diet perfectly for one week, and then began to cheat. When she did so, she noticed that certain foods caused symptoms. In particular, she thought that dairy and sugary foods significantly worsened her afternoon fatigue.

CK's diet consisted primarily of organic or cleaner sources of protein (lean meats, fish, eggs, and protein powder), low glycemic snack bars, nuts, seeds, legumes, fresh fruit, vegetables, and some whole grains. When she started the program, she was inspired to clean out her kitchen cabinets of all unhealthy foods. She then stocked up at the natural foods market, buying a greater variety of foods. CK admitted that she followed the diet perfectly for one week, and then began to cheat. When she did so, she noticed that certain foods caused symptoms. In particular, she thought that dairy and sugary foods significantly worsened her afternoon fatigue.

She reported that it was difficult to maintain dietary changes when traveling, and noticed that her blood sugar was significantly higher after flying, reaching 180 on a recent trip. CK also confessed to being addicted to buffet foods, and decided to limit eating out.

CK's physical exam findings showed great improvement: blood pressure: 127/79, left arm seated (previous reading: 160/104); heart rate: 79 beats per minute (previous rate: 94); weight 170 lbs (previous weight: 190 lbs); BMI: 32.66 (previously: 34.7); waist-to-hip ratio: 0.86 (previous ratio: 0.89).

## Four-Month Follow-up Laboratory Testing

| | | Results | Reference Limits |
|---|---|---|---|
| Fasting blood glucose | H | 124 (previous level: 312) | 65–99 mg/dL |
| Hemoglobin A1C | H | 6.4% (previous level: 9.9%) | 0.0–5.9% non-diabetic range |

**Figure 9. Follow-up glucose and A1C.** Significant improvements in blood glucose and A1C values were demonstrated.

# Four-Month Follow-up Plan

- Dietary Intervention
  - Keep daily food journal
  - Include Brassica vegetables at least 3 times per week; daily is best. Examples: arugula, watercress, cabbage, radish, broccoli sprouts, broccoli, and Brussels sprouts
  - 15 minutes walking if she overeats in a restaurant, followed by blood sugar check
  - Travel food suggestions:
    - Dehydrated bean soups
    - Canned wild salmon (www.vitalchoice.com)
    - Fresh fruit
    - Nuts/seeds
    - Organic fiber bars
    - Medicinal food: store individual servings in plastic bags for easy access
- Medications and nutrient therapy
  - Continue supplements as directed
  - Reduce metformin dosage to 500 mg BID
  - Discontinue glyburide
  - Discontinue metoprolol (has been shown to raise blood glucose[24])
  - Continue to monitor blood sugar
- Laboratory tests ordered (to be completed prior to next office visit):
  - Hemoglobin A1C, metabolic panel, thyroid panel
  - Lipids, lipoprotein subclasses and lipoprotein (a)
  - Vitamin D
  - Organic acids

**Treatment plan rationale:** Dietary suggestions for travel were given. Hypoglycemic medications were reduced based on laboratory findings that demonstrated significant improvement in glucose control. Metoprolol was stopped because it has been shown to elevate blood glucose, and CK's blood pressure was significantly improved.[24]

## Nine-Month Follow-up

CK reported a 30 lb weight loss and stated that her average fasting blood sugar was 91. Her cravings were minimal. She reported no sleep apnea and no colds or other health problems since the start of treatment. She wanted to lose another 15 lbs, after which she would completely discontinue glyburide and metformin. She started working with a trainer on interval and strength training two times a week. CK complained of being very busy with work-related travel, though in general she felt empowered in life and health. She described herself as being at a magical point, happy and enjoying her life.

CK reported a 30 lb weight loss and stated that her average fasting blood sugar was 91. Her cravings were minimal.

### Nine-Month Follow-up Laboratory Testing

| | | Results | Reference Limits |
|---|---|---|---|
| Fasting blood glucose | H | 111 (1st 312; 2nd 124) | 65–99 mg/dL |
| Hemoglobin A1C | | 5.9% (1st 9.9; 2nd 6.4) | 0.0–5.9% |
| Alanine aminotransferase (ALT) | | 29 (previous level: 56) | 6–40 U/L |
| Aspartate aminotransferase (AST) | | 20 | 10–35 U/L |
| TSH | | 1.6 (previous level: 2.6) | 0.3–5.5 µIU/mL OR 0.3–2.0 |
| T4 | | 1.1 (previous level: 1.1) | 0.8–1.8 ng/dL |
| T3 | | 261 (previous level: 286) | 230–420 pg/dL |

**Figure 10. Metabolic panel, A1C, and thyroid panel.** Blood glucose and A1C continued to improve. ALT and AST were within normal limits. TSH had improved, although free T3 was lower than previously.

| | | Results | Reference Limits |
|---|---|---|---|
| LDL | | 75 (previous level: 100) | < 100 mg/dL |
| HDL | | 68 (previous level: 64) | > 40 mg/dL |
| Triglycerides | | 44 (previous level: 101) | < 150 mg/dL |
| LDL particles | | 698 (previous level: 1608) | < 1000 nmol/L |
| Small LDL particles | H | 615 | < 600 nmol/L |
| LDL size | | 20.9 (previous level: 20.3) | 20.6–23.0 nm |
| Small HDL particles | L | 8.8 (previous level: 6.9) | > 9.0 µmol/L |
| Lipoprotein(a) | H | 288 (previous level: 423) | 0–74 nmol/L |

**Figure 11. Lipids, lipoprotein subclasses and Lp(a).** Lipid analytes had greatly improved, although Lp(a), despite a significant reduction, was still quite elevated.

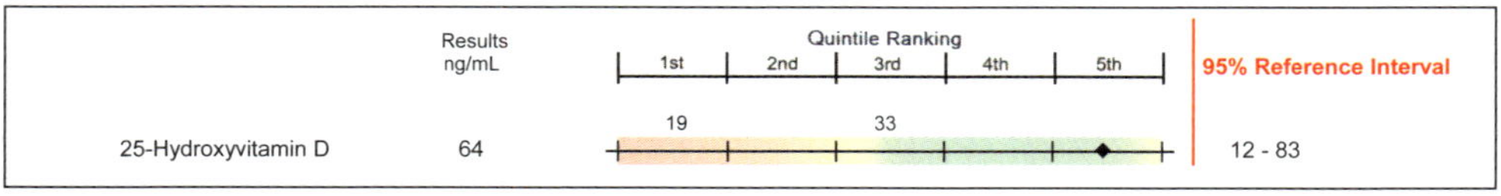


**Figure 12. Serum vitamin D.** Follow-up results demonstrated sufficiency.

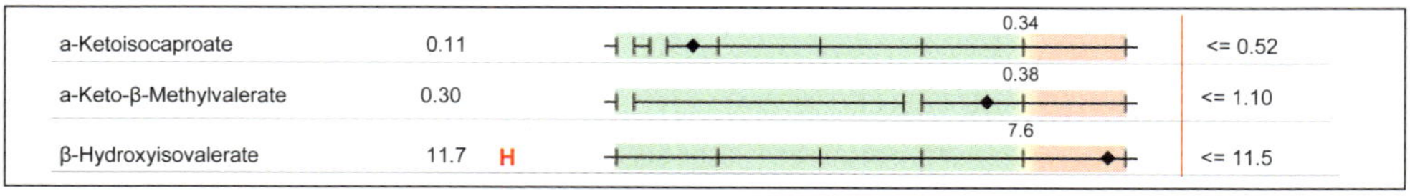


**Figure 13. Organic acid B vitamin markers.** Beta-Hydroxyisovalerate continued to be elevated, despite high-dose supplementation. The alpha-keto acid levels were within normal limits. (Units: µg/mg creatinine)

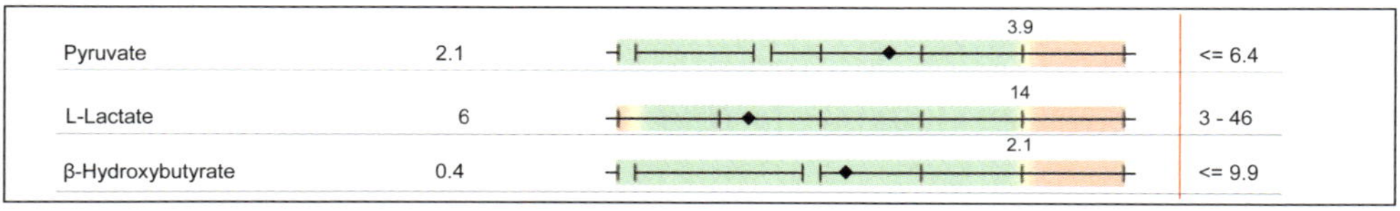


**Figure 14. Organic acid mitochondrial markers.** Lactate and β-Hydroxybutyrate were both within normal range, suggesting improved insulin sensitivity and mitochondrial function. (Units: µg/mg creatinine)

## Nine-Month Follow-up Plan

- Increase exercise as planned
- Continue interventions as directed

# DISCUSSION

Diabetes, an epidemic disease, is a disorder of glucose metabolism that is damaging to every tissue in the body. As such, diabetes is a gateway disease, being associated with cardiovascular and kidney disease, dementia, retinopathy and numerous other conditions. Not surprisingly, morbidity, mortality and cost to society of this preventable illness are extremely high.

> **Organotoxin exposures, including persistent organic pollutants (POPs), polychlorinated biphenyls and bisphenol A, among others, have also been associated with DMII, and individuals eating a typical diabetogenic diet of highly refined, processed foods are at particular risk for exposure.**

As with most complex, chronic conditions, the development of DMII involves environmental exposure coupled with genetic predisposition. It is clear that DMII is strongly associated with physical inactivity, obesity, low HDL levels, excessive alcohol intake,[25] stress[26] and poor dietary choices. Organotoxin exposures, including persistent organic pollutants (POPs), polychlorinated biphenyls and bisphenol A, among others, have also been associated with DMII, and individuals eating a typical diabetogenic diet of highly refined, processed foods are at particular risk for exposure.[27] Identifying genetics has been a more elusive path; however, variants in the transcription factor 7-like 2 (TCF7L2) gene, involved in insulin exocytosis, have been shown to be associated with an almost 30% increased risk of DMII in certain populations.[28-30]

As shown in her family history, CK demonstrated a strong genetic predisposition toward heart disease and diabetes. Environmental risk factors antecedent to her diagnoses included a high-stress, sedentary lifestyle with excessive sugar and alcohol intake. Further, her waist-hip ratio, considered to be a more sensitive marker of cardiovascular risk than body-mass index, was mildly elevated at 0.89.[31]

As indicated in Figure 1, hemoglobin A1C, blood and urinary glucose were all markedly elevated despite being on glyburide and metformin. Looking at the high-normal insulin level in relation to the pronounced elevation of blood and urinary glucose suggested that the pancreas was unable to produce enough insulin to overcome resistance. Allowed to continue, CK would likely have required exogenous insulin at some point in the future. CK's use of the beta-blocker metoprolol could also have been contributing to the dysglycemia.[32] BUN, creatinine, and urinary microalbumin were within normal limits, demonstrating intact kidney function.

Lp(a) is not controlled by statin therapy. Thus, individuals with type 2 diabetes with pharmaceutically controlled levels of total cholesterol may continue to have an increased risk of cardiac and cerebrovascular events based on size, quantity and type of lipoproteins present.

An elevated ALT and an ALT/AST ratio of > 1 (Figure 1) may be early indications of non-alcoholic fatty liver disease (NASH), which is associated with type 2 diabetes.[33,34] Medications including atorvastatin also may increase liver enzymes. While the thyroid panel findings were within normal limits, a TSH > 2.5 has been considered indicative of subclinical hypothyroidism.[35] Subclinical hypothyroidism occurs with significantly greater frequency in type 2 diabetics, and may contribute to dyslipidemia.[36]

The lipid panel (Figure 2), including LDL, HDL, and triglycerides, was within normal limits. However, a closer inspection of cholesterol particle quantity and size demonstrated a significantly different risk picture. Elevated total LDL particle quantity, despite normal LDL-C, is associated with increased risk for cardiovascular disease in type 2 diabetics.[5] The small size of LDL and HDL particles is associated with atherosclerosis in type 2 diabetics.[6] The markedly elevated lipoprotein(a) is indicative of increased risk for vascular disease, particularly in diabetics.[7] Further, Lp(a) is not controlled by statin therapy.[22] Thus, individuals with type 2 diabetes with pharmaceutically controlled levels of total cholesterol may continue to have an increased risk of cardiac and cerebrovascular events based on size, quantity, and type of lipoproteins present.[5]

Figure 3 demonstrated hypovitaminosis D. Vitamin D has been found lower in type 2 diabetics as compared to type 1, and inversely correlated with BMI.[37]

Figure 4 demonstrated functional evidence of biotin deficiency (elevated beta-hydroxyisovalerate). Biotin deficiency is associated with impaired glucose tolerance and utilization of glucose. Biotin upregulates genes involved in lowering blood sugar, including pancreatic and hepatic glucokinase enzymes.[11] CK also demonstrated significant elevation of two alpha-keto acids, both of which have been shown to normalize in some cases with high-dose thiamine, and may be lowered with pantothenic acid, niacin, riboflavin, and alpha-lipoic acid. Finally, while the level of the $B_{12}$ functional marker methylmalonic acid was normal, $B_{12}$ should be periodically monitored because CK was taking metformin, which has been shown to deplete this nutrient in certain individuals.[38]

Figure 5: There are several possible reasons for CK's lactate elevation. An elevated blood lactate/pyruvate ratio was shown to occur in individuals on statin therapy, demonstrating a mitochondropathy and compromised cellular respiration.[39] It is hypothesized that urinary lactate is likely elevated in diabetic patients, as plasma lactate has been shown to be.[40] Furthermore, metformin has been shown to increase serum lactate levels.[41]

Also found in Figure 5 were high urinary ketones (β-Hydroxybutyrate), evidence for increased fatty acid beta oxidation due to insulin resistance. HMG was also mildly elevated, suggesting inhibition of HMG-CoA reductase enzyme, which was expected given CK's use of the pharmaceutical inhibitor, atorvastatin. HMG-CoA reductase is the rate-limiting enzyme in cholesterol and CoQ10 synthesis. CoQ10 deficiency has been shown to occur in statin users.[39, 42] In cell studies, statin exposure causes increased oxidative DNA damage, early cell death, decreased ATP production and CoQ10 deficiency.[43] Taken together, the elevated lactate along with the HMG elevation may have been associated with inadequate CoQ10 availability compromising cellular respiration, causing subclinical mitochondropathy. As discussed below (Figure 8), the high level of lipid peroxidation is further evidence for mitochondrial dysfunction.

**Taken together, the elevated lactate along with the HMG elevation may have been associated with inadequate CoQ10 availability compromising cellular respiration, causing subclinical mitochondropathy.**

Figure 6: Omega-3 fatty acids EPA and DHA were within normal limits, but the omega-6 fatty acid AA was elevated, providing the substrate for eicosanoid inflammatory compounds. Insulin stimulates the production of AA[44] through up-regulation of delta-5-desaturase. AA elevation has been associated with insulin resistance.[45, 46]

The element insufficiencies shown in Figure 7 may have contributed to the pathogenesis of CK's complaints. In brief, chromium is involved in cellular glucose uptake via potentiating insulin receptor tyrosine kinase. Indeed, elevated blood sugar itself has been proposed as a surrogate marker for chromium deficiency.[47] Vanadium is believed to be involved in lipid and glucose metabolism.[47] Selenium is a cofactor in multiple enzymes involved in glutathione and thyroid metabolism, and thus low selenium status may be contributing to increased oxidative stress (see below) as well as the mild thyroid dysfunction. Magnesium is a cofactor for some 375 enzymes, including those involved in glucose and insulin regulation. It also plays a role in modulating blood pressure by supporting smooth muscle relaxation.[47] Magnesium is frequently found to be low in diabetics.[48] Multiple essential element deficiencies also suggest compromised digestion and absorption in addition to poor dietary intake.

The elevated lipid peroxides (Figure 8) were indicative of oxidative damage to cell membranes, which occurs with greater frequency in diabetic individuals. An association between glycemic control, A1C and lipid peroxides has been demonstrated in individuals with type 2 diabetes.[49] Mitochondropathy has also been associated with increased reactive oxidative species and CoQ10 deficiency.[50, 51]

As discussed above, the plan for CK was based on the laboratory findings and included aggressive nutrient intervention with attention to glucose metabolism, oxidative stress, lipid abnormalities, nutrient deficiencies, and subclinical mitochondropathy. Diet and exercise were important components of the plan.

On follow-up, CK presented with improved energy, reduced sugar cravings, decreased blood pressure, and a 20-pound weight-loss. She was inspired by her progress to continue exercising consistently and to focus on a healthy diet. Her follow-up laboratory data (Figure 9) reflected her commitment: glucose and A1C were both significantly improved. Though not yet in the normal range, A1C did meet guidelines for those with type 2 diabetes. Her follow-up plan included stopping glyburide, metoprolol (which has been shown to contribute to dysglycemia[24]) and reducing metformin.

**The relatively slow rate of weight loss by CK may have minimized exposure to stored organotoxins liberated from adipose, making the process of weight reduction safer.**

At her nine-month follow-up visit, CK reported her average blood sugar to be 91 and total weight loss of 30 pounds. Her sleep apnea was resolved. She was pleased with her progress, and inspired to lose 15 additional pounds, which she intended to do by increasing her exercise routine with a personal trainer. She would continue to work with the clinician to achieve her goals.

It is important to note that CK's weight loss may have been assisted by the resolution of her sleep apnea, as poor sleep quality is associated with weight gain or difficulty in losing weight.[52, 53] Also, the relatively slow rate of weight loss (30 pounds over nine months) by CK may have minimized exposure to stored organotoxins liberated from adipose tissue, making the process of weight reduction safer.[54, 55] Recent research has demonstrated a highly significant increase in the blood level of key fat-soluble toxins normally stored in adipose tissue during weight loss. The rate of release parallels the rate of weight loss, suggesting that a slower pace of weight loss may reduce toxic exposure.[54] These toxins, including polychlorinated biphenyls (PCBs), hexachlorobenzene (HCB), and p,p'-dichlorophenyldichloroethylene (DDE) are ubiquitous microcontaminants that are lipid soluble and accumulate in stored fat. Assessment of organotoxin status may be indicated prior to and during weight reduction programs.

CK's nine-month follow-up laboratory data continued to reflect improvement (Figure 10). Blood sugar was at 111, down from an original 312. Liver enzymes were at normal levels, and her TSH was also improved at 1.6. Figure 11 showed significant improvement in lipids, with HDL at a robust 68. While still elevated at 288, Lp(a) had dropped considerably from the original measurement of 423. Vitamin D was sufficient, as shown in Figure 12. Urinary organic acids in Figure 13 also showed improvement, although beta-Hydroxyisovalerate continued to be elevated, despite aggressive supplementation. Biotin is primarily produced by bacteria in the GI tract. Ongoing deficiency despite supplementation suggested possible GI imbalance. Lactate and β-Hydroxybutyrate were both within normal ranges (Figure 14), suggesting improved insulin sensitivity and mitochondrial function.

# CONCLUSION

It is difficult to overstate the diabetes epidemic and its associated ramifications. Diabetes is one of the top seven causes of death in the United States, and is associated with six of the top ten causes of death. In 2007, one of every five U.S. healthcare dollars was spent caring for someone diagnosed with diabetes. According to the World Health Organization, over 220 million people worldwide now have diabetes, and deaths from diabetes are expected to double by the year 2030. However, 90% of DMII is likely preventable through lifestyle changes alone.[1, 56-58]

Excess body weight is a strong independent risk factor in diabetes, and some one in three Americans (including children) is obese or overweight.[1] Obesity and DMII have been closely linked to organotoxins, exposure to which is greatly increased in those who follow the typical standard American diet.[27] Successful pharmacological control of DMII is achieved in fewer than 50% of all patients.[1] Alternatives in combating this disease are therefore urgently needed.

> **It is well-established that lifestyle intervention can significantly reduce the incidence of DMII, however, these interventions go largely untried.**

It is well-established that lifestyle intervention can significantly reduce the incidence of DMII. As evidenced by the above statistics, however, these interventions are infrequently used. DMII might be considered a socio-political disease, since the advent of government-subsidized foods such as wheat, soy, and high-fructose corn syrup has led to increased consumption of processed foods and simple carbohydrates, resulting in the twin epidemics of obesity and DMII.[59] This suggests that the solution to the epidemic will require government involvement not dissimilar to that which occurred with the tobacco industry. Moreover, the technological revolution has contributed to the onset of a more sedentary lifestyle, also contributing to the disease incidence.[60]

As in the case of CK, patient education, inspiration and self-awareness are essential factors needed to alter the diabetes epidemic. Laboratory assessment of disease risk and nutrient status guided the development of safe interventions that involved individualized diet, nutrient and lifestyle changes. Individualized therapies, education and empowerment may be the key inspirational tools required to turn around the epidemic of DMII. Innovations in group treatment and sustainable behavior change are critical to help stem the rising tide of cost and suffering attributable to type 2 diabetes.

---

**Authors: Kara Fitzgerald, ND; Mark Hyman, MD**

**Case Clinicians: Mark Hyman, MD, Chairman, Institute for Functional Medicine; Kathie Swift, MS, RD**

## References


1. Campbell RK, Martin TM. The chronic burden of diabetes. *Am J Manag Care.* Sep 2009;15(9 Suppl):S248-254.
2. Nissen SE, Wolski K. Effect of rosiglitazone on the risk of myocardial infarction and death from cardiovascular causes. *N Engl J Med.* Jun 14 2007;356(24):2457-2471.
3. Diabetes Statistics. http://www.diabetes.org/diabetes-basics/diabetes-statistics/. Accessed 9/16/2010, 2010.
4. Diabetes Public Health Resource - 2007 National Diabetes Fact Sheet. http://www.cdc.gov/diabetes/pubs/general07.htm#gen_a, 2010.
5. Cromwell WC, Otvos JD. Heterogeneity of low-density lipoprotein particle number in patients with type 2 diabetes mellitus and low-density lipoprotein cholesterol <100 mg/dl. *Am J Cardiol.* Dec 15 2006;98(12):1599-1602.
6. Hayashi Y, Okumura K, Matsui H, et al. Impact of low-density lipoprotein particle size on carotid intima-media thickness in patients with type 2 diabetes mellitus. *Metabolism.* May 2007;56(5):608-613.
7. Kubo M, Takami S, Matsuzawa Y. Contribution of Lp(a) to the occurrence of vascular diseases: correlation of several risk factors including diabetes mellitus. *J Atheroscler Thromb.* 1995;2 Suppl 1:S22-25.
8. Holick MF. Vitamin D deficiency. *N Engl J Med.* Jul 19 2007;357(3):266-281.
9. Membrez M, Blancher F, Jaquet M, et al. Gut microbiota modulation with norfloxacin and ampicillin enhances glucose tolerance in mice. *Faseb J.* Mar 7 2008.
10. Mock DM, Henrich CL, Carnell N, Mock NI. Indicators of marginal biotin deficiency and repletion in humans: validation of 3-hydroxyisovaleric acid excretion and a leucine challenge. *Am J Clin Nutr.* Nov 2002;76(5):1061-1068.
11. Fernandez-Mejia C. Pharmacological effects of biotin. *J Nutr Biochem.* Jul 2005;16(7):424-427.
12. Wang ZQ, Cefalu WT. Current concepts about chromium supplementation in type 2 diabetes and insulin resistance. *Curr Diab Rep.* Apr 2010;10(2):145-151.
13. Muramatsu T, Yatsuya H, Toyoshima H, et al. Higher dietary intake of alpha-linolenic acid is associated with lower insulin resistance in middle-aged Japanese. *Prev Med.* May-Jun 2010;50(5-6):272-276.
14. Klein G, Kim J, Himmeldirk K, Cao Y, Chen X. Antidiabetes and Anti-obesity Activity of Lagerstroemia speciosa. *Evid Based Complement Alternat Med.* Dec 2007;4(4):401-407.
15. Al-Romaiyan A, Liu B, Asare-Anane H, et al. A novel Gymnema sylvestre extract stimulates insulin secretion from human islets in vivo and in vitro. *Phytother Res.* Sep 2010;24(9):1370-1376.
16. Martina V, Masha A, Gigliardi VR, et al. Long-term N-acetylcysteine and L-arginine administration reduces endothelial activation and systolic blood pressure in hypertensive patients with type 2 diabetes. *Diabetes Care.* May 2008;31(5):940-944.
17. Streeper RS, Henriksen EJ, Jacob S, Hokama JY, Fogt DL, Tritschler HJ. Differential effects of lipoic acid stereoisomers on glucose metabolism in insulin-resistant skeletal muscle. *Am J Physiol.* 1997;273(1 Pt 1):E185-191.
18. Vuksan V, Sievenpiper JL, Xu Z, et al. Konjac-Mannan and American ginsing: emerging alternative therapies for type 2 diabetes mellitus. *J Am Coll Nutr.* Oct 2001;20(5 Suppl):370S-380S; discussion 381S-383S.
19. Anderson JW, Allgood LD, Lawrence A, et al. Cholesterol-lowering effects of psyllium intake adjunctive to diet therapy in men and women with hypercholesterolemia: meta-analysis of 8 controlled trials. *Am J Clin Nutr.* Feb 2000;71(2):472-479.
20. Bland J, Barrager E, Reedy R, Bland K. A Medical Food-Supplemented Detoxification Program in the Management of Chronic Health Problems. *Altern Ther Health Med.* 1995;1(5):62-71.
21. Fedor D, Kelley DS. Prevention of insulin resistance by n-3 polyunsaturated fatty acids. *Curr Opin Clin Nutr Metab Care.* Mar 2009;12(2):138-146.
22. Scanu AM, Hinman J. Issues concerning the monitoring of statin therapy in hypercholesterolemic subjects with high plasma lipoprotein(a) levels. *Lipids.* May 2002;37(5):439-444.
23. Hoogwerf BJ, Sprecher DL, Pearce GL, et al. Blood glucose concentrations < or = 125 mg/dl and coronary heart disease risk. *Am J Cardiol.* Mar 1 2002;89(5):596-599.
24. Fonseca VA. Effects of beta-blockers on glucose and lipid metabolism. *Curr Med Res Opin.* Mar 2010;26(3):615-629.

25. van de Wiel A. Diabetes mellitus and alcohol. *Diabetes Metab Res Rev.* Jul-Aug 2004;20(4):263-267.

26. Wellen KE, Hotamisligil GS. Inflammation, stress, and diabetes. *J Clin Invest.* May 2005;115(5):1111-1119.

27. Porta M. Persistent organic pollutants and the burden of diabetes. *Lancet.* Aug 12 2006;368(9535):558-559.

28. da Silva Xavier G, Loder MK, McDonald A, et al. TCF7L2 regulates late events in insulin secretion from pancreatic islet beta-cells. *Diabetes.* Apr 2009;58(4):894-905.

29. Owen KR, McCarthy MI. Genetics of type 2 diabetes. *Curr Opin Genet Dev.* Jun 2007;17(3):239-244.

30. Yan Y, North KE, Ballantyne CM, et al. Transcription factor 7-like 2 (TCF7L2) polymorphism and context-specific risk of type 2 diabetes in African American and Caucasian adults: the Atherosclerosis Risk in Communities study. *Diabetes.* Jan 2009;58(1):285-289.

31. Dobbelsteyn CJ, Joffres MR, MacLean DR, Flowerdew G. A comparative evaluation of waist circumference, waist-to-hip ratio and body mass index as indicators of cardiovascular risk factors. The Canadian Heart Health Surveys. *Int J Obes Relat Metab Disord.* May 2001;25(5):652-661.

32. Fonseca V, Bakris GL, Bell DS, et al. Differential effect of beta-blocker therapy on insulin resistance as a function of insulin sensitizer use: results from GEMINI. *Diabet Med.* Jul 2007;24(7):759-763.

33. Schindhelm RK, Diamant M, Dekker JM, Tushuizen ME, Teerlink T, Heine RJ. Alanine aminotransferase as a marker of non-alcoholic fatty liver disease in relation to type 2 diabetes mellitus and cardiovascular disease. *Diabetes Metab Res Rev.* Nov-Dec 2006;22(6):437-443.

34. Clark JM. The epidemiology of nonalcoholic fatty liver disease in adults. *J Clin Gastroenterol.* Mar 2006;40(3 Suppl 1):S5-10.

35. Wartofsky L, Dickey RA. The evidence for a narrower thyrotropin reference range is compelling. *J Clin Endocrinol Metab.* Sep 2005;90(9):5483-5488.

36. Wu P. Thyroid disorders and diabetes. It is common for a person to be affected by both thyroid disease and diabetes. *Diabetes Self Manag.* Sep-Oct 2007;24(5):80-82, 85-87.

37. Di Cesar DJ, Ploutz-Snyder R, Weinstock RS, Moses AM. Vitamin D deficiency is more common in type 2 than in type 1 diabetes. *Diabetes Care.* Jan 2006;29(1):174.

38. Buvat DR. Use of metformin is a cause of vitamin $B_{12}$ deficiency. *Am Fam Physician.* Jan 15 2004;69(2):264; author reply 264, 266.

39. De Pinieux G, Chariot P, Ammi-Said M, et al. Lipid-lowering drugs and mitochondrial function: effects of HMG-CoA reductase inhibitors on serum ubiquinone and blood lactate/pyruvate ratio. *Br J Clin Pharmacol.* Sep 1996;42(3):333-337.

40. Cameron MA, Maalouf NM, Adams-Huet B, Moe OW, Sakhaee K. Urine composition in type 2 diabetes: predisposition to uric acid nephrolithiasis. *J Am Soc Nephrol.* May 2006;17(5):1422-1428.

41. Davis TM, Jackson D, Davis WA, Bruce DG, Chubb P. The relationship between metformin therapy and the fasting plasma lactate in type 2 diabetes: The Fremantle Diabetes Study. *Br J Clin Pharmacol.* Aug 2001;52(2):137-144.

42. Rundek T, Naini A, Sacco R, Coates K, DiMauro S. Atorvastatin decreases the coenzyme Q10 level in the blood of patients at risk for cardiovascular disease and stroke. *Arch Neurol.* Jun 2004;61(6):889-892.

43. Tavintharan S, Ong CN, Jeyaseelan K, Sivakumar M, Lim SC, Sum CF. Reduced mitochondrial coenzyme Q10 levels in HepG2 cells treated with high-dose simvastatin: a possible role in statin-induced hepatotoxicity? *Toxicol Appl Pharmacol.* Sep 1 2007;223(2):173-179.

44. Das UN. Is obesity an inflammatory condition? *Nutrition.* Nov-Dec 2001;17(11-12):953-966.

45. Aldamiz-Echevarria L, Prieto JA, Andrade F, Elorz J, Sanjurjo P, Rodriguez Soriano J. Arachidonic acid content in adipose tissue is associated with insulin resistance in healthy children. *J Pediatr Gastroenterol Nutr.* Jan 2007;44(1):77-83.

46. Galgani JE, Aguirre CA, Uauy RD, Diaz EO. Plasma arachidonic acid influences insulin-stimulated glucose uptake in healthy adult women. *Ann Nutr Metab.* 2007;51(5):482-489.

47. *Laboratory Evaluations for Integrative and Functional Medicine.* Atlanta: Metametrix Institute; 2008.

48. Sales CH, Pedrosa Lde F. Magnesium and diabetes mellitus: their relation. *Clin Nutr.* Aug 2006;25(4):554-562.

49. Lawrence JR, Campbell GR, Barrington H, et al. Clinical and biochemical determinants of plasma lipid peroxide levels in type 2 diabetes. *Ann Clin Biochem.* May 1998;35 ( Pt 3):387-392.

**50.** Addabbo F, Montagnani M, Goligorsky MS. Mitochondria and reactive oxygen species. *Hypertension.* Jun 2009;53(6):885-892.

**51.** Quinzii CM, Lopez LC, Gilkerson RW, et al. Reactive oxygen species, oxidative stress, and cell death correlate with level of CoQ10 deficiency. *Faseb J.* Oct 2010;24(10):3733-3743.

**52.** Carter R, 3rd, Watenpaugh DE. Obesity and obstructive sleep apnea: Or is it OSA and obesity? *Pathophysiology.* Aug 2008;15(2):71-77.

**53.** Patel SR. Reduced sleep as an obesity risk factor. *Obes Rev.* Nov 2009;10 Suppl 2:61-68.

**54.** Chevrier J, Dewailly E, Ayotte P, Mauriege P, Despres JP, Tremblay A. Body weight loss increases plasma and adipose tissue concentrations of potentially toxic pollutants in obese individuals. *Int J Obes Relat Metab Disord.* Oct 2000;24(10):1272-1278.

**55.** Hue O, Marcotte J, Berrigan F, et al. Increased plasma levels of toxic pollutants accompanying weight loss induced by hypocaloric diet or by bariatric surgery. *Obes Surg.* Sep 2006;16(9):1145-1154.

**56.** Pradhan A. Obesity, Metabolic Syndrome, and Type 2 Diabetes: Inflammatory Basis of Glucose Metabolic Disorders. *Nutr Rev.* 2007;65(12 Pt 2):S152-156.

**57.** WHO. Diabetes Key Facts. http://www.who.int/mediacentre/factsheets/fs312/en/. Accessed 9/20/2010, 2010.

**58.** Willett WC. Balancing life-style and genomics research for disease prevention. *Science.* Apr 26 2002;296(5568):695-698.

**59.** Muller M, Schoonover H, Wallinga D. *Considering the Contribution of U.S. Food and Agricultural Policy to the Obesity Epidemic: Overview and Opportunities.* Minneapolis: Institute for Agriculture and Trade Policy; 2007.

**60.** Hu FB. Sedentary lifestyle and risk of obesity and type 2 diabetes. *Lipids.* Feb 2003;38(2):103-108.

# 6 Gastrointestinal Disorders

## Inflammatory Bowel Disease

*Ulcerative colitis (UC) and Crohn disease are the principal constituents of the gastrointestinal inflammatory condition group known as Inflammatory Bowel Disease (IBD). IBD is one of the five most common gastrointestinal diseases in the United States. Because there is no recognized cure, patients require a lifetime of care. Annually, the health care cost of IBD exceeds $1.7 billion and more than 115,000 patients are placed on disability.[1] IBD is associated with an increased risk for intestinal cancers.[2] Up to 75% of Crohn disease patients and 33% of UC patients will require surgery (colectomy).[1] The case below describes a patient with pancolitis, a severe form of UC that involves the whole colon. Pancolitis that is non-responsive to medication, as was the case with this individual, frequently requires surgical intervention.[3]*

### 29-Year-Old Female with Ulcerative Colitis/Pancolitis

| | |
|---|---|
| **Additional Symptoms and Conditions** | Chronic diarrhea, erythema nodosum, weight loss, fatigue; medications ineffective |
| **Lifestyle Factors** | Standard American diet, high stress due to illness |
| **Medications** | Mesalamine (Asocol®), azathioprine (Imuran®), prednisone |
| **Tests Used** | Food-specific IgG antibodies, microbial stool analysis using DNA identification; celiac genes and serology |
| **Imbalances Identified** | Elevated food-specific IgG antibodies, intestinal dysbiosis and parasitosis |
| **Treatments** | Diet modification, albendazole, digestive enzymes, antimicrobial and nutritive botanicals, probiotics |
| **Outcome** | Weight normalization (gain), significant resolution of symptoms, improved energy, daily use of medications no longer required |
| **Significance** | Because this patient's pancolitis could not be medically managed using prednisone, mesalamine and azathioprine, it is likely that surgery would have been her next step. The testing and treatment used in this case resulted in dramatic clinical improvement and enhanced quality of life. It is probable that the treatment prevented the need for surgical intervention. Given the grim epidemiological statistics of IBD, research investigating the efficacy of the cost-saving, multifactorial, integrative approach used in this case is highly recommended. |

# CASE HISTORY

EM was a 29-year-old female presenting with extremely active ulcerative colitis (UC). Colonoscopy had detected pancolitis. She was at her lowest body weight since entering adulthood. She was taking prednisone, mesalamine (a cyclooxygenase and prostaglandin blocker), and azathioprine (an immunosuppressive drug with unknown mechanism), but these medications were not bringing her relief. She had chronic diarrhea and severe fatigue. She also had erythema nodosum (nodular erythematous eruptions on the lower legs) which presented as large, multiple oozing lesions which were preceded by bruises. For the erythema nodosum, she was prescribed a two-month course of the antibiotic cephalexin. Because of the debility of her illness, EM stated that she couldn't be a mother to her two children.

For most of her life, EM had eaten a standard American diet (SAD) characterized by high intake of red meat, sugary desserts and drinks, high-fat foods, dairy products, eggs, and refined grains. Ten months before her initial visit, an IgG food antibody test reported significant reactions to yeast, gluten, and dairy, so she eliminated foods containing these components from her diet. Tests for celiac serology and genes turned out negative. Even with the adoption of this oligoantigenic diet based on her specific reactions, however, she noted no significant change to her condition at the time of her initial visit.

> Because this patient's pancolitis could not be medically managed using prednisone, mesalamine and azathioprine, it is likely that surgery would have been her next step.

EM's family history did not include inflammatory bowel disease or other autoimmune conditions. Her husband had irritable bowel syndrome. Although EM was under a great deal of stress because of her condition and had eaten the SAD for most of her life, there were no other contributing lifestyle factors apparent.

## Initial Laboratory Results

**Laboratory tests ordered and rationale:**

1. **Previous testing:** Tests for celiac serology and celiac genes turned out negative. IgG food-specific antibody testing identified significant antibody elevations to yeast, gluten and dairy. Adverse food reactions, including an association with celiac disease, have been identified in IBD.[4-5] Removal of offending foods has been noted to improve symptoms. Note that laboratory findings demonstrated a positive gluten IgG reaction, but frank celiac disease (gluten intolerance) was ruled out, suggesting an alternative inflammatory response to gluten.
2. **Microbial stool analysis using DNA identification:** Gastrointestinal microbiota imbalance (dysbiosis) is a common and significant finding in inflammatory bowel disease.[6] Dysbiosis was suspected to be a significant etiopathogenic factor in this case, particularly given the lack of favorable response to the removal of potential antigenic foods.

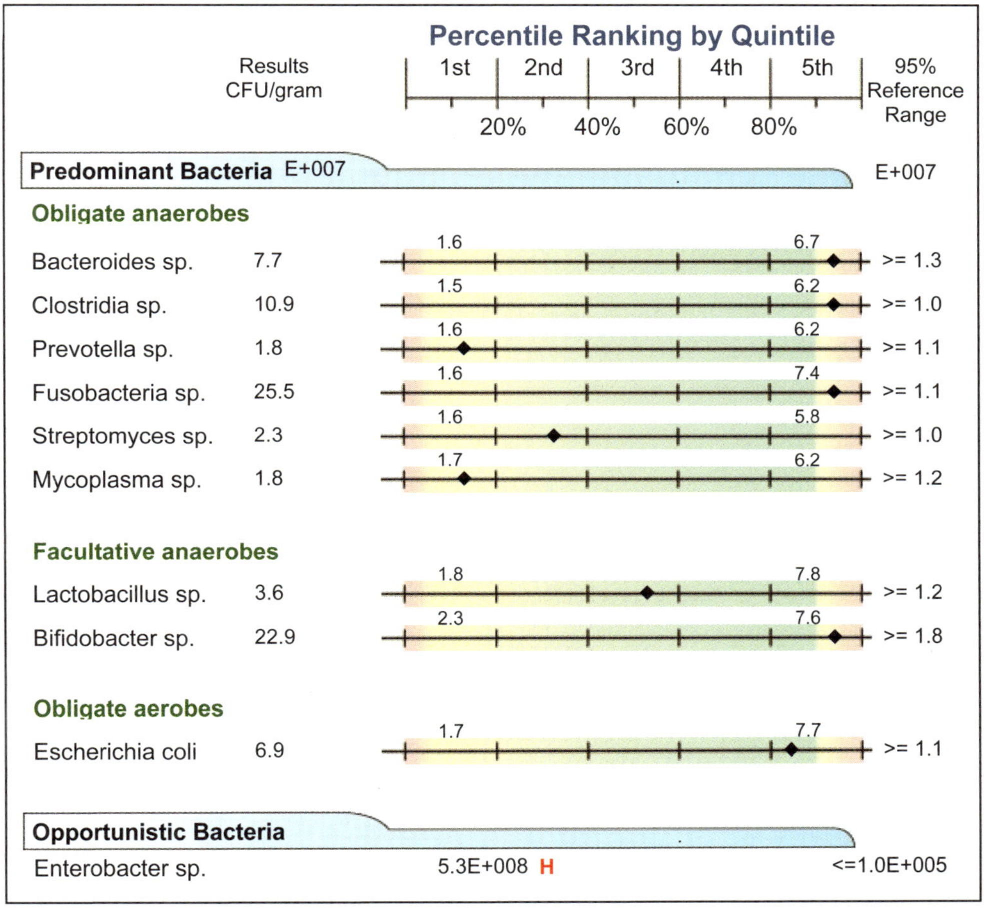


**Figure 1. Microbial stool analysis using DNA identification.** Opportunistic bacteria present. Imbalance in the pattern of predominant bacteria suggested dysbiosis.

| Pathogenic Bacteria | | 95% Reference Range |
|---|---|---|
| Helicobacter pylori | <0.01 | <=1.0E+005 |
| Campylobacter sp. | 5.5E+008 **H** | <=1.0E+005 |
| Clostridium difficile | <0.01 | <=1.0E+005 |
| E.H.E. coli | 5.9E+008 **H** | <=1.0E+005 |
| ***Parasites*** | | |
| Necator americanus (hookworm) | **Positive** | Neg |

**Figure 2. Microbial stool analysis using DNA identification.** Pathogenic bacteria and a parasite detected in patient's stool.

| Pharmaceuticals | S | R |
|---|---|---|
| Amoxicillin | | R |
| Ampicillin | | R |
| Cefuroxime | | R |
| Ciprofloxacin | S | |
| Clindamycin | S | |
| Erythromycin | | R |
| Levofloxacin | S | |
| Penicillin | | R |
| Potassium Clavula | | R |
| Sulfamethoxazole | S | |
| Tetracyclin | S | |
| Trimethoprim-Sulfa | S | |

| Botanicals | S | R |
|---|---|---|
| 5-Hydroxy-1,4-naphthoquinone<br>Black Walnut | S | |
| Alliin<br>Garlic | | R |
| Arbutin<br>Uva Ursi | | R |
| Artemisinin<br>Wormwood | | R |
| Berberine<br>Goldenseal | S | |
| Caprylic acid<br>Octanoic acid | S | |
| Carvacrol<br>Oregano | S | |
| Oleuropein<br>Olive Leaf | | R |
| Quinic Acid<br>Cats Claw | S | |
| Thymol<br>Oil of Thyme | S | |
| Undecylenic acid<br>Undecylenic acid | S | |

**Figure 3. Bacterial sensitivities to pharmaceutical and botanical interventions.** Findings suggested that bacteria detected in stool may have resistance to cefuroxime, among other antibiotics and botanicals. S = sensitive; R = resistant.

# Assessment

- Pancolitis with associated weight loss, fatigue and diarrhea
- Erythema nodosum
- Dysbiosis
- Antibiotic resistance

# Treatment Plan

- Albendazole 250 mg, 1 tab PO BID for 3 days; then 1 tab on day 8, day 30, and day 90
- Berberine (botanical antimicrobial formula), 1 tab PO BID
- Multi-botanical antimicrobial formula, 2 caps PO BID (Contains: bilberry extract (25% anthocyanosides), Noni, Milk Thistle, Echinacea (purpurea & angustifolia), Goldenseal, Shiitake, White Willow (bark), Garlic, Grapeseed extract, Black Walnut (hull and leaf), Raspberry, Fumitory, Gentian, Tea Tree oil, Galbanum oil, Lavender oil (plant and flower), Oregano oil)
- Deglycyrrhizinated licorice (DGL), 2 tabs PO TID AC
- Aloe vera capsules, 2 caps PO BID
- Vegetable greens powder, 1 scoop PO QD
- *Lactobacillus rhamnosus* strain GG
- *Saccharomyces boulardii*
- *Lactobacillus sp.*, *Bifidobacter sp.*, and *Streptococcus thermophilus*
- Digestive enzymes, 2 tabs PO TID AC
- Continue:
  - Diet: Eliminate gluten, dairy, and yeast
  - Mesalamine (COX/PG blocker) 400 mg, 1 tab PO TID

**Treatment plan rationale:** It was decided that the parasite would be treated with albendazole and the pathogenic and opportunistic bacteria would be addressed using a combination of antimicrobial botanicals that were identified as sensitive on laboratory testing (Figure 3). Botanicals were chosen because the patient had a history of extensive exposure to antibiotics. Botanicals may be less disruptive to the predominant flora for a number of reasons. For example, some antimicrobial botanicals contain prebiotic substances such as polysaccharides.[7] Botanicals are also suggested to be less likely to contribute to antibiotic resistance.[8] The mucilaginous botanicals, aloe vera and licorice (DGL), were used to reduce GI inflammation and support healing of the mucosa.[9-10] A vegetable-greens powder was employed with the expectation that it would provide bioavailable nutritional support. Comprehensive probiotics, including *Saccharomyes boulardii*, were used to normalize microflora, reduce inflammation and support intestinal health.[11] Digestive enzymes were given to optimize macronutrient breakdown to facilitate improved bioavailability and absorption of micronutrients. The dietary restrictions and mesalamine were continued. Note that this relatively low-risk protocol was directed at addressing the suspected causal factors of EM's IBD as identified on laboratory analysis, rather than suppressing the symptoms and pathogenic mechanisms, as the higher-risk medications were designed to do.

## Ten-Month Follow-Up

EM gained weight and the erythema nodosum resolved. Her energy level increased. She had stopped the azathioprine and had been titrated off the steroids. Her dose of mesalamine was reduced and then discontinued, although she occasionally used it for flare-ups. The flare-ups were mostly caused by inadvertent exposure to foods to which she was reactive. Although exposures to such foods would throw her off track for a few days, she recovered more quickly than she had in the past. She thought that if she were successful in avoidance of all reactive foods, her recovery would be 100%. The most important benefit of her healing was, to EM, that she could once again be a mother to her two children. As she herself said, she was doing "incredibly well." For maintenance treatment, it was recommended that EM continue with dietary restrictions, probiotics and digestive enzymes; periodic clinical and laboratory assessments would determine need for additional interventions. See Figure 4.

> **To EM, the greatest benefit of her healing was that she could once again be a mother to her two children.**

# DISCUSSION

EM's pancolitis and erythema nodosum were evidence of an intense systemic inflammatory reaction. Factors involved in the pathogenesis of inflammatory bowel disease (IBD) include the host's intestinal microflora, the host's genetic and immune predisposition, infection, psychological stress, environmental stimuli, and intestinal barrier permeability.[12-14] Immunological reactivity to foods, including gluten intolerance, have been reported as causes of colonic inflammation and IBD.[4-5]

EM did not have a family history of IBD, but she was under a good deal of stress caused by her limited ability to care for her children, on account of her illness. While this particular stressor was not a causative factor, it may have exacerbated her IBD. Components of the SAD she followed for most of her life were very antigenic for her, as identified on IgG testing. The severe reactions, while not numerous enough to indicate intestinal hyperpermeability, did reflect a pronounced inflammatory response. The IgG class is comprised of a group of four immunoglobulins. IgG1 and IgG4 can form complexes with the offending food protein. Only IgG4 subclass elevation is associated with chronic exposure.The antigen-antibody complex may initiate an immune response, leading to a wide variety of symptoms, ranging from gastrointestinal symptoms including diarrhea, to

> **This patient's laboratory results point to several factors that may have contributed to the etiopathogenesis of ulcerative colitis.**

## Ten-Month Follow-up Laboratory Results

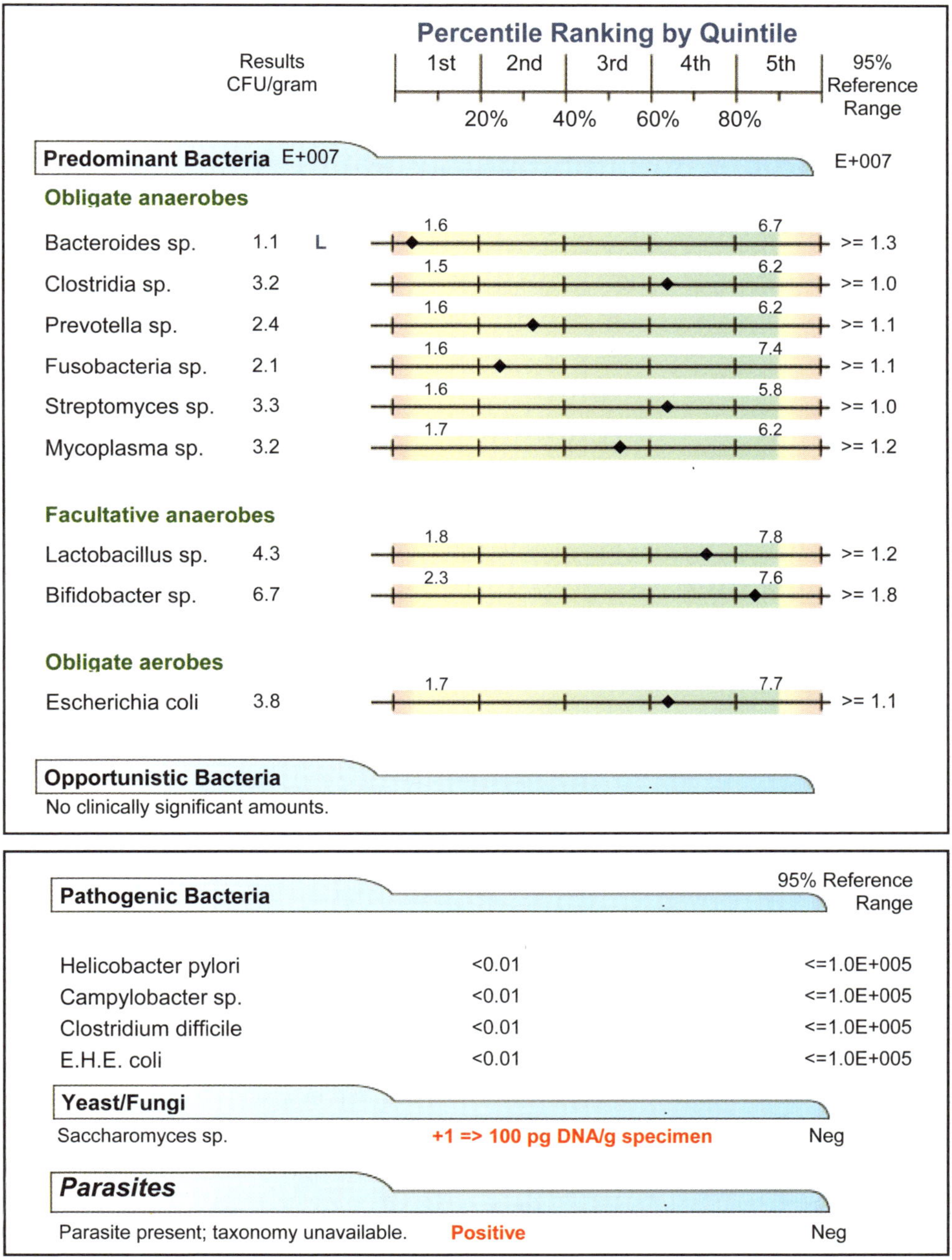


**Figure 4. Follow-up microbial stool analysis using DNA identification.** Findings were negative for *Enterobacter sp., Campylobacter sp.*, *EHEC*, and hookworm. *Saccharomyces* species were detected, probably as a result of supplementation. Parasite was detected; taxonomy was unavailable but was probably dietary exposure to parasitic DNA rather than a pathogen. Predominant bacteria were more balanced, although *Bacteroides* species were low.

skin changes, headaches or joint inflammation and myopathy. Indeed, symptoms associated with IgG reactions are found associated with most organ systems.[15] It is interesting to note that EM had a severe reaction on IgG testing to gluten, but was negative for celiac disease (and celiac genes), suggesting that an inflammatory response to foods in UC is not limited to a single pathogenic mechanism.

This patient's laboratory results pointed to several factors that may have contributed to the pathogenesis of UC. As shown in Figure 1, very high levels of predominant bacteria spp. *(Bacteroides sp., Clostridia sp., Fusobacteria sp., and Bifidobacter sp.)* and *Enterobacter sp.* (an opportunistic bacterium) demonstrated significantly altered microflora (dysbiosis). Imbalances of predominant anaerobic bacteria (both high and low) have been reported in IBD. Specifically, *Bacteroides*, *Eubacterium* (such as *E. coli*, *Enterobacter*, *Shigella*, *Salmonella*, *Yersinia*, etc.), and *Lactobacillus* have been identified.[16] Similar to EM's findings, studies have also shown increased anaerobes (especially gram-negative anaerobes such as *Bacteroides*) in Crohn disease (CD), UC, and pouchitis. In one study, 50% of CD patients had either *E. coli* or *Bacteroides* as the predominant GI bacterial group.[17]

*Enterobacter spp,* the opportunistic bacteria shown in Figure 1, are asymptomatic in healthy individuals but are a leading cause of nosocomial bacterial infections, including urinary tract infections, bacteremia, skin and soft tissue infections, and septic arthritis.[18] However, there are not many cases in the literature of *Enterobacter*-induced colitis or gastroenteritis.

Two pathogens, *Campylobacter sp.* and *Enterohemorrhagic Escherichia coli* (EHEC), were also detected (Figure 2), illustrating the severity of dysbiosis. Bacterial enteritis can induce or exacerbate IBD.[13] *Campylobacter sp.* and *EHEC* have been reported as causes of bacterial colitis.[14,19-20] *Campylobacter* specifically has been detected in IBD,[21] and has been cited as a rare cause of pancolitis.[19]

**_Campylobacter_ specifically has been detected in IBD, and has been cited as a rare cause of pancolitis.**

Erythema nodosum is the most common dermatologic manifestation of IBD, and UC specifically is known to trigger this condition, especially with flare-ups.[22] Further, it can be caused by bacterial or fungal infection, and *Campylobacter sp.* has been specifically implicated.[22] Erythema nodosum has also been associated with celiac disease.[23] In this case, it may be that the combination of immunosuppressive steroids, IBD, GI *Campylobacter,* and gluten sensitivity led to the expression of this condition.

Hookworm, *Necator americanus*, was detected (Figure 2). UC has been exacerbated or even caused by helminth infections, specifically *Strongyloides* species.[24-25] However, "worm therapy" using the helminth *Trichuris suis* has been reported to significantly improve IBD symptoms.[26] It is unclear whether EM's infection with the helminth *Necator americanus* was a significant factor in her UC.

Based on research findings, *Campylobacter sp.* and *EHEC* were most likely involved in the pathogenesis of EM's pancolitis. Given the dearth of evidence connecting *Enterobacter sp.* and *Necator americanus* to pancolitis, it is not clear the contribution these played in EM's condition, although they may have added to her overall inflammatory burden.

It is noteworthy that the bacterial culture and sensitivity (Figure 3) showed resistance to cefuroxime, a second generation cephalosporin antibiotic. At the time of her first visit, EM had been on two months of cephalexin which is a first-generation cephalosporin antibiotic. Resistance to this class of antibiotics could explain why she had high predominant bacteria, opportunistic bacteria, and pathogenic bacteria even after two months of cephalexin. Because of her history of antibiotic use, this patient was a candidate for antimicrobial botanicals, to which microbes may have more difficulty developing resistance.[27]

**In this case, it may be that the combination of immunosuppressive steroids, IBD, GI *Campylobacter*, and gluten sensitivity led to the expression of erythema nodosum.**

As EM's remarkable clinical response and normalized follow-up laboratory results in Figure 4 demonstrated, she responded favorably to treatment with albendazole, antimicrobial herbal formulas, digestive enzymes, DGL, aloe vera, vegetable greens powder, and a variety of probiotics. This relatively low-risk protocol addressed the suspected causal factors of IBD, rather than inhibiting symptoms and pathogenic mechanisms as her high-risk medication was designed to do. Consistent with published research, the aggressive protocol of probiotics appears to have been quite therapeutic in EM's case.[16-17, 28] Certain species of *Lactobacillus* and *Bifidobacteria* have been shown to attenuate colitis in animal models.[28] Treatments with *Lactobacillus sp.*, *Bifidobacteria sp.*, and *Saccharomyces boulardii* have been shown to bring about remission in UC.[16]

The presence of taxonomically unidentified parasitic DNA (Figure 4) was considered to be clinically irrelevant, as evidenced by her significant improvement. It is suggested that if the major pathogenic parasites in humans have been tested for using PCR technology and ruled out, the finding of parasitic DNA is likely from a transient, food-based exposure and not indicative of parasitic infection. The *Saccharomyces* species detected on follow-up was most likely from supplementation of *Saccharmyces boulardii*. The predominant *Bacteroides sp.* count, while low after treatment, may have actually been a desirable finding. It has been shown that *Bacteroides vulgatus* causes inflammation and that increased *Bacteroides fragilis* may be involved with CD.[16] The fact that her *Bacteroides sp.* count was high when she was symptomatic and lower after treatment that resulted in clinical improvement suggests that the *Bacteroides* in her stool included *B. vulgatus* or *B. fragilis*.

A comprehensive protocol designed to remove GI microbial imbalances and antigenic foods, replace digestive enzymes and nutrients, repair the intestinal lining, and reinoculate with beneficial microflora resulted in almost a full recovery from the initial presentation. The patient experienced a significant improvement or resolution of all of her major symptoms, including diarrhea, erythema nodosum, fatigue and weight loss, and was able to stop regular use of all medications. She observed that it was likely that hidden exposure to antigenic foods resulted in the periodic flare-ups that kept her from a full, 100% recovery.

It is interesting to note that the removal of antigenic foods from EM's diet appears to have clearly contributed to her improvement, as evidenced by the fact that accidental ingestion of those substances triggered symptomatic flare-ups. However, it was only after normalization of bowel microbial status that the effect of antigenic foods was experienced, suggesting that the GI microbial imbalances in EM were the significant underlying etiological factors.

# CONCLUSION

Pancolitis that is non-responsive to medications frequently requires surgical intervention (colectomy), resulting in significant quality-of-life issues.[3] Because this patient's condition could not be medically managed using the high-risk, immunosuppressive combination of prednisone, mesalamine and azathioprine, colectomy would most probably have been her next step.

Laboratory testing identified IgG food reactions and severe gastrointestinal microbial imbalances, including disruption of the predominant flora, the presence of opportunistic and pathogenic bacteria and a parasite. The low-risk and non-invasive protocol employed was designed to address underlying causes of the patient's IBD, dramatically reduced GI inflammation and may have prevented the need for surgical intervention.

**The fact that this UC case showed such dramatic improvements once the microbiota were normalized, strongly suggests that this approach may have benefit for any IBD case.**

The fact that this UC case showed such dramatic improvements once the microbiota were normalized strongly suggests that this approach might have great benefit for any inflammatory bowel case, particularly in light of the numerous reports in the literature that significant microbial imbalances are associated with the etiopathogenesis of inflammatory bowel diseases. Given the epidemiological statistics of IBD, research investigating the efficacy of this cost-saving, safe, multifactorial and integrative approach is highly recommended.

---

**Authors: Kara Fitzgerald, ND; Cass Nelson-Dooley, MS**

**Case Clinician: Kathleen Janel, ND**

## References

1. Hanauer SB. Inflammatory bowel disease: epidemiology, pathogenesis, and therapeutic opportunities. *Inflammatory bowel diseases.* Jan 2006;12 Suppl 1:S3-9.
2. O'Connor PM, Lapointe TK, Beck PL, Buret AG. Mechanisms by which inflammation may increase intestinal cancer risk in inflammatory bowel disease. *Inflamm Bowel Dis.* Feb 12 2010.
3. Cuffari C, Present DH, Bayless TM, Lichtenstein GR. Optimizing therapy in patients with pancolitis. *Inflammatory bowel diseases.* Oct 2005;11(10):937-946.
4. Yang A, Chen Y, Scherl E, Neugut AI, Bhagat G, Green PH. Inflammatory bowel disease in patients with celiac disease. *Inflamm Bowel Dis.* Jun 2005;11(6):528-532.
5. MacDermott RP. Treatment of irritable bowel syndrome in outpatients with inflammatory bowel disease using a food and beverage intolerance, food and beverage avoidance diet. *Inflamm Bowel Dis.* Jan 2007;13(1):91-96.
6. Marteau P. Bacterial flora in inflammatory bowel disease. *Dig Dis.* 2009;27 Suppl 1:99-103.
7. Guo FC, Williams BA, Kwakkel RP, et al. Effects of mushroom and herb polysaccharides, as alternatives for an antibiotic, on the cecal microbial ecosystem in broiler chickens. *Poult Sci.* Feb 2004;83(2):175-182.
8. Abascal K YE. Herbs and Drug Resistance: Part 1—Herbs and Microbial Resistance to Antibiotics. *Alternative and Complementary Therapies.* August 2002 2002 8(4):237-241.
9. Davis RH, Donato JJ, Hartman GM, Haas RC. Anti-inflammatory and wound healing activity of a growth substance in Aloe vera. *J Am Podiatr Med Assoc.* Feb 1994;84(2):77-81.

10. Stewart PM, Prescott SM. Can licorice lick colon cancer? *J Clin Invest.* Apr 2009;119(4):760-763.

11. Mengheri E. Health, probiotics, and inflammation. *J Clin Gastroenterol.* Sep 2008;42 Suppl 3 Pt 2:S177-178.

12. Goodhand JR, Wahed M, Rampton DS. Management of stress in inflammatory bowel disease: a therapeutic option? *Expert review of gastroenterology & hepatology.* Dec 2009;3(6):661-679.

13. Kalischuk LD, Buret AG. A role for Campylobacter jejuni-induced enteritis in inflammatory bowel disease? *American journal of physiology.* Oct 29 2009.

14. Singh J. Colitis. *emedicine from WebMD* 2009; http://emedicine.medscape.com/article/927845-overview. Accessed 12/31/09, 2009.

15. Lord RS BJ. Laboratory Evaluations for Integrative and Functional Medicine. Atlanta: Metametrix Institute; 2008:435-437.

16. Ott SJ, Musfeldt M, Wenderoth DF, et al. Reduction in diversity of the colonic mucosa associated bacterial microflora in patients with active inflammatory bowel disease. *Gut.* May 2004;53(5):685-693.

17. Tamboli CP, Neut C, Desreumaux P, Colombel JF. Dysbiosis in inflammatory bowel disease. *Gut.* Jan 2004;53(1):1-4.

18. Fraser SL, Arnett M. Enterobacter infections. *emedicine from WebMD* 2009; http://emedicine.medscape.com/article/216845-overview. Accessed 1/05/2010, 2010.

19. Siegal D, Syed F, Hamid N, Cunha BA. Campylobacter jejuni pancolitis mimicking idiopathic ulcerative colitis. *Heart Lung.* Jul-Aug 2005;34(4):288-290.

20. Sumrall A, McMullan L, Abrasley C, East H. A case of severe hemorrhagic diarrhea. *Journal of the Mississippi State Medical Association.* Dec 2007;48(12):366-369.

21. Gradel KO, Nielsen HL, Schonheyder HC, Ejlertsen T, Kristensen B, Nielsen H. Increased short- and long-term risk of inflammatory bowel disease after salmonella or campylobacter gastroenteritis. *Gastroenterology.* Aug 2009;137(2):495-501.

22. Hebel JL, Habif T. Erythema Nodosum. *emedicine from WebMD* 2009; http://emedicine.medscape.com/article/1081633-overview. Accessed 12/31/09, 2009.

23. Bartyik K, Varkonyi A, Kirschner A, Endreffy E, Turi S, Karg E. Erythema nodosum in association with celiac disease. *Pediatric dermatology.* May-Jun 2004;21(3):227-230.

24. Ghoshal UC, Alexender G, Ghoshal U, Tripathi S, Krishnani N. Strongyloides stercoralis infestation in a patient with severe ulcerative colitis. *Indian journal of medical sciences.* Mar 2006;60(3):106-110.

25. Weight SC, Barrie WW. Colonic Strongyloides stercoralis infection masquerading as ulcerative colitis. *Journal of the Royal College of Surgeons of Edinburgh.* Jun 1997;42(3):202-203.

26. Summers RW, Elliott DE, Urban JF, Jr., Thompson RA, Weinstock JV. Trichuris suis therapy for active ulcerative colitis: a randomized controlled trial. *Gastroenterology.* Apr 2005;128(4):825-832.

27. Sibanda T, Okoh A. The challenges of overcoming antibiotic resistance: plant extracts as potential sources of antimicrobial and resistance modifying agents. *African J of Biotechnology.* December 2007;6(25):2886-2896.

28. Sheil B, Shanahan F, O'Mahony L. Probiotic effects on inflammatory bowel disease. *J Nutr.* Mar 2007;137(3 Suppl 2):819S-824S.

# Parasitic Gastroenteritis

*In the United States, the Centers for Disease Control recognizes about 13 million newly diagnosed parasitic infections per year, with the most common being Trichomoniasis.*[1] *However, chronic, idiopathic gastrointestinal complaints are a common and expensive public health concern.*[2] *A portion of these cases may involve undiagnosed parasitic infections, which would increase current CDC estimates. For example, D. fragilis, identified in the case below, is considered to be fairly rare in the United States; however, the incidence may be higher than reported because, until recently, identification techniques have been fairly insensitive.*[3, 4] *Parasitic gastroenteritis can become a chronic problem, presenting with symptoms such as diarrhea, abdominal pain, anorexia, nausea, vomiting, fatigue, and weight loss. GI inflammation and alternating diarrhea and constipation are not unusual.*[5] *The case below describes a patient with chronic, idiopathic gastrointestinal pain that was later identified as being caused by D. fragilis and food sensitivities. It is hypothesized that the latter complaint may be resultant from intestinal damage incurred by the chronic parasitic infection. Appropriate testing allowed for accurate diagnosis and successful treatment.*

## 38-Year-Old Male with Idiopathic Gastrointestinal Pain

| | |
|---|---|
| **Additional Symptoms and Conditions** | Diarrhea alternating with constipation, weight loss, severe bloating, reflux, flatulence |
| **Tests Used** | Microbial stool analysis using DNA identification, food-specific IgG4 antibodies, urinary organic acids |
| **Imbalances Identified** | *Dientamoeba fragilis,* intestinal hyperpermeability, multiple IgG4 food sensitivities, oxidative stress |
| **Treatments** | Metronidazole, anti-inflammatory GI medicinal food, probiotics, deglycyrrhized licorice, cabbage juice, elimination diet |
| **Outcome** | Three month follow-up visit: significant improvement in, or resolution of, all symptoms |
| **Discussion/ Significance** | In this case, the appropriate battery of testing allowed the correct diagnosis to be made. The insensitivity of current technology may limit the positive identification of parasites, resulting in an underreporting of their true prevalence. Mucosal damage from chronic parasitosis may result in intestinal hyperpermeability, food sensitivities, and the systemic oxidative stress seen in this case. Microbial stool analysis using DNA identification and testing of IgG4 food-specific antibodies in cases of idiopathic gastrointestinal complaints may aid in identification of causal factors. |

## CASE HISTORY

JC was 38 years old when he presented with a complaint of severe, dull, upper right and left quadrant pain. On the visual analogue scale (VAS) rating pain severity, his was at the highest levels (9 to 10 on a scale of 0 to 10) for one year. He used antispasmodic medications, but only infrequently, as they brought only marginal relief. Occasionally, the recurrent abdominal pains radiated to the lower abdomen and back. Since the onset of the pain, JC experienced abdominal bloating, reflux, and flatulence after eating. As a result, he greatly curtailed the amount of food he ate and had lost 20 pounds over one year. He had frequent bouts of diarrhea alternating with occasional constipation. There was no apparent causative factor. JC had not traveled, nor were his wife or two children symptomatic. JC worked at an assisted living facility as a physical therapist, where there was no apparent outbreak of enteritis. JC noted that when he took antibiotics for a sinus infection, he experienced some improvement in his GI symptoms. Concurrently, JC became oliguric, with increased urgency to void, a weak stream, and incomplete emptying. He denied experiencing dehydration, fever, pubic pain, hematuria, or dysuria. Urology and multiple gastroenterology assessments, including physical examination, urinalysis, complete blood count and blood chemistry, colonoscopy, and endoscopy, gave normal results. JC drank unsweetened cranberry juice daily for the urinary tract complaints.

JC's medical history was unremarkable except for a history of chronic sinusitis, for which he took regular antibiotics. JC had been a vegetarian for more than five years. Upon physical examination, JC presented as thin, but was normal weight-for-height. On resisted range of motion, he demonstrated sufficient muscle tone. His skin was pale. He had hyperactive bowel sounds in all four abdominal quadrants with mild distention and mild, diffuse tenderness in the upper quadrants. There was no hepatosplenomegaly noted. Rebound tenderness and McBurney's point were both negative; costovertebral angle tenderness was negative. His lungs were clear to auscultation bilaterally, and his heart sounds were of a regular rate and rhythm. A urinalysis completed during the first office visit showed results that were unremarkable.

> Parasitic gastroenteritis can become a chronic problem, presenting with symptoms such as diarrhea, abdominal pain, anorexia, nausea, vomiting, fatigue, and weight loss. GI inflammation and alternating diarrhea and constipation are not unusual.

# Initial Laboratory Results

**Laboratory tests ordered and rationale**

1. **Microbial stool analysis using DNA identification** : The sensitivity of DNA testing may allow for identification of GI pathogenic agents not readily seen using older technologies. Chemistries in this test include biomarkers of inflammation, digestion and absorption.
2. **Food-specific IgG4 antibodies**: Food sensitivities may be associated with the gastrointestinal complaints seen in this case.
3. **Organic acids**: A functional assessment of systemic nutrient status, mitochondrial function, oxidative and inflammatory stress. Chronic GI imbalance may compromise digestion and absorption, potentially contributing to nutrient deficiencies, systemic inflammation and oxidative stress.

| Parasites | | | |
|---|---|---|---|
| Dientamoeba fragilis | | Positive | Neg |
| Endolimax nana | | Positive | Neg |
| WBCs | Few | | Neg-Rare |
| Mucus | Pos | | Neg |

**Figure 1. Baseline DNA parasitology.** Stool analysis demonstrated the presence of two protozoa parasites. *D. fragilis* is pathogenic in most individuals regardless of immune status, whereas *E. nana* is generally asymptomatic. Evidence of inflammation was also present with the positive findings of white blood cells and mucus.

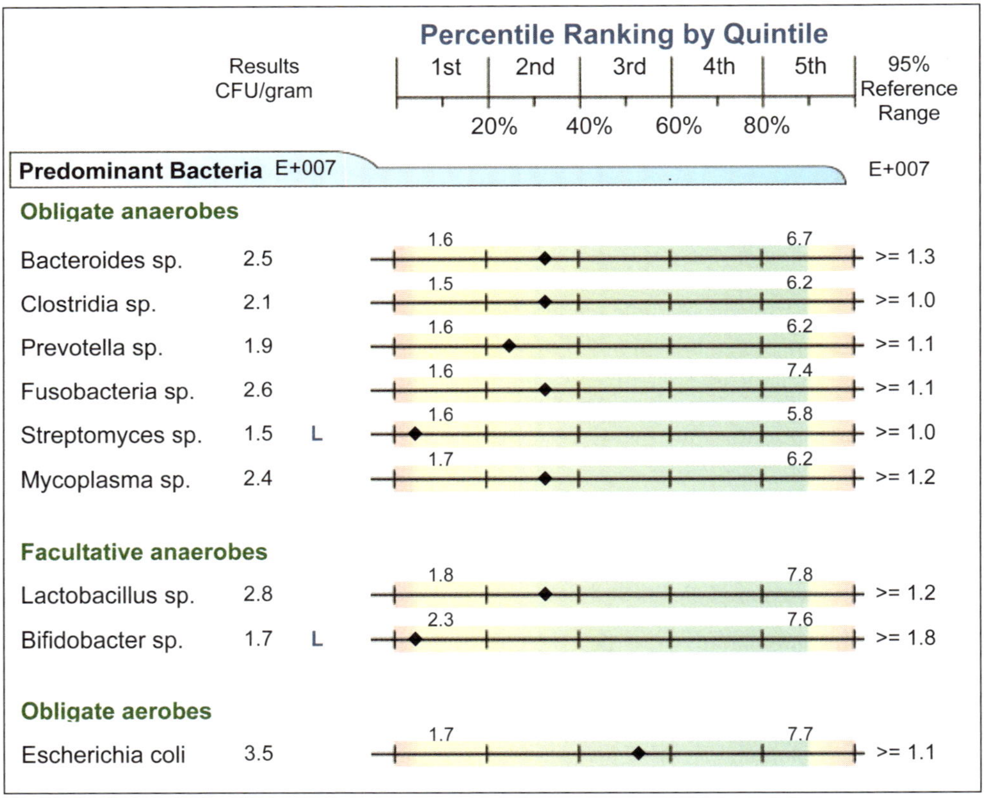


**Figure 2. Baseline microbial DNA stool analysis.** Predominant bacteria in the lower GI tract demonstrated low to low-normal values.

**0075 IgG4 Food Antibodies (90 Antigens)** — *Methodology: ELISA*

| | Results ng/mL | Response | Class |
|---|---|---|---|
| **Dairy/Meat/Poultry** | | | |
| Beef | <10 | | |
| Casein | >2000 | Severe | +5 |
| Chicken | 624 | Mod | +4 |
| Egg, White | >2000 | Severe | +5 |
| Egg, Yolk | >2000 | Severe | +5 |
| Lamb | <10 | | |
| Milk | >2000 | Severe | +5 |
| Pork | <10 | | |
| Turkey | 586 | Mod | +4 |
| **Fish/Shellfish** | | | |
| Clam | 9 | | |
| Codfish | <10 | | |
| Crab | <10 | | |
| Flounder | 13 | | |
| Halibut | <10 | | |
| Lobster | <10 | | |
| Mackerel | <10 | | |
| Oyster | <10 | | |
| Salmon | <10 | | |
| Shrimp | <10 | | |
| Trout | <10 | | |
| Tuna | <10 | | |
| **Fruits** | | | |
| Apple | <10 | | |
| Apricot | <10 | | |
| Banana | <10 | | |
| Blueberry | 52 | Mild | +1 |

| | Results ng/mL | Response | Class |
|---|---|---|---|
| Cantaloupe | 13 | | |
| Cranberry | 8 | | |
| Grape | <10 | | |
| Grapefruit | 9 | | |
| Honeydew | <10 | | |
| Lemon | <10 | | |
| Orange | <10 | | |
| Peach | 10 | | |
| Pear | <10 | | |
| Pineapple | <10 | | |
| Strawberry | <10 | | |
| Watermelon | <10 | | |
| **Grains** | | | |
| Barley | 262 | Mod | +3 |
| Corn | <10 | | |
| Oat | <10 | | |
| Rice | 14 | | |
| Rye | 1510 | Severe | +5 |
| Wheat | 562 | Mod | +4 |
| **Legumes** | | | |
| Bean, String | <10 | | |
| Lentil | 938 | Severe | +5 |
| Lima Bean | 627 | Mod | +4 |
| Navy Bean | 900 | Mod | +4 |
| Pea, Green | <10 | | |
| Peanut | 221 | Mod | +3 |
| Pinto Bean | 847 | Mod | +4 |
| Soybean | 1892 | Severe | +5 |

**Class Definitions:**

| Class | Cutoffs |
|---|---|
| Negative | 0-40 |
| Mild (+1/+2) | 80/150 |
| Moderate (+3/+4) | 500/900 |
| Severe (+5) | > 900 |

**0075 IgG4 Food Antibodies (90 Antigens)** — *Methodology: ELISA*

| | Results ng/mL | Response | Class |
|---|---|---|---|
| **Miscellaneous** | | | |
| Aspergillus | <10 | | |
| Black Pepper | <10 | | |
| Chocolate | <10 | | |
| Cinnamon | <10 | | |
| Coffee | <10 | | |
| Ginger | 902 | Severe | +5 |
| Malt | 305 | Mod | +3 |
| Tea | <10 | | |
| Vanilla | <10 | | |
| Yeast, Baker's | <10 | | |
| Yeast, Brewer's | <10 | | |
| **Nuts/Seeds** | | | |
| Almond | 1046 | Severe | +5 |
| Cashew | 74 | Mild | +1 |
| Coconut | <10 | | |
| Pecan | 9 | | |
| Pistachio | <10 | | |
| Sesame | 64 | Mild | +1 |
| Sunflower | 100 | Mild | +2 |
| Walnut | <10 | | |
| **Vegetables** | | | |
| Asparagus | 22 | | |
| Avocado | 104 | Mild | +2 |
| Broccoli | 59 | Mild | +1 |
| Cabbage | 14 | | |
| Carrot | <10 | | |
| Cauliflower | 74 | Mild | +1 |
| Celery | 15 | | |
| Cucumber | 74 | Mild | +1 |
| Garlic | 58 | Mild | +1 |
| Lettuce | 26 | | |
| Mushroom | <10 | | |
| Mustard | 106 | Mild | +2 |
| Olive | <10 | | |
| Onion | <10 | | |
| Pepper, Green | <10 | | |
| Potato | 8 | | |
| Spinach | 13 | | |
| Sweet Potato | 12 | | |
| Tomato | <10 | | |
| Zucchini | 347 | Mod | +3 |

**Figure 3. Food-specific IgG4 antibody test.** Multiple severe food sensitivities were detected, suggesting intestinal hyperpermeability. It was thought that the GI damage from the parasite may have contributed to the intestinal hyperpermeability. The negative and mild findings helped guide the design of a rotation diet.

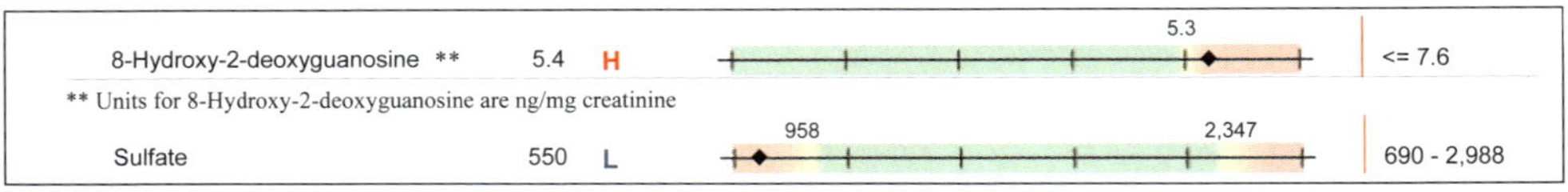


**Figure 4. 8OHdG and sulfate.** Urinary organic acid test revealed increased oxidative stress and a very low sulfate level. (Units: 8OHdG ng/mg creatinine; sulfate µg/mg creatinine)

# Initial Assessment

- Parasitic gastroenteritis
- Intestinal hyperpermeability
- Multiple food sensitivity reactions
- Oxidative stress

# Initial Plan

- Metronidazole 500 mg, 1 tab PO TID for 10 days
- Gastrointestinal medicinal food, 2 scoops with juice daily (includes glutamine, anti-inflammatory botanicals, B vitamins, essential minerals)
- Probiotic powder, ½ tsp PO BID (providing 200 billion mixed genus CFU per day)
- Deglycyrrhizinated licorice (DGL), chew 2 tablets with meals
- Cabbage juice, consume 1–2 liters/day
- Eliminate all +3, +4, and +5 foods. Rotate +1 and +2 foods every four days. Strongly recommend reintroduction of animal and fish proteins
- Follow-up microbial stool analysis using DNA identification and IgG4 test in three months

**Treatment plan rationale:** The first priority was treating the parasitic infection, followed by restoration of the intestinal mucosa with a protein-based medicinal food. Probiotics were employed to restore the intestinal microbiota.[6] Deglycyrrhized licorice, which was used to support mucosal regeneration, has been shown to minimize pathogenic infections.[7] Cabbage juice has a long history of traditional use in treating gastrointestinal disorders including, most famously, peptic ulcers.[8] Rich in sulfur and methyl compounds, both are required for restoring mucosal function.

The elimination diet—removing the foods to which JC had a significant IgG4 reaction—was also a priority intervention. These foods were stimulating pronounced inflammation that probably contributed to his GI complaints, including reflux, bloating, and recurrent abdominal pains. Following food-specific IgG4 antibody-guided exclusion diets has been effective in improving symptoms in irritable bowel syndrome patients.[9-11] JC was also urged to introduce some low reactivity animal and fish protein, because protein is a required macronutrient for mucosal restoration.[12]

## Three-Month Follow-up

JC responded very favorably to treatment. His GI symptoms were largely resolved, with the exception of some residual gas, bloating and occasional pain. He rated his pain level at 3 out of 10, 10 as the most severe pain possible. Previously, it had been 9 to 10 out of 10. The urinary tract complaints had diminished as well. He had no sinus infections in the three months between office visits. He continued to take cranberry juice, stating that it was still helpful for his urinary tract. JC stated that the diet was very difficult to follow, given the number of food reactions he had. He was looking forward to reintroducing some foods.

### Three-Month Follow-up Laboratory Testing

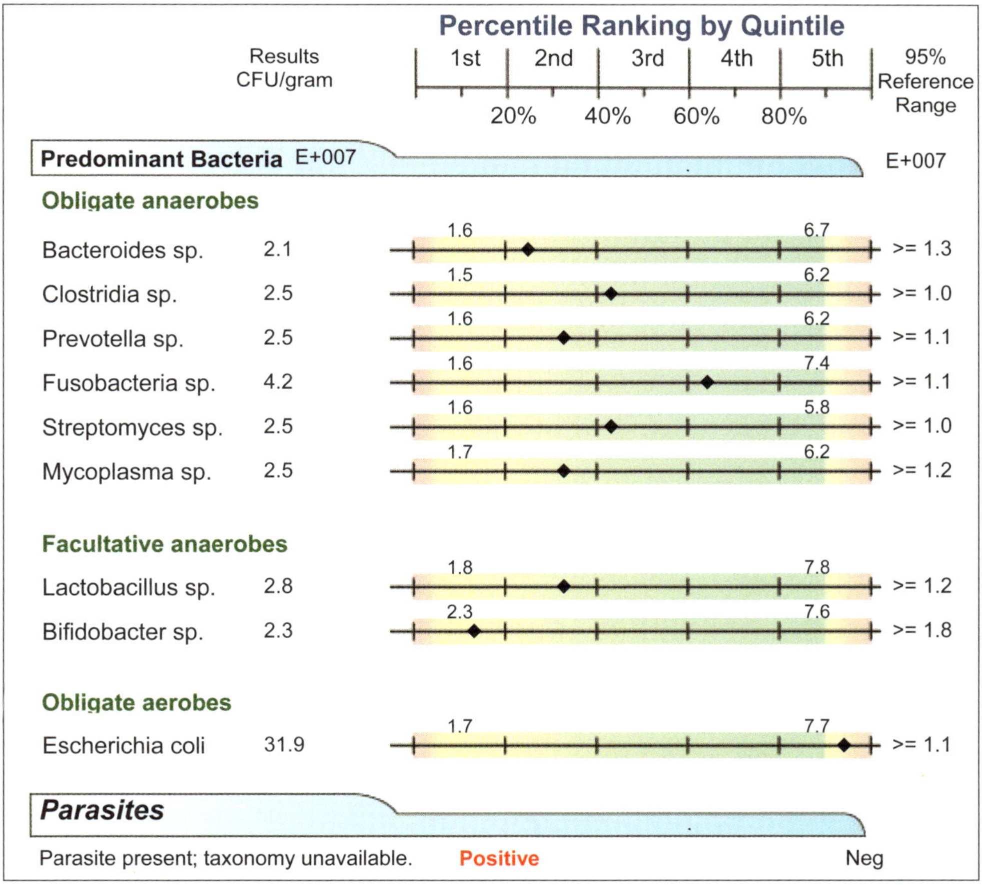


**Figure 5. Follow-up microbial DNA stool analysis.** Some improvement was noted in the predominant flora, although the level of *Bifidobacter* was still considered suboptimal and that of *E. coli* was high relative to the others. *D. fragilis* and *E. nana* had been effectively eradicated. It was thought that the taxonomically unidentified parasite was probably not a significant presence.

**0075 IgG4 Food Antibodies (90 Antigens)** *Methodology: ELISA*

| | Results ng/mL | Response | Class |
|---|---|---|---|
| **Dairy/Meat/Poultry** | | | |
| Beef | <10 | | |
| Casein | 821 | Mod | +4 |
| Chicken | 52 | Mild | +1 |
| Egg, White | 755 | Mod | +4 |
| Egg, Yolk | 1165 | Severe | +5 |
| Lamb | <10 | | |
| Milk | 555 | Mod | +4 |
| Pork | <10 | | |
| Turkey | <10 | | |
| **Fish/Shellfish** | | | |
| Clam | <10 | | |
| Codfish | <10 | | |
| Crab | <10 | | |
| Flounder | <10 | | |
| Halibut | <10 | | |
| Lobster | <10 | | |
| Mackerel | <10 | | |
| Oyster | <10 | | |
| Salmon | <10 | | |
| Shrimp | <10 | | |
| Trout | <10 | | |
| Tuna | <10 | | |
| **Fruits** | | | |
| Apple | <10 | | |
| Apricot | <10 | | |
| Banana | <10 | | |
| Blueberry | <10 | | |

| | Results ng/mL | Response | Class |
|---|---|---|---|
| Cantaloupe | <10 | | |
| Cranberry | <10 | | |
| Grape | <10 | | |
| Grapefruit | <10 | | |
| Honeydew | <10 | | |
| Lemon | <10 | | |
| Orange | <10 | | |
| Peach | <10 | | |
| Pear | <10 | | |
| Pineapple | <10 | | |
| Strawberry | <10 | | |
| Watermelon | <10 | | |
| **Grains** | | | |
| Barley | 46 | Mild | +1 |
| Corn | <10 | | |
| Oat | <10 | | |
| Rice | <10 | | |
| Rye | 78 | Mild | +1 |
| Wheat | 155 | Mod | +3 |
| **Legumes** | | | |
| Bean, String | 11 | | |
| Lentil | 103 | Mild | +2 |
| Lima Bean | <10 | | |
| Navy Bean | 52 | Mild | +1 |
| Pea, Green | <10 | | |
| Peanut | 56 | Mild | +1 |
| Pinto Bean | 41 | Mild | +1 |
| Soybean | 66 | Mild | +1 |

**Class Definitions:**

| Class | Cutoffs |
|---|---|
| Negative | 0-40 |
| Mild (+1/+2) | 80/150 |
| Moderate (+3/+4) | 500/900 |
| Severe (+5) | > 900 |

**0075 IgG4 Food Antibodies (90 Antigens)** *Methodology: ELISA*

| | Results ng/mL | Response | Class |
|---|---|---|---|
| **Miscellaneous** | | | |
| Aspergillus | 8 | | |
| Black Pepper | <10 | | |
| Chocolate | 16 | | |
| Cinnamon | <10 | | |
| Coffee | 12 | | |
| Ginger | 52 | Mild | +1 |
| Malt | 11 | | |
| Tea | <10 | | |
| Vanilla | <10 | | |
| Yeast, Baker's | <10 | | |
| Yeast, Brewer's | <10 | | |
| **Nuts/Seeds** | | | |
| Almond | 419 | Mod | +3 |
| Cashew | <10 | | |
| Coconut | <10 | | |
| Pecan | <10 | | |
| Pistachio | <10 | | |
| Sesame | 143 | Mild | +2 |
| Sunflower | 170 | Mod | +3 |
| Walnut | <10 | | |

| | Results ng/mL | Response | Class |
|---|---|---|---|
| **Vegetables** | | | |
| Asparagus | 10 | | |
| Avocado | <10 | | |
| Broccoli | 17 | | |
| Cabbage | 14 | | |
| Carrot | <10 | | |
| Cauliflower | 42 | Mild | +1 |
| Celery | <10 | | |
| Garlic | <10 | | |
| Lettuce | <10 | | |
| Mushroom | <10 | | |
| Mustard | 9 | | |
| Olive | <10 | | |
| Onion | <10 | | |
| Pepper, Green | <10 | | |
| Potato | 25 | | |
| Spinach | 18 | | |
| Sweet Potato | <10 | | |
| Tomato | <10 | | |
| Zucchini | <10 | | |

**Figure 6. Food-specific IgG4 antibody follow-up test.** General reduction in the severity and number of reactions. The continued +4 and +5 reaction to dairy and eggs may have been due to occult exposure. Complete avoidance of those and the remaining +3 foods would be required.

## Three-Month Follow-up Plan

- Continue medicinal food, probiotics, DGL, and cabbage juice
- Add botanical antimicrobial formula that includes berberine, oregano, wormwood, barberry, black walnut, and olive leaf, 4 caps PO BID × 2 months
- Continue elimination of all +3 to +5 foods. Add animal and fish protein as tolerated
- Read food labels very closely to ensure avoidance of severely antigenic foods. Re-evaluate IgG4 and microbial stool analysis using DNA identification in 6 months

**Treatment plan rationale:** The antimicrobial botanicals and continued probiotic supplementation were prescribed to normalize the predominant flora dysbiosis. A hypoallergenic diet with rotation of the less reactive foods was prescribed. JC was educated on reading food and supplement labels closely to identify exposures to dairy, eggs and wheat. A high-dose, bioavailable multivitamin mineral supplement was planned for introduction at a later time, when GI restoration would allow for optimal absorption.

# DISCUSSION

The patient in this case presented with severe idiopathic gastrointestinal pain (VAS 9 to 10 out of 10) of one year's duration. He also complained of diarrhea alternating with constipation, weight loss, bloating, reflux and flatulence. Standard laboratory testing and diagnostic imaging yielded no significant findings. Antispasmodics were of little relief. Laboratory evaluations including a microbial stool analysis, food-specific antibody testing and urinary organic acids were undertaken.

Figure 1 identified the presence of *D. fragilis* and *E. nana*. *E. nana* is not generally associated with gastroenteritis, whereas *D. fragilis* is almost always problematic. However, since identifying *D. fragilis* has historically been challenging, it is likely under-diagnosed. The most commonly employed diagnostic method remains microscopy, which has low sensitivity and specificity even with multiple specimens.[3,4] DNA analysis improves sensitivity of a single specimen significantly.[13,14] Regarding exposure, it was believed that the assisted living facility at which he worked could have been the source, despite the absence of any recognized outbreak of gastroenteritis. *D fragilis* is found in increased incidence in communal settings.[15]

Figure 2 illustrated the predominant anaerobic flora found in JC's stool specimen. Since the vast majority of the microbiota in the lower GI is anaerobic, DNA analysis, rather than culture technique, was used for identification and quantification.[16-18] JC demonstrated low *Bifidobacterium* species, which may have multiple causes, including antibiotic use for chronic sinusitis and/or diarrhea from the parasitic infection.[19] Supplementation with probiotics has been shown to relieve gastrointestinal symptoms.[6] The parasitic infection may also have contributed to GI bacterial imbalance via immune reactions.[20]

Figure 3 demonstrated mild to severe IgG4 reactions to 28 foods. JC was reacting to most foods he commonly ate in his vegetarian diet, suggesting significant mucosal permeability.[21-24] Intestinal hyperpermeability has also been known to result from gastrointestinal damage due to parasitic infection.[25-27] It is possible that mucosal damage second to parasitosis contributed to the IgG reaction to the foods he ate. It is also possible that he had some of these reactions prior to the parasitic infection, as sinusitis has been associated with immunological food reactions.[28]

Figure 4 depicted the sulfate deficiency and oxidative stress detected upon evaluation of urinary organic acids. Low sulfate suggests a deficiency of total body sulfur compounds.[29,30] Such a finding may be indicative of poor or imbalanced diet and/or insufficient sulfur amino acid intake. Hypothetically, low sulfur status may contribute to insufficiency of endogenous sulfur-based antioxidant compounds such as glutathione, which could contribute to increased oxidative stress.

As discussed, treatment for JC included eliminating the parasitic infection, removing the antigenic foods and restoring GI mucosal and microbiota health with the appropriate nutrients and probiotics. He was advised to eat healthy sources of hypoallergenic meat and fish protein to further support gut restoration.

**At his three-month follow-up visit, JC noted significant improvement in, or resolution of, all symptoms, including diarrhea alternating with constipation, severe bloating, reflux and flatulence.**

Follow-up testing corroborated the significant clinical improvements experienced by the patient. As shown in Figure 5, JC's microbiota was more robust and *D. fragilis* was no longer present. However, he had a markedly elevated *E. coli* level, suggesting imbalance of a single genus. Researchers have found that some elimination diets can lead to increases in fecal *E. coli* counts and reduce other predominant bacteria, thus ongoing probiotic support was recommended.[31] The taxonomically unidentified parasite was likely a "passer-by" not associated with any pathology. If JC had not been improving clinically, use of a broad spectrum anti-protozoan agent might have been indicated.

Figure 6 demonstrated significant improvements in immunological food reactions, but the continued presence of numerous mild-to-moderate sensitivities indicated that mucosal restoration was still needed. Additionally, the moderate-to-severe elevation in antibodies to dairy, eggs, and wheat indicated that continued total avoidance of those foods was required. Indeed, occult exposure may have been responsible for his remaining complaints of mild gas, bloating and pain. Low-grade antigen exposure has been associated with chronic elevation of IgG4 antibodies, and may be evidence of a blocking effect against a more severe IgE response.[32,33]

The follow-up treatment plan was designed to continue mucosal restoration and support microbiota balance. Guidance was provided on identifying occult exposures to antigenic foods.

---

NOTES

# CONCLUSION

After one year of severe gastrointestinal pain, for which no clear cause could be identified, the patient was diagnosed with what was likely a chronic GI protozoal infection. He was also found to have severe IgG4 reactions to many foods he commonly consumed. It was suspected that the food reactions resulted from the intestinal hyperpermeability caused by a parasitic infection.

The treatment for this individual was very straightforward: eradicate the parasitic infection, remove antigenic foods and restore the mucosa. Response to the treatment was swift: at the three-month follow-up visit, it was reported that all symptoms were resolved or significantly alleviated. His pain was reduced from a VAS score of 9 to 3 on a scaled of 0 to 10.

In this case, the appropriate battery of testing allowed the correct diagnosis to be made. The insensitivity of microscopy may falsely reduce positive identification of parasites, causing an underreporting of their true prevalence.

Chronic, idiopathic gastrointestinal complaints are a common and expensive public health concern.[2] Microbial stool analysis using DNA identification along with food-specific IgG4 antibody testing may be effective tools for identifying causal factors for this challenging clinical presentation.

---

**Author: Kara Fitzgerald, ND**
**Case Clinician: Kara Fitzgerald, ND**

## References

1. National Center for Zoonotic V-b, and Enteric Diseases (ZVED), Center for Disease Control and Prevention, CDC. About Parasites and Parasitic Diseases. http://www.cdc.gov/ncidod/dpd/aboutparasites.htm
2. IFFGD. Reporter's Guide to Functional Gastrointestinal Disorders: International Foundation for Functional Gastrointestinal Disorders; 2009.
3. Prevention CfDCa. *National Center for for Zoonotic V-B, and Enteric Diseases V-B, and Enteric Diseases, Diseases DoP. Dientaomeba fragilis infection.*
4. Hiatt RA, Markell EK, Ng E. How many stool examinations are necessary to detect pathogenic intestinal protozoa? *Am J Trop Med Hyg.* Jul 1995;53(1):36-39.
5. Merck. Gastroenteritis. https://www.merck.com/mmpe/sec02/ch016/ch016a.html. Accessed 7/19/2010, 2010.
6. Kajander K, Myllyluoma E, Rajilic-Stojanovic M, et al. Clinical trial: multispecies probiotic supplementation alleviates the symptoms of irritable bowel syndrome and stabilizes intestinal microbiota. *Aliment Pharmacol Ther.* Jan 1 2008;27(1):48-57.
7. Wittschier N, Faller G, Hensel A. Aqueous extracts and polysaccharides from liquorice roots (Glycyrrhiza glabra L.) inhibit adhesion of Helicobacter pylori to human gastric mucosa. *J Ethnopharmacol.* Sep 7 2009;125(2):218-223.
8. Miron A, Hancianu M, Aprotosoaie AC, Gacea O, Stanescu U. [Contributions to chemical study of the raw polysaccharide isolated from the fresh pressed juice of white cabbage leaves]. *Rev Med Chir Soc Med Nat Iasi.* Oct-Dec 2006;110(4):1020-1026.
9. Zar S, Benson MJ, Kumar D. Food-specific serum IgG4 and IgE titers to common food antigens in irritable bowel syndrome. *Am J Gastroenterol.* Jul 2005;100(7):1550-1557.

10. Zar S, Mincher L, Benson MJ, Kumar D. Food-specific IgG4 antibody-guided exclusion diet improves symptoms and rectal compliance in irritable bowel syndrome. *Scand J Gastroenterol.* Jul 2005;40(7):800-807.

11. Anthoni S, Savilahti E, Rautelin H, Kolho KL. Milk protein IgG and IgA: the association with milk-induced gastrointestinal symptoms in adults. *World J Gastroenterol.* Oct 21 2009;15(39):4915-4918.

12. Shyntum Y, Iyer SS, Tian J, et al. Dietary sulfur amino acid supplementation reduces small bowel thiol/disulfide redox state and stimulates ileal mucosal growth after massive small bowel resection in rats. *J Nutr.* Dec 2009;139(12):2272-2278.

13. Verweij JJ, Mulder B, Poell B, van Middelkoop D, Brienen EA, van Lieshout L. Real-time PCR for the detection of Dientamoeba fragilis in fecal samples. *Mol Cell Probes.* Oct-Dec 2007;21(5-6):400-404.

14. Bruijnesteijn van Coppenraet LE, Wallinga JA, Ruijs GJ, Bruins MJ, Verweij JJ. Parasitological diagnosis combining an internally controlled real-time PCR assay for the detection of four protozoa in stool samples with a testing algorithm for microscopy. *Clin Microbiol Infect.* Sep 2009;15(9):869-874.

15. Mack D. Dientamoeba Fragilis Infection. *Medscape's continually updated clinical reference* [http://emedicine.medscape.com/article/997239-overview

16. Ventura M, Turroni F, Canchaya C, Vaughan EE, O'Toole PW, van Sinderen D. Microbial diversity in the human intestine and novel insights from metagenomics. *Front Biosci.* 2009;14:3214-3221.

17. Zoetendal EG, Cheng B, Koike S, Mackie RI. Molecular microbial ecology of the gastrointestinal tract: from phylogeny to function. *Curr Issues Intest Microbiol.* Sep 2004;5(2):31-47.

18. Zoetendal EG, Rajilic-Stojanovic M, de Vos WM. High-throughput diversity and functionality analysis of the gastrointestinal tract microbiota. *Gut.* Nov 2008;57(11):1605-1615.

19. Engelbrektson A, Korzenik JR, Pittler A, et al. Probiotics to minimize the disruption of faecal microbiota in healthy subjects undergoing antibiotic therapy. *J Med Microbiol.* May 2009;58(Pt 5):663-670.

20. Guarner F. Prebiotics, probiotics and helminths: the 'natural' solution? *Dig Dis.* 2009;27(3):412-417.

21. Sabra A, Bellanti JA, Rais JM, Castro HJ, de Inocencio JM, Sabra S. IgE and non-IgE food allergy. *Ann Allergy Asthma Immunol.* Jun 2003;90(6 Suppl 3):71-76.

22. Shah U, Walker WA. Pathophysiology of intestinal food allergy. *Adv Pediatr.* 2002;49:299-316.

23. Yu LC. The epithelial gatekeeper against food allergy. *Pediatr Neonatol.* Dec 2009;50(6):247-254.

24. Bischoff SC. Physiological and pathophysiological functions of intestinal mast cells. *Semin Immunopathol.* Jul 2009;31(2):185-205.

25. Baumgart DC, Dignass AU. Intestinal barrier function. *Curr Opin Clin Nutr Metab Care.* Nov 2002;5(6):685-694.

26. Turner JR. Intestinal mucosal barrier function in health and disease. *Nat Rev Immunol.* Nov 2009;9(11):799-809.

27. Visser J, Rozing J, Sapone A, Lammers K, Fasano A. Tight junctions, intestinal permeability, and autoimmunity: celiac disease and type 1 diabetes paradigms. *Ann N Y Acad Sci.* May 2009;1165:195-205.

28. Chester AC. Chronic sinusitis. *Am Fam Physician.* Feb 15 1996;53(3):877-887.

29. Curno R, Magee EA, Edmond LM, Cummings JH. Studies of a urinary biomarker of dietary inorganic sulphur in subjects on diets containing 1-38 mmol sulphur/day and of the half-life of ingested 34SO4(2-). *Eur J Clin Nutr.* Sep 2008;62(9):1106-1115.

30. Magee EA, Curno R, Edmond LM, Cummings JH. Contribution of dietary protein and inorganic sulfur to urinary sulfate: toward a biomarker of inorganic sulfur intake. *Am J Clin Nutr.* Jul 2004;80(1):137-142.

31. De Palma G, Nadal I, Collado MC, Sanz Y. Effects of a gluten-free diet on gut microbiota and immune function in healthy adult human subjects. *Br J Nutr.* Oct 2009;102(8):1154-1160.

32. Savilahti E, Kuitunen M, Vaarala O. Pre and probiotics in the prevention and treatment of food allergy. *Curr Opin Allergy Clin Immunol.* Jun 2008;8(3):243-248.

33. Noh G, Ahn HS, Cho NY, Lee S, Oh JW. The clinical significance of food specific IgE/IgG4 in food specific atopic dermatitis. *Pediatr Allergy Immunol.* Feb 2007;18(1):63-70.

# 7 Genetic Diseases

## Hemochromatosis

*Hereditary hemochromatosis is one of the most common genetic disorders in the United States. Although it most often affects Caucasians of Northern European descent, other ethnic groups are also affected. About 1 in 200 of the U.S. Caucasian population carries two copies of the hemochromatosis gene and is susceptible to developing the disease.[1] Hemochromatosis is a condition of high intestinal iron absorption resulting in accumulations of iron system-wide; primary affected areas include the liver, heart, and pancreas. If left untreated, it results in death from cirrhosis, liver cancer, or cardiomyopathy.[2] Hemochromatosis is characterized by a variety of seemingly unrelated symptoms and conditions, including severe fatigue (74%), arthralgia, cardiomyopathy, diabetes (65%), and hyperpigmentation or skin bronzing. (70%).[3] Increased toxic metal uptake has also been associated with the disease.[3-8] About 1 in 10 persons in the U.S. is heterozygous for the hemochromatosis mutation in the HFE gene that, while it might not result in a frank disease state, can cause increased iron absorption.[9] Given the high incidence of hemochromatosis in the U.S., routine screening for evidence of iron and toxic metal accumulation in vulnerable populations is prudent.*

### 58-Year-Old Female with Hemochromatosis

| | |
|---|---|
| **Symptoms and Conditions** | Fatigue, leg pain, and varicose veins; reduced mental clarity; nausea, heart flutters, cold intolerance, light-headedness, hypertension |
| **Tests Used** | Iron panel, hemochromatosis gene *C282Y*, urine toxic elements, blood chemistries |
| **Imbalances Identified** | Iron and toxic metal overload; homozygous for hemochromatosis gene *C282Y* |
| **Treatments** | Phlebotomy, intravenous EDTA (ethylenediaminetetraacetic acid) chelation therapy |
| **Outcome** | Improved energy, mood, and blood pressure; resolution of leg pain |
| **Discussion/ Significance** | This case illustrated the importance of using multiple specimen types for accurate and early detection of imbalances in total body iron status. Disruption in iron homeostatic mechanisms may explain parallel accumulations of iron and toxic metals. Management of the iron overload patient should therefore include an evaluation of toxic metals. Early identification of iron and toxic metal overload in this patient allowed for early treatment with positive clinical outcome, significantly reducing the likelihood of long-term complications. |

# CASE HISTORY

JR was 58 years old when she presented with complaints of leg pain, poor mental clarity, fatigue that became worse in the afternoon, and nausea. She experienced light-headedness when standing for too long. She was intolerant to cold and experienced occasional heart flutters. She had large, painful, chronic leg varicosities, which had been stripped and ligated twice, at ages 25 and 57.

Hemochromatosis is a condition of high intestinal iron absorption resulting in accumulations of iron system-wide; primary affected areas include the liver, heart, and pancreas. If left untreated, it results in death from cirrhosis, liver cancer, or cardiomyopathy.

She occasionally drank wine to excess. JR was a non-smoker and worked as a real estate agent. JR's father died at age 87, but was generally well throughout his life. Her mother died of skin cancer at age 83. JR had 10 siblings, one of whom died at age 52 of complications related to multiple sclerosis.

Upon examination, her blood pressure was 150/100; her pulse was 84 beats per minute and quality was regular. She had trophic changes in her lower legs with varicosities. Her fingers and toes had a bluish color. Pedal pulses were diminished bilaterally and feet were cool to the touch. Delayed capillary refill was demonstrated in bilateral hands and feet. All other findings on physical exam were unremarkable.

## Initial Laboratory Results

**Laboratory tests ordered and rationale:**

1. **Iron panel**: A standard laboratory assessment
2. **Hemochromatosis gene *C282Y***: Confirmatory test for hereditary hemochromatosis
3. **Urine toxic elements**: Increased toxic element uptake is not an uncommon finding in hemochromatosis patients, and therefore should be assessed. The patient's associated clinical symptoms also suggested heavy metal toxicity.
4. **Complete blood count and comprehensive metabolic panel**: Routine general health assessments. Hemoglobin used to monitor hemochromatosis treatment

| | | Pre-Treatment Results | Normal Range |
|---|---|---|---|
| Hemoglobin | | 14.3 | 12.0–15.0 g/dL |
| Serum Ferritin | H | 482 | 40–200 µg/L |
| Iron | | 28 | 10–30 µmol/L |
| TIBC | L | 41 | 45–75 µmol/L |
| Transferrin Saturation | H | 68% | 14–50 |

| Genetic Study | Results |
|---|---|
| Hemochromatosis gene *C282Y* | Homozygous positive |

**Figure 1. Hemoglobin, iron indices and hemochromatosis gene *C282Y*.** Findings before treatment.

# Errata Sheet

www.metametrix.com • 800.221.4640

For document titled **CASE STUDIES in Integrative and Functional Medicine** published April 2011. Revised 5/25/2011.

Errata posted 5/25/2011.

| Page | Erratum | |
|---|---|---|
| 159 | In the "Initial Plan" section, replace text up to "Treatment plan rationale" with the following three bullets: | **Initial Plan**<br>• Weekly phlebotomy treatments (After three weekly phlebotomy procedures, hemoglobin decreased from 14.3 g/dL to 11.3 g/dL, which was low. Phlebotomy procedures were then reduced to every other week.)<br>• Weekly intravenous EDTA chelation therapy × 20 weeks<br>• Laboratory tests: Iron panel, CBC, urinary toxic element test (UTE) after 20 EDTA treatments (and then reduce EDTA treatments as UTE results dictate) |

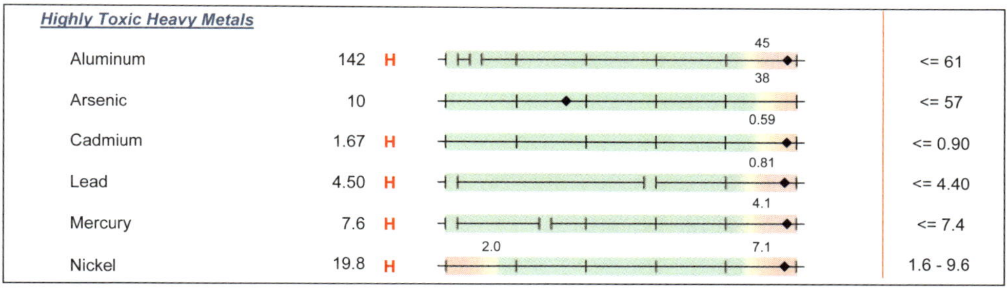


**Figure 2. Urinary toxic elements with provocation (EDTA).** Multiple elevations are shown. (Units: µg/g creatinine)

# Initial Assessment

- Hemochromatosis
- Elevated body burden of multiple toxic elements

# Initial Plan

**Elimination/Rotation Diet:** Eliminate all foods with $IgG_4$ levels of +4 and +5 for one month. Foods with +1 to +3 reactions should be consumed no more often than twice per week. Reintroduction phase: after one month of avoidance, rotate $IgG_4$ +4 and +5 foods into diet no more than twice per week.

- *Lactobacillus* and *Bifidobacterium* species 20 billion CFU, 1 capsule PO QD
- Glutamine 5000 mg, 1 tsp PO BID
- Custom amino acids (10 g per 1 tsp):
  - Start with 0.25 tsp PO QAM and increase dose by 0.25 tsp until reaching 1.5 tsp QAM
- Fish oil, 1 capsule PO BID
- Women's specific multivitamin and mineral supplement taken as directed

**Treatment plan rationale:** Phlebotomy is the treatment of choice for hemochromatosis. IV EDTA is an effective protocol for reducing toxic metals. EDTA may also support the reduction of iron, although it is not a main therapy.[10]

# One-Year Follow-up

After approximately one year of therapy, JR reported an increased sense of well-being and improved energy. She had good mental clarity and her leg pain resolved. She no longer complained of heart flutters, cold intolerance, nausea, and lightheadedness. Her blood pressure dropped from an initial high of 150/100 to 130/78.

JR did observe that she needed to be consistent with phlebotomy in order to maintain the positive changes. She stated that when she neglected phlebotomy and her iron stores rose, she would first experience leg pain, followed by nausea and lastly, a decline in mental clarity. Because of these symptoms, she was generally consistent with therapy. JR did not complete the follow-up urine toxic element test.

> **JR reported an increased sense of well-being and improved energy... good mental clarity and her leg pain resolved. She no longer complained of heart flutters, cold intolerance, nausea, and lightheadedness.**

After JR's experience, her family members were screened for hemochromatosis. Of her 10 siblings, one was homozygous and four were heterozygous for the hemochromatosis gene. JR's children were also heterozygous for the *C282Y* gene. JR's deceased sister's son was homozygous. Given the family genetic presentation, her mother and father must have been heterozygous carriers of the hemochromatosis gene mutation.

## Follow-up Laboratory Results

| | Pre-Treatment Results | | Normal Range |
|---|---|---|---|
| Hemoglobin | L | 11.3 | 12.0–15.0 g/dL |
| Serum Ferritin | L | 16 | 40–200 µg/L |
| Iron | | 24 | 10–30 µmol/L |
| TIBC | L | 43 | 45–75 µmol/L |
| Transferrin Saturation | H | 56% | 14–50 |

**Figure 3. Hemoglobin and iron indices.** Hemoglobin findings after three weeks of weekly phlebotomy treatment; iron indices after 47 weeks of biweekly phlebotomy treatments and IV EDTA chelation treatments (weekly and then monthly).

# Follow-up Plan

- Continue monthly EDTA chelation
- Phlebotomy every two months
- Repeat iron panel, CBC, and urine toxic elements

**Treatment rational:** EDTA and phlebotomy treatments were to be continued as needed, and laboratories monitored regularly.

# DISCUSSION

JR's baseline iron indices demonstrated that serum ferritin and transferrin saturation were high (Figure 1). Her standard chemistries, including liver function tests and hemoglobin, were within normal limits. Because of the elevated ferritin and transferrin saturation, JR was tested for the hemochromatosis gene *C282Y* and found to be homozygous positive (Figure 1). Because JR's cardiovascular symptoms might have been associated with toxic elements and iron burden, an IV EDTA urinary provocation test was ordered. The results demonstrated elevations in cadmium, lead, mercury, aluminum and nickel (Figure 2). After three weeks of phlebotomy treatments, hemoglobin was reduced from 14.3 g/dL to 11.3 g/dL (Figure 3). Because of the low hemoglobin findings, phlebotomy frequency was reduced to once every other week. After approximately one year of phlebotomy therapy and IV EDTA chelation, the patient reported significant clinical improvement. Follow-up indices of iron and hemoglobin, while abnormal, were much improved (Figure 3). Phlebotomy frequency was then reduced to a maintenance protocol of once every two months, while IV EDTA was continued monthly. JR's presenting complaints were resolved with consistent treatment. If she neglected therapy, and iron stores accumulated, she experienced a recurrence of leg pain, followed by nausea and poor mental clarity. Hereditary hemochromatosis is an autosomal recessive trait. The most prevalent form of hereditary hemochromatosis is caused by a mutation of the *HFE* gene, either *C282Y* or *H63D*. The incidence of hemochromatosis is approximately 1:200 to 250, and *HFE* variants are found in as many as 1:10 individuals in the United States.[11]

Signs and symptoms of hemochromatosis include fatigue, arthralgia, diabetes, heart disease and hyperpigmentation.[2] JR's signs and symptoms of hypertension, heart flutters, cold intolerance, light-headedness and varicosities could have resulted from either iron overload or toxic metal overload; it was therefore important that both potential causes be investigated. Free metal ions in the tissues will increase the rate of free radical generation, which may account for much of the tissue damage seen in hemochromatosis and toxic metal overload.[12]

Toxic metal accumulation with hemochromatosis is not uncommon, as gastrointestinal uptake may occur via shared transport proteins, such as divalent metal transporter 1 (DMT1), which is significantly increased in the disease. DMT1 is also found in the blood brain barrier and thus accumulation of iron and toxic metals may be seen in the central nervous system as well, contributing to neurodegenerative conditions.[5,7,13] Excessive consumption of alcohol is often associated with hemochromatosis for unknown reasons, and alcohol increases iron uptake.[14] JR's consumption of alcohol probably increased her absorption of iron.

**Toxic metal accumulation with hemochromatosis is not uncommon, as gastrointestinal uptake may occur via shared transport proteins, such as divalent metal transporter 1 (DMT1), which is significantly increased in the disease. DMT1 is also found in the blood brain barrier and thus accumulation of iron and toxic metals may be seen in the central nervous system as well, contributing to neurodegenerative conditions.**

# CONCLUSION

This case illustrates the importance of using multiple specimen types for accurate and early detection of imbalances in total-body iron status. At initial evaluation, serum ferritin and transferrin saturation were elevated; transferrin iron binding capacity (TIBC) was low. Transferrin saturation is considered to be the best marker for detecting hemochromatosis; its continued elevation even after phlebotomy is notable.[15] JR's post-treatment results show low hemoglobin and low serum ferritin, which would normally suggest iron deficiency, but iron therapy would be contraindicated in this case.

Genetic abnormalities in iron regulation allow for parallel accumulations of iron and toxic metals.[3-8] Management of the iron overload patient should include an evaluation of toxic metals.

Early identification of iron and toxic metal overload in this patient enabled early treatment and a very favorable clinical outcome, significantly reducing the likelihood of long-term complications.

---

**Authors: Cass Nelson-Dooley, MS; Kara Fitzgerald, ND**

**Case Clinician: John Cline, MD**

## References

1. NIH. Hemochromatosis. http://digestive.niddk.nih.gov/ddiseases/pubs/hemochromatosis/index.htm. Accessed 7/6/2010, 2010.
2. Fauci AS. *Harrison's principles of internal medicine / editors, Anthony S. Fauci ... [et al.]*. 17th ed. New York: McGraw-Hill Medical; 2008. pgs. 2429-2433.
3. Sfeir HE, Klachko DM. Hemochromatosis. *emedicine from WebMD*; 2006:12.
4. Heeney MM, Andrews NC. Iron homeostasis and inherited iron overload disorders: an overview. *Hematol Oncol Clin North Am.* Dec 2004;18(6):1379-1403, ix.
5. Conrad ME, Umbreit JN. Pathways of iron absorption. *Blood Cells Mol Dis.* Nov-Dec 2002;29(3):336-355.
6. Fleming RE, Migas MC, Zhou X, et al. Mechanism of increased iron absorption in murine model of hereditary hemochromatosis: increased duodenal expression of the iron transporter DMT1. *Proc Natl Acad Sci U S A.* Mar 16 1999;96(6):3143-3148.
7. Morgan EH, Oates PS. Mechanisms and regulation of intestinal iron absorption. *Blood Cells Mol Dis.* Nov-Dec 2002;29(3):384-399.
8. Rolfs A, Bonkovsky HL, Kohlroser JG, et al. Intestinal expression of genes involved in iron absorption in humans. *Am J Physiol Gastrointest Liver Physiol.* Apr 2002;282(4):G598-607.
9. Fuchs J, Podda M, Packer L, Kaufmann R. Morbidity risk in HFE associated hereditary hemochromatosis C282Y heterozygotes. *Toxicology.* Nov 15 2002;180(2):169-181.
10. NIH. Questions and Answers: The NIH Trial of EDTA Chelation Therapy for Coronary Artery Disease. http://nccam.nih.gov/health/chelation/. Accessed 7/6/2010, 2010.
11. Sheahan O, O'Connell E. Hereditary haemochromatosis: patient support and education. *Nurs Stand.* Sep 23-29 2009;24(3):49-56.
12. Weiss G. Genetic mechanisms and modifying factors in hereditary hemochromatosis. *Nat Rev Gastroenterol Hepatol.* Jan;7(1):50-58.
13. Fauci AS. *Harrison's principles of internal medicine / editors, Anthony S. Fauci ... [et al.]*. 17th ed. New York: McGraw-Hill Medical; 2008. p.2086.
14. Chapman RW, Morgan MY, Boss AM, Sherlock S. Acute and chronic effects of alcohol on iron absorption. *Dig Dis Sci.* Apr 1983;28(4):321-327.
15. Medscape. Clinical Aspects of Hemochromatosis. http://www.medscape.com/viewarticle/518662. Accessed 7/6/2010, 2010.

# Mitochondrial Disease

*Mitochondrial disease (MD) comprises a heterogeneous group of genetic conditions that affect the composition and function of the electron transport chain.[1] The underlying pathophysiology of MD involves compromised oxidative phosphorylation, resulting in reduced energy production (ATP).[1] Clinical presentation of MD is highly variable, but symptoms may be more often associated with energy demanding organ systems such as muscle (skeletal and cardiac), the gastrointestinal tract and the central nervous system. Annually, one newborn in 5,000 is diagnosed with mitochondrial disease.[1] The expression of milder forms may not be perceived until later in life, often precipitated by an energy-demanding event, such as an illness, certain medications or toxic exposures. Because of the variability in presentation and the delayed expression of disease, the true incidence of MD is higher than previously believed, and is a common cause of chronic morbidity, contributing to the pathogenesis of many diseases.[2, 3]*

## 2-Year-Old Male with Mitochondrial Disease

| | |
|---|---|
| **Symptoms and Conditions** | Failure to thrive, gastroesophageal reflux disease (GERD) |
| **Tests Used** | Urinary organic acids |
| **Imbalances Identified** | Elevated urinary lactic acid and other mitochondrial metabolites, elevated dysbiosis markers including D-arabinitol |
| **Treatments** | Carnitine, creatinine monophosphate, high-dose B-complex vitamins, CoQ10, alpha lipoic acid, vitamin E<br>Anti-*Candida* diet (very low in sugars and other simple carbohydrates) |
| **Outcome** | Growth and development were described as being significantly improved. While the GERD was also improved, allowing him to tolerate the nutrients, parents were not consistent in following the dietary recommendations, and he continued to have some gastrointestinal complaints. |
| **Discussion/ Significance** | Assays of urinary organic acids may be a useful way to measure mitochondrial and gastrointestinal function.[4] Using ranges set on a healthy population (in this case, a healthy pediatric population) that include quintile rankings in addition to the standard 95$^{th}$ reference interval allows for the identification of subtle perturbations in addition to more significant elevations. In this case, treatment based on the findings of subclinical mitochondropathy and GI fungal dysbiosis yielded good clinical outcome. These laboratory findings would have likely been missed in an organic acids test with reference ranges set to identify only severe forms of MD. The broad spectrum of mitochondrial genetic lesions suggests that organic acid analysis with more sensitive ranges may be beneficial in identifying subtle MD variations. |

# CASE HISTORY

DR was 2 years old when he presented with a diagnosis of mitochondrial disease (complex I and II deficiencies). As a result of the inborn error of metabolism, he had severe gastroesophageal reflux disease (GERD) with a failure to thrive. As part of a general evaluation, the clinician ordered a urinary organic acid test to assess mitochondrial function and gastrointestinal microbiota.

## Initial Laboratory Results

**Laboratory tests ordered and rationale:**

1. **Urine organic acids**: Assessment of mitochondrial and gastrointestinal function. Also useful for functional assessment of nutrient insufficiencies

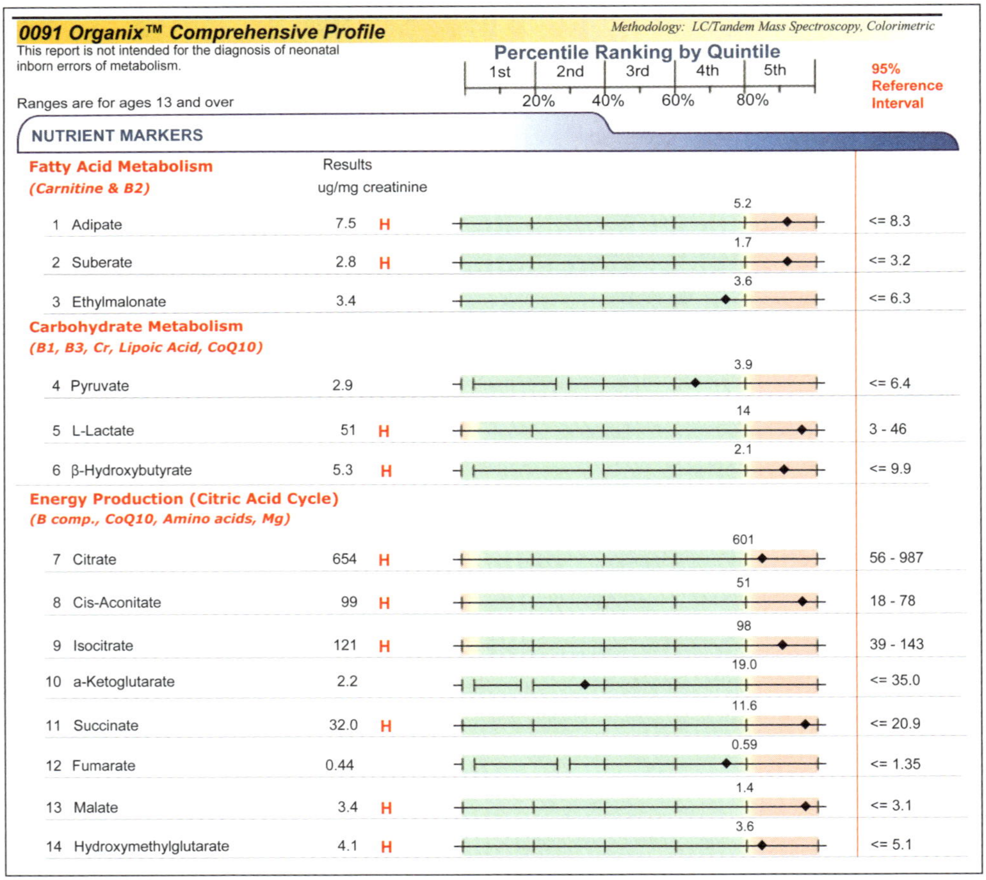
**0091 Organix™ Comprehensive Profile**

*Methodology: LC/Tandem Mass Spectroscopy, Colorimetric*

This report is not intended for the diagnosis of neonatal inborn errors of metabolism.

Ranges are for ages 13 and over

Percentile Ranking by Quintile: 1st | 2nd | 3rd | 4th | 5th (20% 40% 60% 80%)

NUTRIENT MARKERS

| | Results ug/mg creatinine | | Quintile marker value | 95% Reference Interval |
|---|---|---|---|---|
| **Fatty Acid Metabolism** *(Carnitine & B2)* | | | | |
| 1 Adipate | 7.5 | H | 5.2 | <= 8.3 |
| 2 Suberate | 2.8 | H | 1.7 | <= 3.2 |
| 3 Ethylmalonate | 3.4 | | 3.6 | <= 6.3 |
| **Carbohydrate Metabolism** *(B1, B3, Cr, Lipoic Acid, CoQ10)* | | | | |
| 4 Pyruvate | 2.9 | | 3.9 | <= 6.4 |
| 5 L-Lactate | 51 | H | 14 | 3 - 46 |
| 6 β-Hydroxybutyrate | 5.3 | H | 2.1 | <= 9.9 |
| **Energy Production (Citric Acid Cycle)** *(B comp., CoQ10, Amino acids, Mg)* | | | | |
| 7 Citrate | 654 | H | 601 | 56 - 987 |
| 8 Cis-Aconitate | 99 | H | 51 | 18 - 78 |
| 9 Isocitrate | 121 | H | 98 | 39 - 143 |
| 10 a-Ketoglutarate | 2.2 | | 19.0 | <= 35.0 |
| 11 Succinate | 32.0 | H | 11.6 | <= 20.9 |
| 12 Fumarate | 0.44 | | 0.59 | <= 1.35 |
| 13 Malate | 3.4 | H | 1.4 | <= 3.1 |
| 14 Hydroxymethylglutarate | 4.1 | H | 3.6 | <= 5.1 |

**Figure 1. Baseline urine organic acids.** Assessment of mitochondrial activity demonstrated elevations in fatty acid and carbohydrate metabolism and energy production intermediates. Taken together, these finding suggested mitochondrial dysfunction in multiple central energy pathways.

| No. | Organic acid | Result | Flag | Marker | Reference |
|---|---|---|---|---|---|
| **Bacterial - general** | | | | | |
| 36 | Benzoate | <DL* | | 0.6 | <= 9.3 |
| 37 | Hippurate | 124 | | 594 | <= 1,150 |
| 38 | Phenylacetate | 0.05 | H | 0.04 | <= 0.15 |
| 39 | Phenylpropionate | <DL* | | 0.4 | <= 0.4 |
| 40 | p-Hydroxybenzoate | 0.48 | | 0.99 | <= 2.08 |
| 41 | p-Hydroxyphenylacetate | 23 | H | 19 | <= 34 |
| 42 | Indican | 75 | H | 40 | <= 74 |
| 43 | Tricarballylate | 0.79 | H | 0.73 | <= 1.41 |
| **L. acidophilus / general bacterial** | | | | | |
| 44 | D-Lactate | 0.8 | | 2.3 | <= 7.0 |
| **Clostridial species** | | | | | |
| 45 | 3,4-Dihydroxyphenylpropionate | <DL* | | 0.12 | <= 0.12 |
| **Yeast / Fungal** | | | | | |
| 46 | D-Arabinitol | 68 | H | 36 | <= 73 |

*Creatinine = 100 mg/dL*

* <DL = less than detection limit

**Figure 2. Baseline urine organic acids.** Assessment of gastrointestinal microbial activity demonstrated elevated production of a number of metabolites, suggesting bacterial and fungal imbalances. (Units: µg/mg creatinine)

# Initial Assessment

- Mitochondrial myopathy, presenting with GERD and failure to thrive
- Metabolic imbalances in central energy pathway intermediates relating to mitochondrial myopathy, including:
    - Citric acid cycle intermediate accumulation
    - Lactic aciduria
    - Mild HMG-CoA pathway inhibition
    - Mild inhibition of beta oxidation of fatty acids
- Gastrointestinal microbial overgrowth

# Initial Plan

- Carnitine 250 mg, 1 tablet PO BID
- Creatine monophosphate, 2 g PO QD
- B-complex, 1 tablet PO QD
- CoQ10 250 mg, 1 tablet PO QD
- Alpha lipoic acid 250 mg, 1 tablet PO BID
- Vitamin E (mixed tocopherols) 200 IU, 1 capsule PO QD

- Anti-*Candida* diet (Animal and vegetable protein, healthy unsaturated fats, fruits and vegetables. Very low in simple carbohydrates. Foods should be organic when possible)
- Organic acid follow-up testing recommended after six months

**Treatment plan rationale:** Treatment in this case focused on supporting mitochondrial function, including increasing energy production (carnitine, creatine, and CoQ10) and quenching oxidative stress (alpha lipoic acid, vitamin E).[5] Several high-quality studies have shown an increase in muscle mass with the use of creatine. Numerous studies suggest that creatine may help treat various neuromuscular diseases and may delay the onset of symptoms when used with standard treatment.[6] B vitamins were also used, as they are coenzymes required at multiple steps in the central energy pathways. Riboflavin and nicotinamide have been shown to improve outcomes in certain cases of mitochondrial dysfunction.[7,8] The GI microbial imbalances were addressed in this case using dietary changes only. Specifically, a diet low in simple carbohydrates was prescribed to minimize fungal overgrowth, which the clinician determined to be a significant issue.

**The expression of milder forms of mitochondrial disease may not be perceived until later in life, often precipitated by an energy-demanding event, such as an illness, certain medications or toxic exposures.**

## Two-Year Follow-up

The parents reported that DR responded very well to the nutrients, and they continued to give them to him over the two-year period. They stated that they did not follow up as directed, because he was doing so well. His growth and development were described as being significantly improved. While the GERD was also improved, allowing him to tolerate the nutrients, the parents did not consistently follow the anti-*Candida* dietary recommendations, and he continued to have some gastrointestinal complaints.

NOTES

# Two-Year Follow-Up Laboratory Results

Percentile Ranking by Quintile: 1st | 2nd | 3rd | 4th | 5th (20% / 40% / 60% / 80%)

Ranges are for ages 13 and over

**NUTRIENT MARKERS**

| # | Marker | Results ug/mg creatinine | Flag | Value above bar | 95% Reference Interval |
|---|---|---|---|---|---|
| | **Fatty Acid Metabolism** *(Carnitine & B2)* | | | | |
| 1 | Adipate | 2.4 | | 5.2 | <= 8.3 |
| 2 | Suberate | 1.1 | | 1.7 | <= 3.2 |
| 3 | Ethylmalonate | 2.9 | | 3.6 | <= 6.3 |
| | **Carbohydrate Metabolism** *(B1, B3, Cr, Lipoic Acid, CoQ10)* | | | | |
| 4 | Pyruvate | <DL* | | 3.9 | <= 6.4 |
| 5 | L-Lactate | 15 | H | 14 | 3 - 46 |
| 6 | β-Hydroxybutyrate | <DL* | | 2.1 | <= 9.9 |
| | **Energy Production (Citric Acid Cycle)** *(B comp., CoQ10, Amino acids, Mg)* | | | | |
| 7 | Citrate | 350 | | 601 | 56 - 987 |
| 8 | Cis-Aconitate | 36 | | 51 | 18 - 78 |
| 9 | Isocitrate | 112 | H | 98 | 39 - 143 |
| 10 | a-Ketoglutarate | 4.5 | | 19.0 | <= 35.0 |
| 11 | Succinate | 9.4 | | 11.6 | <= 20.9 |
| 12 | Fumarate | 0.62 | H | 0.59 | <= 1.35 |
| 13 | Malate | 1.0 | | 1.4 | <= 3.1 |
| 14 | Hydroxymethylglutarate | 3.4 | | 3.6 | <= 5.1 |

**Figure 3. Follow-up urine organic acids.** Assessment of mitochondrial function demonstrated overall improvement, but not full resolution of previously detected imbalances.

| # | Marker | Result | Flag | Value above bar | Reference Interval |
|---|---|---|---|---|---|
| | **Bacterial - general** | | | | |
| 36 | Benzoate | <DL* | | 0.6 | <= 9.3 |
| 37 | Hippurate | 277 | | 594 | <= 1,150 |
| 38 | Phenylacetate | <DL* | | 0.04 | <= 0.15 |
| 39 | Phenylpropionate | <DL* | | 0.4 | <= 0.4 |
| 40 | p-Hydroxybenzoate | 0.45 | | 0.99 | <= 2.08 |
| 41 | p-Hydroxyphenylacetate | 17 | | 19 | <= 34 |
| 42 | Indican | 41 | H | 40 | <= 74 |
| 43 | Tricarballylate | 0.35 | | 0.73 | <= 1.41 |
| | **L. acidophilus / general bacterial** | | | | |
| 44 | D-Lactate | 0.8 | | 2.3 | <= 7.0 |
| | **Clostridial species** | | | | |
| 45 | 3,4-Dihydroxyphenylpropionate | <DL* | | 0.12 | <= 0.12 |
| | **Yeast / Fungal** | | | | |
| 46 | D-Arabinitol | 80 | H | 36 | <= 73 |

*Creatinine = 210 mg/dL*

* <DL = less than detection limit

**Figure 4. Follow-up urine organic acids.** Assessment of gastrointestinal microbial activity demonstrated improvement in all markers, with the exception of D-arabinitol, which had significantly worsened. (Units: μg/mg creatinine)

## Follow-up Assessment

- Mitochondrial myopathy (responding to therapy)
- Mild lactic aciduria
- Gastrointestinal candidiasis

## Follow-up Plan

- Continue supplement protocol
- Reintroduce anti-*Candida* diet
- Consider antifungal medication

**Treatment plan rationale:** Because the patient was diagnosed with MD rather than a resolvable nutrient deficiency, it was determined that the supplements would likely be required for life, with periodic re-evaluation of organic acids. On follow-up, the D-arabinitol level lay above baseline, demonstrating the need for stronger intervention (antifungal medication) and a reintroduction/review of the anti-*Candida* diet.

# DISCUSSION

DR presented with failure to thrive and GERD as the chief complaints of MD. GERD is a fairly common symptom in MD,[1] caused by GI dysmotility, and failure to thrive is a common end result of GERD.[9] In Figure 1, the evidence of mitochondrial dysfunction is noted in the accumulation of citric acid cycle intermediates.[4] There is some dispute on the efficacy of using urinary CAC for identifying mitochondrial disease.[10] Because of the large continuum of MD presentations, it is possible that mild mitochondrial dysfunction is missed when a large reference interval is employed for organic acid assessment, thereby reducing the sensitivity of the assays.

**The true incidence of mitochondrial disease is higher than previously believed, and is a common cause of chronic morbidity, contributing to the pathogenesis of many diseases.**

Lactic acid was elevated (Figure 1), resulting from impaired cellular respiration, causing an increase in anaerobic metabolism. Lactic acid elevation is a common finding in MD.[11-13] Also, a mild deficiency of carnitine is suggested with the 5th quintile accumulation of adipate and suberate. These dicarboxylic acids are spilled into the urine with compromised beta oxidation of fatty acids.[14] Since beta oxidation is a central energy pathway, even mild deficiencies in a patient with MD may have significant clinical ramifications.

Figure 1 demonstrated a mild presence of urinary ketones, as evidenced by the 5th quintile level of β-hydroxybutyrate. Since ketosis is stimulated by glycogen, and glycogen is a potent inhibitor of hydroxymethylglutarate (HMG) CoA reductase, it is not surprising that there was a mild elevation of HMG in the urine as a consequence of ketosis. Cholesterol and

CoQ10 are produced via the HMG pathway; this mild inhibition in HMG may have been causing a CoQ10 insufficiency that further compromised electron transport chain (ETC) function (Figure 5).

Figure 2 revealed gastrointestinal overgrowth as determined by the elevated urinary level of metabolites produced by bacteria as well as D-arabinitol, an alcohol produced by *Candida* species.[4, 15] It is not uncommon for MD to involve gastrointestinal imbalances as a result of the high energy requirements of the GI tract.

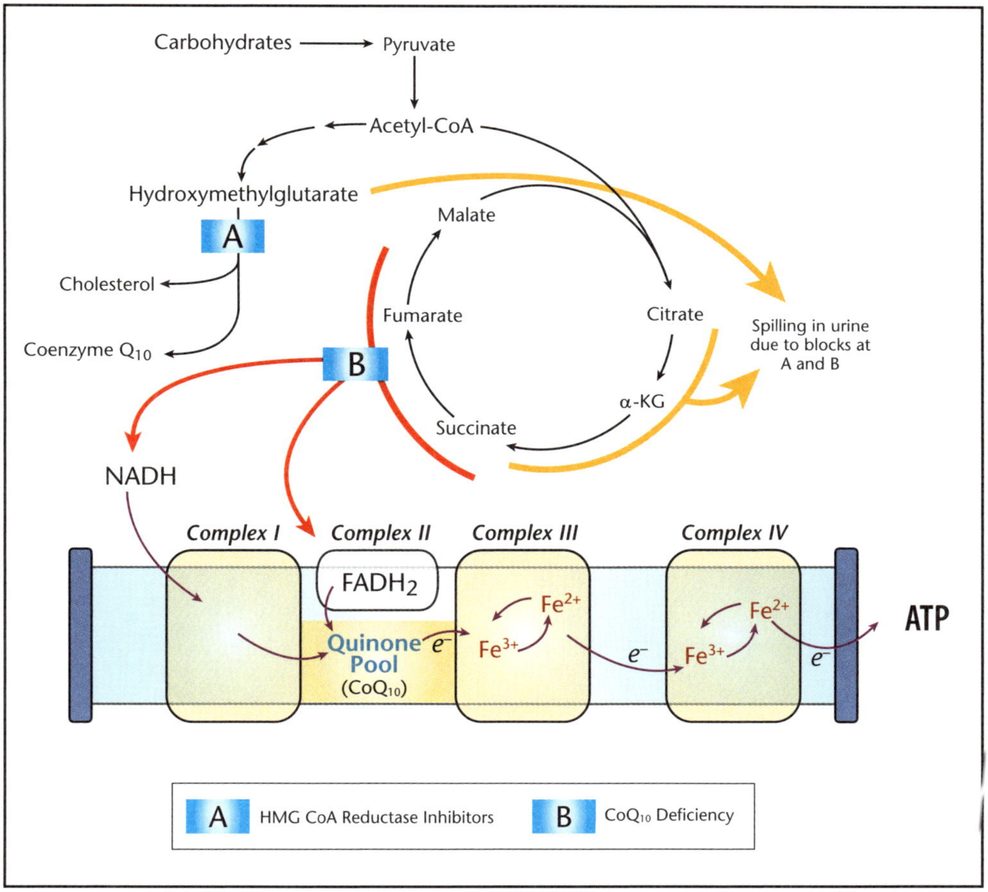


**Figure 5. ATP and the electron transport chain (ETC).** Genetic deficiencies of complexes I-IV, which make up the ETC, may result in insufficient energy production (ATP). Insufficient CoQ10 production secondary to a block in the synthetic pathway (A) may also inhibit energy production by compromising the quinone pool (CoQ10) in the ECT. CoQ10 production may be inhibited by various endogenous regulators or exogenous compounds such as statins. In this case, both an insufficiency in ETC complexes and a block in the CoQ10 synthetic pathway (Figure 1) were present. Both factors likely participated in the urinary accumulation of citric acid cycle intermediates (B) and of lactic acid (Figure 1).

As discussed above, treatment focused on supporting energy production, minimizing the oxidative stress potential and addressing the presence of *Candida* species by minimizing simple carbohydrates, which are its primary growth substrate.

The follow-up visit was greatly delayed, but when the parents returned with DR, he was reported to have thrived, with much improved growth and development over the preceding two years.

The follow-up laboratory data confirmed clinical success (Figures 3 and 4). Mitochondrial markers improved or resolved; he was eliminating only a slightly higher-than-normal amount of lactic acid (Figure 3). The bacterial markers were also better. However, the yeast marker, D-arabinitol, had worsened (Figure 4). Strict adherence to the prescribed diet was recommended. Consideration of an antifungal medication was also recommended.

# CONCLUSION

Mitochondrial disease is much more common than previously thought. Mitochondropathy, of genetic and/or environmental origin is an underlying factor in very different clinical conditions, including autism spectrum disorders, diabetes, statin-induced myopathy (Figure 5), neurodegenerative conditions and ageing.[3, 13, 16-19]

Using an organic acids test with sensitive reference ranges allowed the subtle perturbations in mitochondrial function to be identified and treated in this patient, leading to remarkable clinical improvement.

---

**Author: Kara Fitzgerald, ND**

## References


1. Jeyakumar A, Williamson ME, Brickman TM, Krakovitz P, Parikh S. Otolaryngologic manifestations of mitochondrial cytopathies. *Am J Otolaryngol.* May-Jun 2009;30(3):162-165.
2. DiMauro S, Schon EA. Mitochondrial disorders in the nervous system. *Annu Rev Neurosci.* 2008;31:91-123.
3. Schaefer AM, McFarland R, Blakely EL, et al. Prevalence of mitochondrial DNA disease in adults. *Ann Neurol.* Jan 2008;63(1):35-39.
4. Rogers SA. *Using organic acids to diagnose and manage recalcitrant patients*: Altern Ther Health Med; 2006.
5. Rodriguez MC, MacDonald JR, Mahoney DJ, Parise G, Beal MF, Tarnopolsky MA. Beneficial effects of creatine, CoQ10, and lipoic acid in mitochondrial disorders. *Muscle Nerve.* Feb 2007;35(2):235-242.
6. MedlinePlus. Creatine. http://www.nlm.nih.gov/medlineplus/druginfo/natural/patient-creatine.html. Accessed 6/25/2010, 2010.
7. Ogle RF, Christodoulou J, Fagan E, et al. Mitochondrial myopathy with tRNA(Leu(UUR)) mutation and complex I deficiency responsive to riboflavin. *J Pediatr.* Jan 1997;130(1):138-145.
8. Penn AM, Lee JW, Thuillier P, et al. MELAS syndrome with mitochondrial tRNA(Leu)(UUR) mutation: correlation of clinical state, nerve conduction, and muscle 31P magnetic resonance spectroscopy during treatment with nicotinamide and riboflavin. *Neurology.* Nov 1992;42(11):2147-2152.
9. Armentrout D. Gastroesophageal reflux in infants. *Nurse Pract.* May 1995;20(5):54, 58-60, 62-53.
10. Barshop BA. Metabolomic approaches to mitochondrial disease: correlation of urine organic acids. *Mitochondrion.* Sep 2004;4(5-6):521-527.
11. Canafoglia L, Franceschetti S, Antozzi C, et al. Epileptic phenotypes associated with mitochondrial disorders. *Neurology.* May 22 2001;56(10):1340-1346.
12. Shoffner JM. Mitochondrial myopathy diagnosis. *Neurol Clin.* Feb 2000;18(1):105-123.
13. Weissman JR, Kelley RI, Bauman ML, et al. Mitochondrial disease in autism spectrum disorder patients: a cohort analysis. *PLoS ONE.* 2008;3(11):e3815.
14. Liang Y, Liu L, Wei H, Luo XP, Wang MT. [Late-onset riboflavin-responsive multiple acyl-CoA dehydrogenase deficiency (glutaric aciduria type II)]. *Zhonghua Er Ke Za Zhi.* Dec 2003;41(12):916-920.
15. Lehtonen L, Anttila VJ, Ruutu T, et al. Diagnosis of disseminated candidiasis by measurement of urine D-arabinitol/L-arabinitol ratio. *J Clin Microbiol.* Sep 1996;34(9):2175-2179.
16. Beckman KB, Ames BN. Mitochondrial aging: open questions. *Ann N Y Acad Sci.* Nov 20 1998;854:118-127.
17. Balaban RS, Nemoto S, Finkel T. Mitochondria, oxidants, and aging. *Cell.* Feb 25 2005;120(4):483-495.
18. Golomb BA, Evans MA. Statin adverse effects : a review of the literature and evidence for a mitochondrial mechanism. *Am J Cardiovasc Drugs.* 2008;8(6):373-418.
19. Martin LJ. Mitochondrial pathobiology in Parkinson's disease and amyotrophic lateral sclerosis. *J Alzheimers Dis.* 2010;20 Suppl 2:S335-356.

# 8 Neurodegenerative Diseases

## Amyotrophic Lateral Sclerosis

*There is a significant increase in the incidence of neurodegenerative diseases (NDD) including Alzheimer, Parkinson and amyotrophic lateral sclerosis (ALS) in the United States. While the increase may be attributed to the aging of society, there is a lack of clear genetic pathogenesis of these conditions. As such, environmental factors including toxin exposure and poor dietary habits are strongly implicated.[1, 2, 3] The direct and indirect cost of these diseases is high and is expected to continue to rise. The cost of Alzheimer disease alone currently exceeds 172 billion dollars in the United States annually.[4] In addition to the financial costs, there is a pronounced emotional burden placed on patients and their caregivers that is also expected to increase with the increasing incidence of these diseases.[5, 6]*

### 50-Year-Old Male with Amyotrophic Lateral Sclerosis

| | |
|---|---|
| **Symptoms and Conditions** | Abdominal fasciculations, upper and lower extremity muscle weakness; severe fatigue |
| **Tests Used** | Plasma fatty acids; toxic metal assessments |
| **Imbalances Identified** | Omega-3 and -6 fatty acid imbalance; inflammation |
| **Treatments** | Eicosapentaenoic acid (EPA), docosahexaenoic acid (DHA), coconut oil, organic animal protein |
| **Outcome** | Reduced intensity and severity of abdominal fasciculations; improved energy |
| **Discussion/ Significance** | Lipids are among the most crucial molecules for nervous system function, required both for membrane structure and as signaling molecules. Insufficiencies or imbalances of fatty acids, particularly the omega fatty acids, can have significant negative effect on inflammatory processes and on the structure and function of nervous tissue. Pro-inflammatory eicosanoids produced from arachidonic acid (AA) have been implicated in the pathogenesis of ALS and other neurodegenerative conditions.[7,8] In this case, the level of AA was found to be more than 66 times greater in the plasma than that of anti-inflammatory EPA. With correct diagnosis of the fatty acid imbalance and appropriate supplementation and dietary recommendations, the painful abdominal fasciculations that this ALS patient was experiencing were reduced in intensity and frequency. Further research into the identification and treatment of fatty acid imbalances in ALS patients may demonstrate that it is an important therapy in those with an identified need. |

# CASE HISTORY

AV was 50 years old when he presented with a recent diagnosis of amyotrophic lateral sclerosis (ALS). The diagnosis was made by a neurologist after a comprehensive evaluation that involved a physical exam, nerve conduction and imaging studies, and laboratory evaluations. A western blot assay for Lyme disease was found to be negative. AV's complaints, that he began to experience two years previously, included abdominal fasciculations and upper and lower extremity muscle weakness, which presented primarily as right-sided foot drop and loss of grip strength. He also complained of severe fatigue. Since he had no bulbar muscle involvement, he was able to breath and speak without difficulty. AV noted that the abdominal fasciculations had recently become quite severe and very painful.

AV had researched his condition extensively, and was concerned about the connection between ALS and toxic exposures. Because of this concern, he switched to an organic diet and stopped eating all fish and most animal protein, on account of the risk of contamination with organo- and metallotoxins. Though he took numerous supplements recommended by a nutritionist, fatty acids were not included in his regimen.

> **Insufficiencies or imbalances of fatty acids, particularly the omega fatty acids, can have significant negative effect on inflammatory processes and on the structure and function of nervous tissue.**

There was no family history of ALS or any other neurodegenerative conditions. He grew up in a large agricultural region in the South where numerous pesticides were used. He had a few dental amalgam fillings, which he wanted removed.

Significant physical exam findings included: 1) Lower extremity reflexes were brisk bilaterally, with a positive Babinski sign. 2) Upper extremity reflexes were normal. 3) An abdominal reflex test induced multiple, painful fasciculations. 4) Sensory function was intact. 5) Resisted range of motion was reduced in both upper and lower extremities, but was worse on the right side. 6) Right foot drop was observed as patient walked. 7) Breathing and speech were normal, and lungs were clear to auscultation bilaterally.

Understandably, AV's situation involved a comprehensive treatment program; for the purpose of this case study, however, the focus will be on the early phase of treatment, which primarily involved the correction of fatty acid imbalances.

## Initial Laboratory Results

**Laboratory tests ordered and rationale:**

1. **Plasma fatty acids**: Fatty acid imbalances have been associated with neurodegenerative conditions. Fatty acids are involved in the inflammatory response and in the structure and function of nervous tissue.
2. **Toxic metals assessments (hair, whole blood, and urine provocation with DMSA)**: A comprehensive work-up was completed, because metallotoxins have been shown to play a role in ALS pathogenesis.

**0040 Fatty Acids - Plasma**

*Methodology: Capillary Gas Chromatography/Mass Spectrometry*

Ranges are for ages 13 and over

Percentile Ranking by Quintile: 1st | 2nd | 3rd | 4th | 5th (20%, 40%, 60%, 80%)

| | Results uM | | Quintile cutoffs (low / high) | 95% Reference Interval |
|---|---|---|---|---|
| ***Polyunsaturated Omega-3*** | | | | |
| 1 Alpha Linolenic (18:3n3) | 25 | | 20 | 13 - 80 |
| 2 Eicosapentaenoic (20:5n3) | 4 | L | 17 | 5 - 210 |
| 3 Docosapentaenoic (22:5n3) | 12 | L | 16 | 11 - 50 |
| 4 Docosahexaenoic (22:6n3) | 13 | L | 59 | 31 - 213 |
| ***Polyunsaturated Omega-6*** | | | | |
| 5 Linoleic (18:2n6) | 1,125 | | 930 / 1,669 | 821 - 2,032 |
| 6 Gamma Linolenic (18:3n6) | 7 | | 7 / 33 | 5 - 46 |
| 7 Eicosadienoic (20:2n6) | 6.9 | | 6.4 / 15.3 | 5.2 - 22.5 |
| 8 Dihomogamma Linolenic (20:3n6) | 21 | L | 34 / 102 | 27 - 140 |
| 9 Arachidonic (20:4n6) | 265 | | 201 / 451 | 158 - 521 |

**Figure 1. Omega-3 and -6 fatty acid assessment.** Multiple deficiencies demonstrated.

| | Result | | Quintile cutoff | Reference Interval |
|---|---|---|---|---|
| AA/EPA | 66 | H | 20 | 1 - 57 |

**Figure 2. AA/EPA ratio.** Very elevated arachidonic acid/eicosapentaenoic acid (AA/EPA) ratio, despite the low-normal AA status shown in Figure 1.

| | Result | | Quintile cutoff | Reference Interval |
|---|---|---|---|---|
| ***Polyunsaturated Omega-9*** | | | | |
| Mead (20:3n9) | 3.1 | | 5.3 | <= 8.3 |

**Figure 3. Mead acid.** Result was within normal limits, ruling out long-term polyunsaturated fatty acid (PUFA) deficiency. (Units: µM)

| | Result | | Quintile cutoffs (low / high) | Reference Interval |
|---|---|---|---|---|
| ***Saturated*** | | | | |
| 19 Capric (10:0) | 1.1 | L | 1.4 / 4.0 | 0.7 - 6.2 |
| 20 Lauric (12:0) | 2.4 | L | 3.3 / 14.5 | 2.2 - 27.3 |
| 21 Myristic (14:0) | 12 | L | 20 / 87 | 15 - 139 |
| 22 Palmitic (16:0) | 1,289 | | 792 / 1,794 | 667 - 2,526 |
| 23 Stearic (18:0) | 496 | | 294 / 511 | 250 - 629 |
| 24 Arachidic (20:0) | 13.7 | H | 1.5 / 3.2 | 1.3 - 4.7 |
| 25 Behenic (22:0) | 0.8 | | 0.8 / 2.0 | 0.6 - 2.9 |
| 26 Lignoceric (24:0) | 0.84 | | 0.84 / 1.66 | 0.63 - 2.45 |
| 27 Hexacosanoic (26:0) | <0.27 | | 0.36 | <= 0.43 |

**Figure 4. Saturated fatty acids (SFA).** Low to low-normal results.(Units: µM)

## Additional Laboratory Results

Whole blood, hair and urinary chelation challenge using oral dimercaptosuccinic acid showed all negative results for elevated toxic metals, including mercury, lead, arsenic and cadmium.

## Initial Assessment

- Amyotrophic lateral sclerosis
- Multiple fatty acid deficiencies
- Relative omega-6 AA excess (elevated AA/EPA ratio)

## Initial Plan

- EPA and DHA concentrate, 6 grams PO QD
- Coconut oil, 1 TBS PO QD
- Introduction of organic animal products including eggs, game meats, and safe fish (refer to www.epa.gov for current list of least toxic fish)

**Treatment plan rationale:** Omega-3 fatty acids and saturated fatty acids were introduced based on laboratory findings. Saturated fats were increased using bioavailable medium chain fatty acids from coconut oil. It was also recommended that AV increase intake of organic, grass fed animal products, which would supply additional saturated fatty acids, protein and other nutrients.

## Three-Month Follow-up

AV reported that the abdominal fasciculations had been reduced significantly in their frequency and intensity after the initiation of the EPA and DHA. He also stated that he had noticed an improvement in his energy. Upon physical exam, the abdominal reflex test elicited fewer fasciculations; they were reported by AV as being less painful. No change in muscle strength was noted.

---

NOTES

# DISCUSSION

Amyotrophic lateral sclerosis is the most common neurodegenerative disease of the motor neuron system. There is no known cure. Median survival time is about 2 to 3 years from onset of symptoms, although there is much inter-patient variability.[9, 10] The majority of cases are nonfamilial; genetics play a primary role only about 10% of the time. ALS is thought to be caused by interactions among environmental, genetic, and age-related risk factors. Oxidative damage, inflammation, mitochondrial dysfunction, and glutamate excitotoxicity of motor neuron cells have all been implicated in the pathogenesis of ALS.[11] Environmental factors implicated in ALS include smoking, pesticide exposure, and toxic metal accumulations.[12-14] Malnutrition has been shown to be a significant prognostic factor in ALS.[15]

AV was very concerned about the connection with ALS and toxin exposure, and he altered his diet radically to minimize exposures. In doing so, he stopped eating most animal products including meat, fish, and eggs. His levels of PUFA and saturated fatty acids (Figures 1 and 4) were low, probably as a result of this change. The normal mead acid level indicated that the reduction of PUFA intake had been of recent origin (Figure 3). Mead acid, a non-essential omega-9 fatty acid, has been shown to rise with long-term omega-3 and -6 PUFA deficiencies. Its elevation is considered to be a compensatory mechanism to maintain membrane fluidity, although the cell signaling ability retained by certain omega-3 and -6 fatty acids is lost with mead elevations.[16] AV reported that the onset of painful abdominal fasciculations occurred after the dietary changes.

**Oxidative damage, inflammation, mitochondrial dysfunction, and glutamate excitotoxicity of motor neuron cells have all been implicated in the pathogenesis of ALS. Environmental factors implicated in ALS include smoking, pesticide exposure, and toxic metal accumulations.**

AV's treatment was based on his laboratory findings. Figures 1 and 4 demonstrated a strong need for omega-3 EPA and DHA and saturated fatty acids. As shown in Figure 2, the AA/EPA ratio was significantly elevated. The ratio was remarkable—the AA level was only in the second quintile (the 20th percentile of the reference population) but was 66.3 times higher than that of EPA. AA is the precursor to pro-inflammatory 2- and 4-series eicosanoid signaling compounds, which have been implicated in the pathogenesis of ALS and other neurodegenerative conditions.[7, 8] It appeared from AV's history and laboratory findings that his radical dietary changes allowed a powerfully pro-inflammatory PUFA imbalance to arise. Altering the PUFA ratio in favor of AA-produced 2- and 4-series eicosanoids may have played a role in the increased abdominal fasciculations. Moreover, the low level of DHA, which is a significant fatty acid in the myelin sheath and neuronal membranes, may have further compromised function by impairing neuronal integrity—a hypothesis likely valid, considering the rapid clinical improvement with the introduction of appropriate fatty acids. While Figure 1 also showed a need for anti-inflammatory DGLA, the precursor fatty acid GLA was not given initially, on account of concern about its possible conversion to AA.[17]

Despite his amalgams and his concern about the role of toxic metals in ALS, AV did not demonstrate significant elevation of toxic metals in multiple specimen assays. It was therefore determined that metallotoxins were less likely to be playing a pathogenic role in AV's presentation. He was advised to avoid the removal of his amalgams, as there was some concern that the process might liberate metals into circulation.

# CONCLUSION

Lipids comprise about 60% of central nervous system tissue, including 70% of the myelin sheath and 50% of neuronal membranes. Lipids are required both for membrane structure and as signaling molecules.[18-21] As signaling molecules, lipids have a high rate of turnover.[21] Insufficiencies or imbalances of fatty acids, particularly the omega fatty acids, can have significant negative effects on inflammatory processes and on the structure and function of nervous tissue. Thus, it is logical that a deficiency of omega-3 fatty acids and a relative excess of AA could contribute to an increase in the neuromotor symptoms of ALS. The prognosis of ALS is generally poor, particularly when malnutrition is present. In this particular case, identifying and treating fatty acid imbalances had immediate clinical benefit. Addressing nutrient insufficiencies in neurodegenerative conditions may be an easy and cost-effective way to improve patient outcome. Moreover, given the growing association of environmental exposures and neurodegenerative conditions, it may also be prudent that this individual, with a history of pesticide exposure, be evaluated for organotoxin exposures as well.

It is logical that a deficiency of omega-3 fatty acids and a relative excess of AA could contribute to an increase in the neuromotor symptoms of ALS.

---

**Author: Kara Fitzgerald, ND**
**Clinician: Kara Fitzgerald, ND**

## References

1. Izzotti A. Gene-environment interactions in non-cancer degenerative diseases. *Mutat Res. Jul 10 2009;667(1-2):1-3.*
2. Cameron A, Rosenfeld J. Nutritional issues and supplements in amyotrophic lateral sclerosis and other neurodegenerative disorders. *Curr Opin Clin Nutr Metab Care. Nov 2002;5(6):631-643.*
3. Kalaria RN. Neurodegenerative disease: Diabetes, microvascular pathology and Alzheimer disease. *Nat Rev Neurol. Jun 2009;5(6):305-306.*
4. Alzheimer's Disease Facts and Figures. http://www.alz.org/documents_custom/report_alzfactsfigures2010.pdf. Accessed 5/23/2010, 2010.
5. Brown RC, Lockwood AH, Sonawane BR. Neurodegenerative diseases: an overview of environmental risk factors. *Environ Health Perspect. Sep 2005;113(9):1250-1256.*
6. Landrigan PJ, Sonawane B, Butler RN, Trasande L, Callan R, Droller D. Early environmental origins of neurodegenerative disease in later life. *Environ Health Perspect. Sep 2005;113(9):1230-1233.*
7. Cimino PJ, Keene CD, Breyer RM, Montine KS, Montine TJ. Therapeutic targets in prostaglandin E2 signaling for neurologic disease. *Curr Med Chem. 2008;15(19):1863-1869.*
8. Liang X, Wang Q, Shi J, et al. The prostaglandin E2 EP2 receptor accelerates disease progression and inflammation in a model of amyotrophic lateral sclerosis. *Ann Neurol. Sep 2008;64(3):304-314.*

9. del Aguila MA, Longstreth WT, Jr., McGuire V, Koepsell TD, van Belle G. Prognosis in amyotrophic lateral sclerosis: a population-based study. *Neurology. Mar 11 2003;60(5):813-819.*

10. Mitchell JD, Borasio GD. Amyotrophic lateral sclerosis. *Lancet. Jun 16 2007;369(9578):2031-2041.*

11. Rothstein JD. Current hypotheses for the underlying biology of amyotrophic lateral sclerosis. *Ann Neurol. Jan 2009;65 Suppl 1:S3-9.*

12. Kamel F, Umbach DM, Hu H, et al. Lead exposure as a risk factor for amyotrophic lateral sclerosis. *Neurodegener Dis. 2005;2(3-4):195-201.*

13. Kamel F, Umbach DM, Munsat TL, Shefner JM, Sandler DP. Association of cigarette smoking with amyotrophic lateral sclerosis. *Neuroepidemiology. 1999;18(4):194-202.*

14. McGuire V, Longstreth WT, Jr., Nelson LM, et al. Occupational exposures and amyotrophic lateral sclerosis. A population-based case-control study. *Am J Epidemiol. Jun 15 1997;145(12):1076-1088.*

15. Desport JC, Preux PM, Truong TC, Vallat JM, Sautereau D, Couratier P. Nutritional status is a prognostic factor for survival in ALS patients. *Neurology. Sep 22 1999;53(5):1059-1063.*

16. *Laboratory Evaluations for Integrative and Functional Medicine. Atlanta: Metametrix Institute; 2008.*

17. Manku MS, Morse-Fisher N, Horrobin DF. Changes in human plasma essential fatty acid levels as a result of administration of linoleic acid and gamma-linolenic acid. *Eur J Clin Nutr. Jan 1988;42(1):55-60.*

18. Bazan NG. Lipid signaling in neural plasticity, brain repair, and neuroprotection. *Mol Neurobiol. Aug 2005;32(1):89-104.*

19. Yao JK, van Kammen DP. Membrane phospholipids and cytokine interaction in schizophrenia. *Int Rev Neurobiol. 2004;59:297-326.*

20. Yehuda S, Rabinovitz S, Carasso RL, Mostofsky DI. Fatty acids and brain peptides. *Peptides. 1998;19(2):407-419.*

21. Yehuda S, Rabinovitz S, Mostofsky DI. Essential fatty acids and the brain: from infancy to aging. *Neurobiol Aging. Dec 2005;26 Suppl 1:98-102.*

# 9 Neuropsychiatric and Neuroinflammatory Conditions

## Migraine Headache

*Among the world's 20 most disabling health problems, the migraine headache ranks 20th (and 9th in women), affecting up to 8% of men and 18% of women in the United States. The headaches are characterized by painful, disabling and recurring symptoms initiated by a variety of environmental triggers. There is a strong genetic association.[1] Select comorbidities associated with migraine include anxiety, depression, dysmenorrhea and fatigue.[2-4] Depression has been reported to occur more than twice as often in migraine sufferers, and the combination is seen with far greater frequency in women.[4] Migraines alone are estimated to cause 112 million sick days to be taken from work or school every year in the US.[5-7] The cost to society of both conditions is estimated conservatively at $100 billion per year.[5, 8]*

### 40-Year-Old Female with Migraine Headaches and Depression

| | |
|---|---|
| **Additional Symptoms and Conditions** | Anxiety, fatigue, mild environmental allergies |
| **Medications** | Eletriptan hydrobromide (Relpax®), ibuprofen, etonogestrel/ethinyl estradiol vaginal ring (NuvaRing®) |
| **Tests Used** | IgG4 food sensitivities, plasma amino acids, urinary organic acids |
| **Imbalances Identified** | Low plasma amino acids, low and low-normal urinary neurotransmitter metabolites, and moderate to severe IgG4 food antibodies |
| **Treatments** | Elimination diet based on food-specific IgG4 antibodies, free-form amino acids, glutamine, probiotics, fish oil, multivitamin and mineral supplement |
| **Outcome** | Migraine headaches significantly reduced in frequency and severity, medication use reduced by ~75%, improved mood, energy and menstrual symptoms |
| **Discussion/ Significance** | The role of food additives, such as MSG and tyramine, in triggering migraine headache is well recognized.[9, 10] The role of IgG4-mediated hypersensitivity food reactions and migraine has been less substantiated but is gaining recognition.[11, 12] Low levels of amino acids, neurotransmitters and their breakdown products have also been found in depression and migraines, and serotonin modulation is used for treatment in both conditions.[13–29] In this case, assessment of food-specific IgG4 antibodies, plasma amino acids, and urinary neurotransmitter metabolites offered clear, successful treatment direction. Given the debility associated with migraine and depression, further research into this low cost, safe and effective approach is warranted. |

# CASE HISTORY

BB, a 40-year-old female, presented with a 20-year history of common migraine (no prodrome), depression, anxiety and fatigue. At the time of her first office visit, she reported having approximately four to six migraines each week. Headaches were worse around the time of her menses, and were also triggered by jogging. BB took eletriptan hydrobromide, a serotonin receptor agonist, and ibuprofen frequently to manage the migraine headaches. They could last up to three days without medication, but resolved within a few hours with medication. She was not taking medication for depression or anxiety.

> At the time of her first office visit, BB reported approximately four to six migraines each week, worse around the time of menses. Jogging also triggered migraines which she reported would last up to three days without medication.

BB reported having mild environmental allergies, for which she received allergy shots as a child. She also experienced significant bloating with her menses. She denied any gastrointestinal complaints. She used an etonogestrel/ethinyl estradiol vaginal ring for birth control. She reported that it did not alter her headache pattern. BB ate a standard American diet (SAD) which is characterized by high intake of red meat, sugary desserts and drinks, high-fat foods, dairy products, eggs and refined grains. Her physical exam was unremarkable. A standard battery of laboratory testing previously ordered included a complete blood count, comprehensive metabolic panel, and thyroid and iron studies that all showed results within normal limits.

## Initial Laboratory Results

**Laboratory tests ordered and rationale:**

1. **Food-specific IgG4 antibodies:** Food reactions, including those involving IgG antibodies, have been identified as an etiologic factor in migraine headaches.[11, 12, 30]
2. **Plasma amino acids:** Amino acid insufficiencies have been identified in depression.[18, 20]
3. **Urinary organic acids:** Neurotransmitter metabolites and functional indicators of nutrient insufficiency may be assessed in an organic acids panel. Imbalances in urinary neurotransmitter metabolites and nutrients such as $B_{12}$ and folic acid have been associated with depression.[31-34]

NOTES

**0075 IgG4 Food Antibodies (90 Antigens)** *Methodology: ELISA*

| | Results ng/mL | Response | Class |
|---|---|---|---|
| **Dairy/Meat/Poultry** | | | |
| Beef | 32 | | |
| Casein | 1101 | Severe | +5 |
| Chicken | 182 | Mod | +3 |
| Egg, White | >2000 | Severe | +5 |
| Egg, Yolk | 667 | Mod | +4 |
| Lamb | 36 | | |
| Milk | 1149 | Severe | +5 |
| Pork | <10 | | |
| Turkey | <10 | | |
| **Fish/Shellfish** | | | |
| Clam | <10 | | |
| Codfish | <10 | | |
| Crab | <10 | | |
| Flounder | 10 | | |
| Halibut | <10 | | |
| Lobster | <10 | | |
| Mackerel | <10 | | |
| Oyster | <10 | | |
| Salmon | <10 | | |
| Shrimp | <10 | | |
| Trout | <10 | | |
| Tuna | <10 | | |
| **Fruits** | | | |
| Apple | <10 | | |
| Apricot | <10 | | |
| Banana | <10 | | |
| Blueberry | <10 | | |
| Cantaloupe | <10 | | |
| Cranberry | <10 | | |
| Grape | <10 | | |
| Grapefruit | <10 | | |
| Honeydew | <10 | | |
| Lemon | <10 | | |
| Orange | <10 | | |
| Peach | 10 | | |
| Pear | <10 | | |
| Pineapple | <10 | | |
| Strawberry | <10 | | |
| Watermelon | <10 | | |
| **Grains** | | | |
| Barley | <10 | | |
| Corn | <10 | | |
| Oat | <10 | | |
| Rice | <10 | | |
| Rye | <10 | | |
| Wheat | <10 | | |
| **Legumes** | | | |
| Bean, String | <10 | | |
| Lentil | <10 | | |
| Lima Bean | 10 | | |
| Navy Bean | 61 | Mild | +1 |
| Pea, Green | <10 | | |
| Peanut | 21 | | |
| Pinto Bean | 127 | Mild | +2 |
| Soybean | <10 | | |

**Class Definitions:**

| Class | Cutoffs |
|---|---|
| Negative | 0-40 |
| Mild (+1/+2) | 80/150 |
| Moderate (+3/+4) | 500/900 |
| Severe (+5) | > 900 |

**0075 IgG4 Food Antibodies (90 Antigens)** *Methodology: ELISA*

| | Results ng/mL | Response | Class |
|---|---|---|---|
| **Miscellaneous** | | | |
| Aspergillus | 12 | | |
| Black Pepper | <10 | | |
| Chocolate | <10 | | |
| Cinnamon | <10 | | |
| Coffee | <10 | | |
| Ginger | <10 | | |
| Malt | <10 | | |
| Tea | <10 | | |
| Vanilla | <10 | | |
| Yeast, Baker's | <10 | | |
| Yeast, Brewer's | <10 | | |
| **Nuts/Seeds** | | | |
| Almond | 234 | Mod | +3 |
| Cashew | 348 | Mod | +3 |
| Coconut | <10 | | |
| Pecan | <10 | | |
| Pistachio | 142 | Mild | +2 |
| Sesame | 26 | | |
| Sunflower | 171 | Mod | +3 |
| Walnut | <10 | | |
| **Vegetables** | | | |
| Asparagus | 154 | Mod | +3 |
| Avocado | 184 | Mod | +3 |
| Broccoli | 66 | Mild | +1 |
| Cabbage | <10 | | |
| Carrot | <10 | | |
| Cauliflower | 199 | Mod | +3 |
| Celery | <10 | | |
| Cucumber | 170 | Mod | +3 |
| Garlic | 203 | Mod | +3 |
| Lettuce | <10 | | |
| Mushroom | <10 | | |
| Mustard | <10 | | |
| Olive | <10 | | |
| Onion | <10 | | |
| Pepper, Green | <10 | | |
| Potato | <10 | | |
| Spinach | 13 | | |
| Sweet Potato | <10 | | |
| Tomato | <10 | | |
| Zucchini | <10 | | |

**Figure 1. Baseline serum IgG4 antibodies.** Findings demonstrated multiple mild to severe reactions consistent with intestinal hyperpermeability.

Ranges are for ages 13 and over

Percentile Ranking by Quintile: 1st | 2nd | 3rd | 4th | 5th (20% | 40% | 60% | 80%)

| | Results umol/L | | 20th percentile | 80th percentile | 95% Reference Interval |
|---|---|---|---|---|---|
| **Essential Amino Acids** | | | | | |
| *Limiting Amino Acids* | | | | | |
| Lysine | 106 | L | 117 | 203 | 99 - 234 |
| Methionine | 12 | L | 16 | 26 | 14 - 30 |
| Tryptophan | 34 | L | 35 | 59 | 30 - 67 |
| *Branched Chain Amino Acids* | | | | | |
| Isoleucine | 36 | L | 40 | 72 | 33 - 89 |
| Leucine | 61 | L | 80 | 137 | 68 - 161 |
| Valine | 135 | L | 143 | 240 | 123 - 282 |
| *Conditionally Essential Amino Acids* | | | | | |
| Taurine | 68 | | 31 | 73 | 26 - 100 |
| Glycine | 244 | | 162 | 348 | 136 - 430 |
| Serine | 62 | L | 66 | 115 | 57 - 133 |
| *Neurotransmitters and Precursors* | | | | | |
| Tyrosine | 30 | L | 38 | 70 | 29 - 80 |

**Figure 2. Baseline plasma amino acids.** Many essential and non-essential amino acids were low. (Units: µmol/L)

| Neurotransmitter Metabolism Markers (*Tyrosine, Tryptophan, B6, antioxidants*) | | | | | |
|---|---|---|---|---|---|
| Vanilmandelate | 1.8 | | 1.8 | 3.9 | 1.3 - 4.9 |
| Homovanillate | 2.1 | | 2.1 | 6.3 | 1.6 - 10.9 |
| 5-Hydroxyindoleacetate | 1.9 | L | 2.1 | 5.6 | 1.6 - 9.8 |

**Figure 3. Baseline urinary neurotransmitter metabolites.** Low and low-normal values indicated low total-body serotonin (5-hydroxyindoleacetate) and catecholamine (vanilmandelate and homovanillate) turnover. The catecholamine neurotransmitters are dopamine, epinephrine and norepinephrine. (Units: µg/mg creatinine)

# Initial Assessment

- Dysmenorrhea
- Depression
- Anxiety
- Fatigue
- Multiple food-specific IgG4 antibodies
- Intestinal hyperpermeability
- Multiple amino acid deficiencies resulting in:
  - Low total-body serotonin turnover
  - Low-normal catecholamine turnover

# Initial Plan

- Elimination/Rotation Diet:
  - Eliminate all foods with IgG4 levels of +4 and +5 for one month
  - Foods with +1 to +3 reactions should be consumed no more often than twice per week
  - Reintroduction phase: after one month of avoidance, rotate IgG4 +4 and +5 foods into diet no more than twice per week
- *Lactobacillus* and *Bifidobacterium* species 20 billion CFU, 1 capsule PO QD
- Glutamine 5000 mg, 1 tsp PO BID
- Custom amino acids (10 g per 1 tsp):
  - Start with 0.25 tsp PO QAM and increase dose by 0.25 tsp until reaching 1.5 tsp QAM
- Fish oil, 1 capsule PO BID
- Women's specific multivitamin and mineral supplement taken as directed

**Treatment plan rationale:** Given that various foods can trigger migraine, it was determined that the numerous IgG4 reactions identified (Figure 1) warranted removal or, in the case of milder reactions, significantly reduced exposure. Thus, an elimination/rotation diet based on the laboratory results was initiated. The number of positive reactions was strongly suggestive of intestinal hyperpermeability, so nutrients involved in reducing inflammation and healing the GI tract were introduced, including probiotics, glutamine and fish oil.[35–37] A customized amino acid blend based on BB's laboratory findings (Figure 2) was also implemented to ensure adequate availability of the essential amino acids necessary for their ubiquitous role in metabolism and, particularly, neurotransmitter production. A multivitamin and mineral supplement designed for women (e.g. increased calcium, magnesium, B vitamins) was introduced to support overall metabolic function.[38]

# Two-Month Follow-up

BB reported that migraine episodes were reduced in intensity and frequency. She had not required medication for the previous three weeks, and did not report any medication withdrawal symptoms. When she did experience a headache, she noted that they were triggered when some of the reactive foods were reintroduced, so she avoided these foods with rare exception. She also noted a change in the pain pattern of her headaches. Previously, they started behind her eyes but, after a month of treatment, they were, as she described them, more diffuse, with the pain spanning her forehead.

## Two-Month Follow-up Plan

- Continue supplements
- Continue to avoid all migraine trigger foods identified on reintroduction phase of elimination diet (primarily eggs and dairy)
- Add anti-inflammatory plant sterol

**Treatment plan rationale:** A plant sterol was introduced with the hypothesis that it could reduce the inflammatory response and, in so doing, minimize migraine reaction to IgG4-positive foods.

## Three-Month Follow-up

BB reported feeling more energetic and happy. She stated that she could "feel the positive effects of the amino acids on mood and energy." She found her mood to be much more even, without the big swings between anxiety and depression she experienced in the past. The frequency of migraine attacks was reduced to once per month, accompanying her menses. When she did experience one, it was reduced in intensity and didn't always require medication. She also reported some improvement in bloating and cramps during menses. Previously, she got migraine attacks "all the time" and took medication at least weekly. She did continue to get occasional exertion-induced migraines during exercise, which required eletriptan. She admitted that the rotation diet (especially avoidance of eggs and dairy) was difficult, but it was a significant factor in minimizing migraine attacks, even those associated with her menstrual cycle and exercise. She believed that, if she could fully comply with the diet, she would reduce the incidence of migraines even further.

BB reported feeling more energetic and happy. She found her mood to be much more even, without the big swings between anxiety and depression she experienced in the past. The frequency of migraine attacks was reduced to once per month, accompanying her menses.

## Three-Month Follow-up Plan

- Continue treatment as directed
- Avoid reactive foods
- Counseling given on identifying occult food exposure

## Three-Month Follow-up Laboratory Testing

***0075 IgG4 Food Antibodies (90 Antigens)*** *Methodology: ELISA*

| | Results ng/mL | Response | Class |
|---|---|---|---|
| **Dairy/Meat/Poultry** | | | |
| Beef | 12 | | |
| Casein | 76 | Mild | +1 |
| Chicken | <10 | | |
| Egg, White | 240 | Mod | +3 |
| Egg, Yolk | 38 | | |
| Lamb | <10 | | |
| Milk | 50 | Mild | +1 |
| Pork | <10 | | |
| Turkey | 18 | | |
| **Fish/Shellfish** | | | |
| Clam | <10 | | |
| Codfish | <10 | | |
| Crab | <10 | | |
| Flounder | <10 | | |
| Halibut | <10 | | |
| Lobster | <10 | | |
| Mackerel | <10 | | |
| Oyster | <10 | | |
| Salmon | <10 | | |
| Shrimp | <10 | | |
| Trout | <10 | | |
| Tuna | <10 | | |
| **Fruits** | | | |
| Apple | <10 | | |
| Apricot | <10 | | |
| Banana | <10 | | |
| Blueberry | <10 | | |
| Cantaloupe | <10 | | |
| Cranberry | <10 | | |
| Grape | <10 | | |
| Grapefruit | <10 | | |
| Honeydew | <10 | | |
| Lemon | <10 | | |
| Orange | <10 | | |
| Peach | <10 | | |
| Pear | <10 | | |
| Pineapple | <10 | | |
| Strawberry | <10 | | |
| Watermelon | <10 | | |
| **Grains** | | | |
| Barley | <10 | | |
| Corn | <10 | | |
| Oat | <10 | | |
| Rice | <10 | | |
| Rye | <10 | | |
| Wheat | <10 | | |
| **Legumes** | | | |
| Bean, String | <10 | | |
| Lentil | <10 | | |
| Lima Bean | <10 | | |
| Navy Bean | <10 | | |
| Pea, Green | <10 | | |
| Peanut | 17 | | |
| Pinto Bean | <10 | | |
| Soybean | <10 | | |

| **Class Definitions:** | |
|---|---|
| Class | Cutoffs |
| Negative | 0-40 |
| Mild (+1/+2) | 80/150 |
| Moderate (+3/+4) | 500/900 |
| Severe (+5) | > 900 |

***0075 IgG4 Food Antibodies (90 Antigens)*** *Methodology: ELISA*

| | Results |
|---|---|
| **Miscellaneous** | |
| Aspergillus | <10 |
| Black Pepper | <10 |
| Chocolate | <10 |
| Cinnamon | <10 |
| Coffee | <10 |
| Ginger | <10 |
| Malt | <10 |
| Tea | <10 |
| Vanilla | <10 |
| Yeast, Baker's | <10 |
| Yeast, Brewer's | <10 |
| **Nuts/Seeds** | |
| Almond | 13 |
| Cashew | <10 |
| Coconut | <10 |
| Pecan | <10 |
| Pistachio | <10 |
| Sesame | <10 |
| Sunflower | 17 |
| Walnut | <10 |
| **Vegetables** | |
| Asparagus | <10 |
| Avocado | <10 |
| Broccoli | <10 |
| Cabbage | <10 |
| Carrot | <10 |
| Cauliflower | 30 |
| Celery | <10 |
| Cucumber | <10 |
| Garlic | <10 |
| Lettuce | <10 |
| Mushroom | <10 |
| Mustard | <10 |
| Olive | <10 |
| Onion | <10 |
| Pepper, Green | <10 |
| Potato | <10 |
| Spinach | 12 |
| Sweet Potato | <10 |
| Tomato | <10 |
| Zucchini | <10 |

**Figure 4. Follow-up serum IgG4 antibodies.** Significant improvement noted in both number and severity of reactive foods.

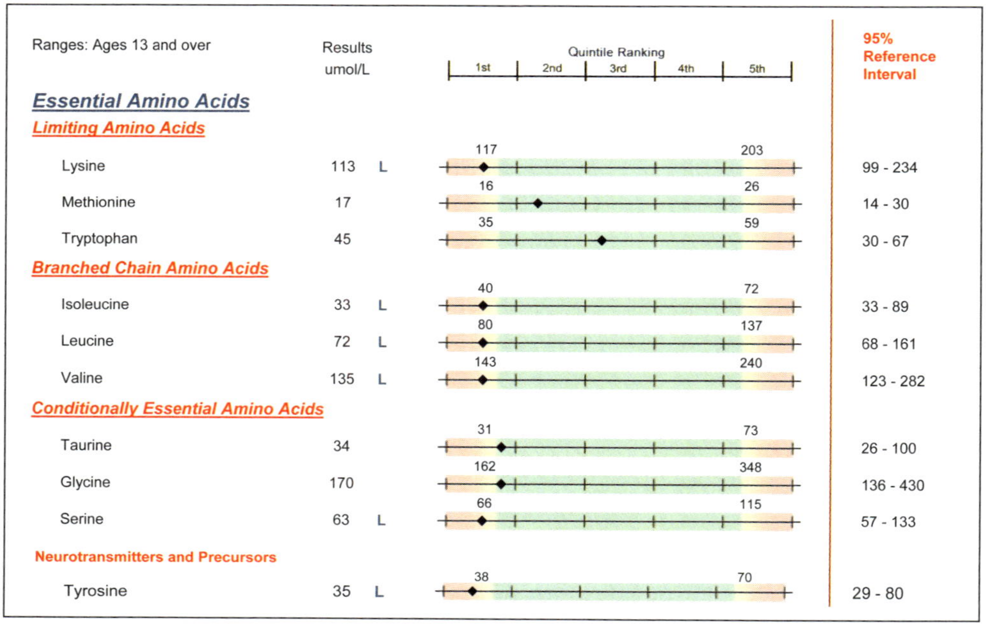

| Ranges: Ages 13 and over | Results umol/L | Flag | Quintile Ranking (1st / 5th) | 95% Reference Interval |
|---|---|---|---|---|
| **Essential Amino Acids** | | | | |
| *Limiting Amino Acids* | | | | |
| Lysine | 113 | L | 117 / 203 | 99 - 234 |
| Methionine | 17 | | 16 / 26 | 14 - 30 |
| Tryptophan | 45 | | 35 / 59 | 30 - 67 |
| *Branched Chain Amino Acids* | | | | |
| Isoleucine | 33 | L | 40 / 72 | 33 - 89 |
| Leucine | 72 | L | 80 / 137 | 68 - 161 |
| Valine | 135 | L | 143 / 240 | 123 - 282 |
| *Conditionally Essential Amino Acids* | | | | |
| Taurine | 34 | | 31 / 73 | 26 - 100 |
| Glycine | 170 | | 162 / 348 | 136 - 430 |
| Serine | 63 | L | 66 / 115 | 57 - 133 |
| Neurotransmitters and Precursors | | | | |
| Tyrosine | 35 | L | 38 / 70 | 29 - 80 |

**Figure 5. Follow-up plasma amino acids.** Many normalized, but some were still low.

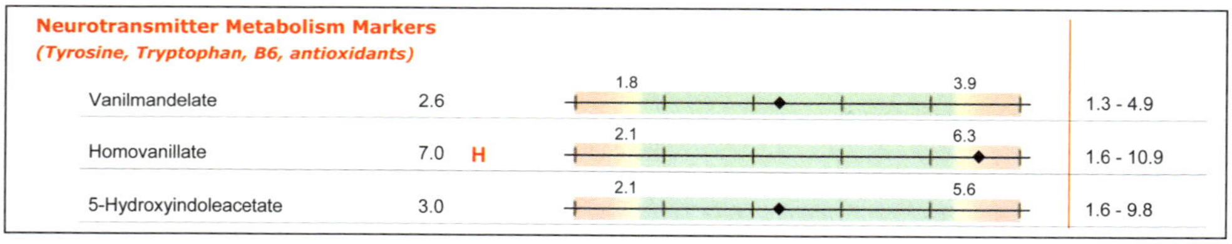

| Neurotransmitter Metabolism Markers (Tyrosine, Tryptophan, B6, antioxidants) | Result | Flag | Quintile Ranking (1st / 5th) | Reference Interval |
|---|---|---|---|---|
| Vanilmandelate | 2.6 | | 1.8 / 3.9 | 1.3 - 4.9 |
| Homovanillate | 7.0 | H | 2.1 / 6.3 | 1.6 - 10.9 |
| 5-Hydroxyindoleacetate | 3.0 | | 2.1 / 5.6 | 1.6 - 9.8 |

**Figure 6. Follow-up urinary neurotransmitter metabolites.** Improvement was noted in all three values.

NOTES

# DISCUSSION

Migraine pathogenesis is believed to involve dysfunction of monoaminergic sensory control systems in the brainstem and thalamus, resulting in increased sensitivity to environmental and sensory input. The monoaminergic system includes the aromatic amino acid-derived neurotransmitters dopamine, epinephrine, norepinephrine and serotonin. Dopamine, epinephrine and norepinephrine are referred to as catecholamines, and serotonin is an indoleamine. A variety of sensory and environmental triggers including light, sounds, exertion, chemicals, foods and hormonal shifts may all lead to migraine attacks. A significant genetic association has also been identified.[1]

The role of foods in triggering migraine headaches is well recognized.[9, 10, 39, 40] Dietary triggers have generally been attributed to specific characteristics such as, tyramine, nitrates or MSG. The majority of studies use migraine frequency to identify specific food triggers. However, newer research has implicated immune reactions to foods as a cause of migraine, as was occurring with this patient. BB's baseline food-specific IgG4 antibody assay revealed many positive findings, including severe reactions to casein, milk and egg white, and mild-to-moderate reactions to numerous other foods (Figure 1). Not surprisingly, an individualized oligoantigenic diet that involved the removal or rotation of reactive foods significantly reduced the incidence and severity of BB's episodes. Oligoantigenic or hypoallergenic diets have shown remarkable success in resolving migraines.[11, 12] A case control study of elimination diets based on IgG response to foods successfully controlled migraines without the need for medications.[30]

**The high number of food reactions suggested intestinal hyperpermeability. Left untreated, larger food peptides are allowed to penetrate the epithelial barrier and form $IgG_4$ antibody/antigen complexes and may be capable of triggering an inflammatory response, which in the case of BB, resulted in migraine attacks.**

The high number of food reactions shown in Figure 1 also suggested intestinal hyperpermeability. Left untreated, larger food peptides are allowed to penetrate the epithelial barrier and form IgG4 antibody/antigen complexes. These complexes may be capable of triggering an inflammatory response, which in the case of BB, resulted in migraine attacks.[41] In addition to an oligoantigenic diet, treatment for the intestinal lining was important for BB, and included glutamine, probiotics, fish oil, amino acids, vitamins and minerals.

BB presented with migraine, depression, anxiety and fatigue. The latter three are recognized migraine comorbidities.[2-4, 42] Monoaminergic dysfunction may be a common pathogenic mechanism in all of these complaints. Serotonin or catecholamine modulation is used for treatment in depression, anxiety, dysmenorrhea and migraines.[17, 21, 23-29, 43]

BB's fasting plasma specimen (Figure 2) revealed a general pattern of low essential and non-essential amino acids, including the aromatic amino acids tryptophan and tyrosine. Phenylalanine, also an aromatic amino acid, was in the second quintile, and therefore on the lower side of a normal finding. The aromatic amino acids are substrates for the monoaminergic neurotransmitters. Urinary organic acid testing demonstrated that the catecholamine metabolites vanilmandelate (VMA) and homovanillate (HVA) were low-normal. 5-Hydroxyindoleacetate (5-HIAA), the serotonin metabolite, was low (Figure 3).

The low to low-normal levels of amino acids, including tryptophan, tyrosine and phenylalanine, were consistent with impaired production of serotonin and the catecholamines and their breakdown products, 5-HIAA, VMA and HVA. Low levels of these amino acids, neurotransmitters and their breakdown products have been found in both depression and migraines.[13-22] Low whole blood serotonin may also be associated with rebound migraine. The low tryptophan and low 5-HIAA suggested that BB's available serotonin pool was also low. With treatment, tryptophan and 5-HIAA normalized (Figures 5 and 6), suggesting that tryptophan levels and serotonin synthesis in the CNS improved.[13, 44] While tryptophan normalization alone could have resulted in improved mood, the patient dramatically reduced her dosage of eletriptan hydrobromide, the serotonin receptor agonist.[18, 28] This change supports the hypothesis that endogenous serotonin production also normalized. Increases in tyrosine (Figure 5), while not enough to be within normal limits, would have increased norepinephrine and dopamine levels and thereby increased VMA and HVA (Figure 6), also contributing to the patient's clinical improvement.[19, 45] It is possible that the small amount of tyrosine being produced from supplementation was being shunted toward production of the catecholamines, and thus was still low in plasma. Regardless, the remaining low amino acids (Figure 5) indicated that supplementation was still required for this patient.

**Low levels of amino acids, neurotransmitters and their breakdown products have been found in both depression and migraines.**

Follow-up IgG4 food antibody production was significantly lower after treatment, both in the number of foods and in the severity of reaction (Figure 4). After three months of treatment, only a moderate reaction to egg and a mild reaction to milk and casein were noted. It is likely that BB was being exposed to small amounts of egg and milk, and therefore generating a slight antibody response. This corroborated her suspicion that occult exposure to dairy and eggs continued to trigger migraine. Since the rest of the reactions were resolved, the intestinal permeability was likely improved.

Laboratory follow-up improvements paralleled those seen clinically. At three months, BB reported increased energy, significantly decreased anxiety and depression, and considerably reduced migraine attacks. Her use of migraine medications was significantly lessened. With poor serotonin synthesis and reliance on eletriptan hydrobromide, BB would have been at risk of developing rebound headaches, which are a difficult-to-treat but relatively common finding with chronic migraine.[46] Complying with the rotation diet was difficult for BB, but she experienced its value in her clinical improvement and was therefore committed to avoiding her known trigger foods.

# CONCLUSION

More than 65 million individuals suffer from either migraine, depression or both conditions in the United States today.[47, 48] However, both conditions are underdiagnosed and undertreated, and therefore the true incidence is likely much higher.[47, 49] The debility of both conditions is also high.[47, 49] For instance: in one study, a full 91% of migraineurs report functional impairment and 53% report severe impairment resulting from their headaches.[47] While migraine medications may be helpful in relieving symptoms after the onset of an attack, regular, frequent use may lead to medication overuse headaches, a challenging-to-treat and painful condition.[46] Antidepressant medication may similarly be quite helpful, although side effects limit tolerance and are the number one reason for cessation.[50] Moreover, while medication is palliative (and likely necessary), it fails to address the underlying causes of the illnesses, and therefore lasting efficacy may be unobtainable.

In this case, laboratory testing uncovered a number of IgG4 food-specific antibodies and amino acid and neurotransmitter imbalances that appeared to be causal factors of migraine, depression and other comorbidities in this patient. The treatment of the patient, which involved removal of the offending foods along with the addition of amino acids and other nutrients, led to a significant reduction in the intensity and frequency of migraine headaches as well as corresponding improvement in mood, energy, and overall quality of life. Medication use was reduced by approximately 75%.

Given the significant debility and cost to society associated with migraine and depression, further investigation into the safe and low-cost approach utilized in this case is warranted.

---

**Authors: Cass Nelson-Dooley, MS; Stephanie Kaplan, ND; J. Alexander Bralley, PhD; Kara Fitzgerald, ND**
**Case Clinician: Stephanie Kaplan, ND**

## References

1. Harrison TR, Fauci AS. Harrison's principles of internal medicine. 17th ed. New York: McGraw-Hill, Health Professions Division; 2008:p 96-99.
2. Peres MF, Zukerman E, Young WB, Silberstein SD. Fatigue in chronic migraine patients. *Cephalalgia*. Nov 2002;22(9):720-724.
3. Tellez-Zenteno JF, Garcia-Ramos G, Zermeno-Pohls F, Velazquez A. Demographic, clinical and comorbidity data in a large sample of 1,147 patients with migraine in Mexico City. *J Headache Pain*. Jun 2005;6(3):128-134.
4. Molgat CV, Patten SB. Comorbidity of major depression and migraine—a Canadian population-based study. *Can J Psychiatry*. Nov 2005;50(13):832-837.
5. Hu XH ea. Burden of migraine in the United States - disability and economic costs, a population based approach. *Abstr Book Assoc Health Serv Res Meet*. 1998(15):272-273.
6. Steiner. Lifting The Burden: the global campaign to reduce the burden of headache worldwide. *J Headache Pain*. 2005;6:373-377.
7. Leonardi M MC. Global burden of migraine in the year 2000: summary of methods and data sources. *WHO health information statistics*. 2000.
8. Scher AI, Bigal ME, Lipton RB. Comorbidity of migraine. *Curr Opin Neurol*. Jun 2005;18(3):305-310.
9. Stang PE, Yanagihara PA, Swanson JW, et al. Incidence of migraine headache: a population-based study in Olmsted County, Minnesota. *Neurology*. Sep 1992;42(9):1657-1662.
10. Van den Bergh V, Amery WK, Waelkens J. Trigger factors in migraine: a study conducted by the Belgian Migraine Society. *Headache*. Apr 1987;27(4):191-196.
11. Egger J, Carter CM, Soothill JF, Wilson J. Oligoantigenic diet treatment of children with epilepsy and migraine. *J Pediatr*. Jan 1989;114(1):51-58.
12. Egger J, Carter CM, Wilson J, Turner MW, Soothill JF. Is migraine food allergy? A double-blind controlled trial of oligoantigenic diet treatment. *Lancet*. Oct 15 1983;2(8355):865-869.

13. Biggio G, Fadda F, Fanni P, Tagliamonte A, Gessa GL. Rapid depletion of serum tryptophan, brain tryptophan, serotonin and 5-hydroxyindoleacetic acid by a tryptophan-free diet. *Life Sci.* Apr 1 1974;14(7):1321-1329.

14. D'Andrea G, Ostuzzi R, Bolner A, et al. Study of tyrosine metabolism in eating disorders. Possible correlation with migraine. *Neurol Sci.* May 2008;29 Suppl 1:S88-92.

15. D'Andrea G, Welch KM, Grunfeld S, Joseph R, Nagel-Leiby S. Platelet norepinephrine and serotonin balance in migraine. *Headache.* Nov 1989;29(10):657-659.

16. Fanciullacci M, Alessandri M, Del Rosso A. Dopamine involvement in the migraine attack. *Funct Neurol.* 2000;15 Suppl 3:171-181.

17. Hamel E. Serotonin and migraine: biology and clinical implications. *Cephalalgia.* Nov 2007;27(11):1293-1300.

18. Ille R, Spona J, Zickl M, et al. "Add-On"-therapy with an individualized preparation consisting of free amino acids for patients with a major depression. *Eur Arch Psychiatry Clin Neurosci.* Jun 2007;257(4):222-229.

19. La Pia S. [Monoamine's role in depression and possible consequences for the clinical management of the core symptoms of major depression]. *Riv Psichiatr.* Jan-Feb 2009;44(1):1-14.

20. Markus CR, Firk C, Gerhardt C, Kloek J, Smolders GF. Effect of different tryptophan sources on amino acids availability to the brain and mood in healthy volunteers. *Psychopharmacology (Berl).* Nov 2008;201(1):107-114.

21. Panconesi A. Serotonin and migraine: a reconsideration of the central theory. *J Headache Pain.* Oct 2008;9(5):267-276.

22. Young SN, Leyton M. The role of serotonin in human mood and social interaction. Insight from altered tryptophan levels. *Pharmacol Biochem Behav.* Apr 2002;71(4):857-865.

23. Ball HA, Samaan Z, Brewster S, et al. Depression, migraine with aura and migraine without aura: their familiality and interrelatedness. *Cephalalgia.* Aug 2009;29(8):848-854.

24. Jurgens TP, Leinisch E, Koch HJ. [A clinical challenge. Pragmatic treatment of migraine and concomitant depression]. *Schmerz.* Feb 2008;22 Suppl 1:11-16.

25. Koch HJ, Jurgens TP. Antidepressants in long-term migraine prevention. *Drugs.* 2009;69(1):1-19.

26. Marino E, Fanny B, Lorenzi C, et al. Genetic bases of comorbidity between mood disorders and migraine: possible role of serotonin transporter gene. *Neurol Sci.* Nov 21 2009.

27. Samaan Z, Farmer A, Craddock N, et al. Migraine in recurrent depression: case-control study. *Br J Psychiatry.* Apr 2009;194(4):350-354.

28. Smith KA, Fairburn CG, Cowen PJ. Relapse of depression after rapid depletion of tryptophan. *Lancet.* Mar 29 1997;349(9056):915-919.

29. Swartz KL, Pratt LA, Armenian HK, Lee LC, Eaton WW. Mental disorders and the incidence of migraine headaches in a community sample: results from the Baltimore Epidemiologic Catchment area follow-up study. *Arch Gen Psychiatry.* Oct 2000;57(10):945-950.

30. Arroyave Hernandez CM, Echevarria Pinto M, Hernandez Montiel HL. Food allergy mediated by IgG antibodies associated with migraine in adults. *Rev Alerg Mex.* Sep-Oct 2007;54(5):162-168.

31. Coppen A, Bolander-Gouaille C. Treatment of depression: time to consider folic acid and vitamin $B_{12}$. *J Psychopharmacol.* Jan 2005;19(1):59-65.

32. Gultepe M, Ozcan O, Avsar K, Cetin M, Ozdemir AS, Gok M. Urine methylmalonic acid measurements for the assessment of cobalamin deficiency related to neuropsychiatric disorders. *Clin Biochem.* Jun 2003;36(4):275-282.

33. Kim JM, Stewart R, Kim SW, Yang SJ, Shin IS, Yoon JS. Predictive value of folate, vitamin $B_{12}$ and homocysteine levels in late-life depression. *Br J Psychiatry.* Apr 2008;192(4):268-274.

34. Ng TP, Feng L, Niti M, Kua EH, Yap KB. Folate, vitamin $B_{12}$, homocysteine, and depressive symptoms in a population sample of older Chinese adults. *J Am Geriatr Soc.* May 2009;57(5):871-876.

35. Hall JC, Heel K, McCauley R. Glutamine. *Br J Surg.* Mar 1996;83(3):305-312.

36. Ohland CL, Macnaughton WK. Probiotic bacteria and intestinal epithelial barrier function. *Am J Physiol Gastrointest Liver Physiol.* Mar 18 2010.

37. Miller AL. The pathogenesis, clinical implications and treatment of intestinal hyperpermeability *Altern Med Rev.* 1997;2(5):330-345.

38. Ames BN. A role for supplements in optimizing health: the metabolic tune-up. *Arch Biochem Biophys*. Mar 1 2004;423(1):227-234.

39. Peatfield RC, Glover V, Littlewood JT, Sandler M, Clifford Rose F. The prevalence of diet-induced migraine. *Cephalalgia*. Sep 1984;4(3):179-183.

40. Robbins L. Precipitating factors in migraine: a retrospective review of 494 patients. *Headache*. Apr 1994;34(4):214-216.

41. Lord RS, Bralley JA. Laboratory Evaluations for Integrative and Functional Medicine. 2nd ed. Duluth, GA: Metametrix Institute; 2008:436.

42. Mannix LK. Menstrual-related pain conditions: dysmenorrhea and migraine. *J Womens Health (Larchmt)*. Jun 2008;17(5):879-891.

43. Clayton AH. Symptoms related to the menstrual cycle: diagnosis, prevalence, and treatment. *J Psychiatr Pract*. Jan 2008;14(1):13-21.

44. Young SN. The use of diet and dietary components in the study of factors controlling affect in humans: a review. *J Psychiatr Neurosci*. 1993;18(5):235-244.

45. Alonso R GC, Wurtman RJ, Agharanya JC, Prieto L. Elevation of urinary catecholamines and their metabolites following tyrosine administration in humans. *Biol Psychiatry*. . 1982;17(7):781-790.

46. Trucco M, Meineri P, Ruiz L. Preliminary results of a withdrawal and detoxification therapeutic regimen in patients with probable chronic migraine and probable medication overuse headache. *J Headache Pain*. Sep 2005;6(4):334-337.

47. Lipton RB, Stewart WF, Diamond S, Diamond ML, Reed M. Prevalence and burden of migraine in the United States: data from the American Migraine Study II. *Headache*. Jul-Aug 2001;41(7):646-657.

48. Health NIMH. The Numbers Count: Mental Disorders in America. http://www.nimh.nih.gov/health/publications/the-numbers-count-mental-disorders-in-america/index.shtml#MajorDepressive, 2010.

49. Sheehan DV. Depression: underdiagnosed, undertreated, underappreciated. *Manag Care*. Jun 2004;13(6 Suppl Depression):6-8.

50. Zimmerman M, Galione JN, Attiullah N, et al. Underrecognition of clinically significant side effects in depressed outpatients. *J Clin Psychiatry*. Apr;71(4):484-490.

# Depression and Inflammatory-Related Disorders

*Sarcoidosis is a granulomatous inflammatory disorder usually involving the lungs, lymph nodes, eyes and skin.[1] Disease mediation includes a powerful inflammatory cascade of cytokines including interferon-γ, tumor necrosis factor-α, interleukins 2 and 8.[1] Depression is also now considered to be an inflammatory disorder.[2] While sarcoidosis is relatively rare, depression affects 1 in 20 individuals, with an annual cost-to-society in the United States exceeding 50 billion dollars.[3] Depression is a common sarcoidosis comorbidity, as are heart disease, diabetes and pulmonary hypertension.[4-6] Inflammation stimulating the tryptophan-depleting kynurenine pathway is a pathogenic mechanism shared among all of these conditions. Interferon-γ is the primary activator of the kynurenine pathway. Evidence of chronic kynurenine pathway stimulation was apparent in the case below and appeared to be a chief causal factor of the patient's refractory depression[7,8] Similar inflammatory molecular underpinnings are shared by many diseases, and the case below identifies biochemical imbalances that may be present in conditions with an inflammatory component.*

## 66-Year-Old Male with Depression and Sarcoidosis

| | |
|---|---|
| **Additional Symptoms and Conditions** | Insomnia, fatigue, hypothyroidism |
| **Medications** | Venlafaxine (Effexor®), levothyroxine (Synthroid®) |
| **Tests Used** | Blood spot amino acids, IgG4 food sensitivities, urine organic acids |
| **Imbalances Identified** | Low urinary 5-HIAA (demonstrating low total body serotonin turnover), high quinolinic acid, low amino acids |
| **Treatments** | Amino acids, 5-hydroxytryptophan, and S-adenosylmethionine |
| **Outcome** | Within two weeks, the patient noticed a dramatic reduction of depressive symptoms, insomnia, and fatigue. At one year, he was off venlafaxine and continued to do well. Chest x-ray revealed no progression of sarcoidosis. |
| **Discussion/ Significance** | Identifying and treating nutrient imbalances caused by the apparent sarcoidosis-mediated inflammation played a central role in resolving this individual's depression, fatigue, and insomnia, suggesting a possible mechanism for the mental health comorbidities often seen with sarcoidosis (inflammation→quinolinic acid production→reduced serotonin synthesis). Evaluation of this effective, nutrient-based approach to treating sarcoidosis-related imbalances is recommended. |

# CASE HISTORY

KM was a 66-year-old Caucasian male who complained of depression for 30 years. While he was prescribed numerous antidepressants over the years he reported that none were effective. He was currently taking venlafaxine, which he also reported as not helping his depression. He also complained of insomnia and nightmares, averaging only three hours of sleep nightly. During severe depressive episodes, he stated that he would spend days at a time in bed.

He reported a history of trauma, which he thought contributed to his depression, but he did not offer details; nor had he attended counseling up to the time of this visit. KM was diagnosed with pulmonary sarcoidosis six years previously, but the granulomas were inactive at time of intake. He also had hypothyroidism, for which he took levothyroxine, although he still complained of extreme fatigue. In addition to his medications, KM took B vitamins, a multivitamin and mineral combination, and omega-3 fatty acids. KM generally adhered to a healthy diet, participated in regular exercise, and had daily bowel movements.

**Depression is an inflammatory disorder, with a chief mechanism being serotonin insufficiency caused by IFN-γ stimulation of the tryptophan-kynurenine pathway. This same mechanism underlies many conditions.**

# Initial Laboratory Results

**Laboratory tests ordered and rationale:**

4. **Urine organic acids**: Imbalances in nutrient status, neurotransmitter turnover, and inflammation could contribute to the patient's complaints.
5. **Blood spot amino acids**: Amino acid imbalances have been associated with depression and fatigue.
6. **Blood spot IgG4 food sensitivities**: Food reactions have been associated with depression and fatigue.

**Neurotransmitter Metabolism Markers**
***(Tyrosine, Tryptophan, B6, antioxidants)***

| Marker | Result | Flag | Quintile markers | Reference range |
|---|---|---|---|---|
| Vanilmandelate | 2.2 | | 1.8 / 3.9 | 1.3 - 4.9 |
| Homovanillate | 2.5 | | 2.1 / 6.3 | 1.6 - 10.9 |
| 5-Hydroxyindoleacetate | 1.0 | L | 2.1 / 5.6 | 1.6 - 9.8 |
| Kynurenate | 2.1 | H | 1.9 | <= 2.7 |
| Quinolinate | 10.8 | H | 4.0 | <= 5.8 |

**Figure 1. Urine organic acids.** Total body serotonin turnover was low, as evidenced by the low level of its chief metabolite, 5-hydroxyindoleacetate. The inflammatory biomarker quinolinate was very high. Kynurenate was mildly elevated. (Units: µg/mg creatinine)

| | Amino acid | Result | Flag | Quintile markers | Reference range |
|---|---|---|---|---|---|
| 11 | Taurine | 135 | L | 145 / 245 | 124 - 282 |
| | Glycine | 233 | L | 243 / 449 | 207 - 559 |
| | Serine | 87 | L | 95 / 219 | 79 - 310 |
| | Glutamine | 294 | L | 307 / 520 | 209 - 573 |
| | Asparagine | 62 | | 49 / 77 | 42 - 88 |
| | Aspartic Acid | 41 | L | 44 / 180 | 26 - 233 |
| | Glutamic Acid | 105 | L | 112 / 207 | 97 - 258 |

**Figure 2. Bloodspot amino acids.** A number of amino acid levels were low (in the first quintile). (Units: µmol/L)

**Pertinent Negative Laboratory Results**

- IgG4 food sensitivities were negative.

# Initial Assessment

- Depression
- Sarcoidosis
- Fatigue
- Low total-body serotonin (low urinary 5-hydroxyindoleacetate)
- Inflammation (high quinolinic acid)
- Amino acid insufficiency

# Initial Plan

- Customized free-form amino acid formula, 5 grams PO BID
- Glycine, 2 grams PO BID
- 5-hydroxytryptophan (5-HTP), 100 mg PO QHS
- S-adenosylmethionine (SAMe), 400 mg PO QD

**Treatment plan rationale:** A customized essential amino acid formula, based on his specific deficiencies, was prescribed. Amino acid blends based on individual needs, as identified using plasma levels, have been successfully employed in fatigue patients.[9] Providing essential amino acids enabled the production of non-essential amino acids, many of which KM also demonstrated a need. While glycine could be made from the essential amino acid precursors given, it was decided to prescribe it specifically because of its role as an inhibitory neurotransmitter.[10] A traditional clinical use of oral glycine is as an anxiolytic agent, suggesting increased glycinergic neurotransmission, either directly or indirectly. 5-HTP was provided to improve serotonin (and melatonin) status, and SAMe was given for depression.[11, 12]

# Two-Week Follow-up

KM responded swiftly to treatment. He reported that his sleep had improved and depressive symptoms were reduced. His nightmares were resolved. With better sleep, his fatigue diminished. He was moved to tears because, in his words, "I've never felt this good in my life." He identified the supplementation protocol as the reason for his improvement. No changes were made to his treatment plan. A blood spot amino acid follow-up test was ordered.

## Six-Month Follow-up

KM continued to do well. He was able to titrate down and eventually withdraw the venlafaxine. His sleep continued to be good, and 5-HTP was taken only as needed. KM began psychological counseling for his past traumas, and noted that his anxiety had increased because of it.

## Six-Month Follow-up Plan

- Decrease SAMe to 200 mg PO QD
- Add:
  - Gamma amino butyric acid (GABA), 500 mg PO BID
  - Valerian standardized extract, 900 mg PO QHS

**Treatment plan rationale:** SAMe was decreased because supplementation has been associated with increased anxiety in some individuals.[13] GABA and valerian were prescribed for anxiety.[14] Research on oral GABA supplementation is lacking, although it has a long clinical tradition as an anxiolytic agent.

| | | | | | |
|---|---|---|---|---|---|
| 11 Taurine | 184 | | 145 | 245 | 124 - 282 |
| Glycine | 223 | L | 243 | 449 | 207 - 559 |
| Serine | 153 | | 95 | 219 | 79 - 310 |
| Tyrosine | 62 | | 44 | 85 | 36 - 99 |
| Citrulline | 32 | | 19 | 41 | 16 - 51 |
| Ornithine | 103 | | 68 | 158 | 50 - 210 |
| Glutamine | 406 | | 307 | 520 | 209 - 573 |
| Asparagine | 67 | | 49 | 77 | 42 - 88 |
| Aspartic Acid | 63 | | 44 | 180 | 26 - 233 |
| Glutamic Acid | 105 | L | 112 | 207 | 97 - 258 |

**Figure 3. Follow-up blood spot amino acids.** Improvement was noted with all amino acids except glycine and glutamic acid. (Units: µmol/L)

## Fourteen-Month Follow-up

KM reported feeling great. He visited the clinic only to pick up his supplements. His recent chest x-ray showed no progression of the sarcoidosis granulomas.

# DISCUSSION

Depression and decreased quality of life are common in sarcoidosis. In one study, 25% of sarcoidosis outpatients met the criteria for Major Depressive Disorder.[15] Other symptoms common in sarcoidosis patients include respiratory complaints, fever, weight loss, night sweats, and severe fatigue. Frequently, however, sarcoidosis is asymptomatic.[1]

Genetic susceptibility is understood to play a role in disease expression, but an environmental trigger is required. Multiple HLA haplotypes such as *DRB1*1101* and *DQB1*0201* are associated with various manifestations of the disease; the latter haplotype is also associated with celiac disease. In the U.S., African Americans are up to 17 times more likely than whites to develop sarcoidosis. Candidate environmental triggers include both infectious agents, such as *Propionibacterium acnes*[16] and *Mycobacterium tuberculosis,*[17] and noninfectious agents, including insecticides and molds.[18] It may be that a genetically vulnerable host response to multiple factors causes a hyper-immune reaction leading to sarcoidosis.

**Identifying and treating nutrient imbalances caused by the apparent sarcoidosis-mediated inflammation played a central role in resolving this individual's depression, fatigue.**

Development of sarcoidosis may have exacerbated KM's long-standing depression; or chronic, subclinical inflammation—perhaps early undiagnosed sarcoidosis— contributed to the development of his depression. Human and animal research has shown that the immune system is often involved in psychiatric disorders (the "cytokine hypothesis of depression").[19] Tryptophan is the precursor of many compounds, including quinolinic acid, kynurenic acid, and serotonin. Pro-inflammatory Th1 cytokines, including interferon-$\gamma$, can activate the enzyme indoleamine 2, 3-dioxygenase of the kynurenin pathway, which alters tryptophan metabolism and can result in high quinolinic acid and low serotonin (Figures 1 and 4). This process has been proposed as a possible mechanism of major depression.[20] Interferon-$\gamma$, among other cytokines, is elevated in sarcoidosis.[1]

Figure 1 demonstrated organic acid findings consistent with inflammation and depression. Quinolinic acid (QUIN) production is stimulated as a result of interferon-$\gamma$ release by macrophages; it is not surprising that KM showed very high levels due to the inflammatory pathophysiology of sarcoidosis. QUIN itself is an excitotoxin that strongly binds N-methyl-D-aspartate (NMDA) receptors.[21] Glutamatergic receptor stimulation from quinolinic acid could have contributed to KM's insomnia or depression. [22] Since kynurenate (KYNA) antagonizes glutamatergic neuronal activity, it is considered to be protective, especially in chronic inflammatory conditions with protracted glutamatergic stimulation.[23] Both QUIN and KYNA are produced via the tryptophan kynurenin pathway (Figure 4).

---

NOTES

5-Hydroxyindoleacetate (5-HIAA) was also shown to be low (Figure 1). As a metabolite of serotonin, low urinary 5-HIAA levels may be associated with low total-body serotonin levels. Serotonin, a product of the tryptophan indolamine pathway, is sacrificed during times of inflammation in favor of the tryptophan kynurenin pathway and QUIN production.[1] Melatonin is also a product of the indolamine pathway. Low levels of these two compounds appear to have been associated with KM's chief complaints of depression (serotonin) and insomnia (melatonin).

With low levels of total body serotonin, selective serotonin reuptake inhibitor (SSRI) antidepressants would have limited effectiveness, which may at least partially explain the so-called "SSRI nonresponder" phenomenon. This hypothesis would also explain why withdrawing the SSRI venlafaxine was relatively easy for the patient and why antidepressant medications in general were not effective for him: modulating serotonin activity is a primary mechanism of action in such drugs.

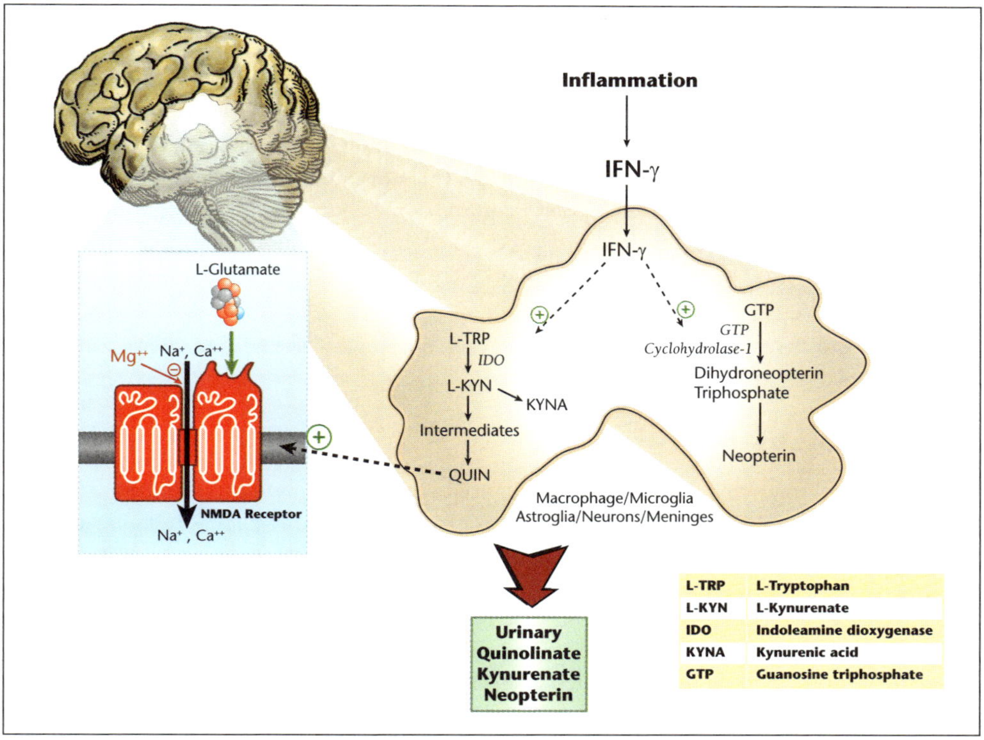


**Figure 4. CNS kynurenin pathway products.** Immune and neuronal cells use the tryptophan kynurenin pathway to produce quinolinate as a way of modulating brain activity. The output of quinolinate interacts with NMDA receptors of the excitatory glutamatergic neurons in the hippocampus and other regions of the brain to increase activity by agonizing response to glutamic acid and glycine. Conversely, kynurenate is antagonistic to glutamatergic neurons, modulating the affects of quinolinate. Inflammatory cascades that involve INF-γ divert tryptophan away from the indolamine pathway (serotonin synthesis) and toward the kynurenin pathway, resulting in increased production of quinolinate and kynurenate and decreased serotonin synthesis. Neopterin is produced separately, from dihydroneopterin triphosphate via the tetrahydrobiopterin synthetic pathway.

Figure 2 demonstrated a number of low amino acids. Low amino acid levels have been associated with depression and can result in reduced neurotransmitter synthesis.[24,25] Low plasma amino acid levels have also been seen in chronic fatigue syndrome.[9] On follow-up, the amino acid levels were largely improved (Figure 3), with the exception of those of glycine and glutamate. Glycine may have been particularly refractory, on account of increased collagen synthesis associated with sarcoidosis.[26] Interestingly, tryptophan level was normal in pre- and post amino acid tests. However, regardless of its status in blood, it was being directed away from serotonin production because of the inflammatory activity.

KM's initial treatment was straightforward, and involved addressing the deficiencies identified on laboratory analysis, including those of amino acids and the serotonin precursor, 5-hydroxytryptophan. SAMe, with good evidence of antidepressant affect, was also included in the plan.[13]

With nutritional treatment of neurotransmitter and amino acid abnormalities, the patient's depression was greatly alleviated and he was able to discontinue the antidepressant medication and initiate psychotherapy. Because psychotherapy was associated initially with anxiety, his follow-up treatment plan included GABA and valerian, nutrients that may have an anxiolytic effect.[10,14] A reduction in SAMe, which has been anecdotally reported to promote anxiety in some cases, was also made. It is not unusual to have obstacles on the road to recovery. His increased anxiety required some short-term intervention, but overall the patient was doing well. His depression lifted, he had more energy, he was sleeping regularly, and his follow-up lab values were normalizing in tandem with the treatment effects.

# CONCLUSION

Identifying and treating the metabolic imbalances apparently caused by sarcoidosis-mediated inflammation played a significant role in improving this patient's reported 30-year depression. He also noted resolution of his fatigue and insomnia. He was able to discontinue the antidepressant medications, which were likely ineffective on account of low serotonin secondary to chronic inflammation. This case illustrates the close mechanistic connection between Th1/INFγ-driven inflammation and depression. Further research into the efficacy of this safe approach to addressing sarcoidosis-associated conditions is warranted.

---

**Authors: Cass Nelson-Dooley, MS; Kara Fitzgerald, ND**

**Case Clinician: Stephanie Tuss;** **Acknowledgement: Eve Bralley, PhD**

## References


1. Fauci AS. *Harrison's principles of internal medicine / editors, Anthony S. Fauci ... [et al.]*. 17th ed. New York: McGraw-Hill Medical; 2008 pgs. 2135-2147.
2. Maes M. Depression is an inflammatory disease, but cell-mediated immune activation is the key component of depression. *Prog Neuropsychopharmacol Biol Psychiatry.* Jun 20.
3. Greenberg PE, Birnbaum SA. Cost of depression: current assessment and future directions. *Expert Rev Pharmacoecon Outcomes Res.* Oct 2001;1(1):69-76.
4. Alhamad EH, Idrees MM, Alanezi MO, Alboukai AA, Shaik SA. Sarcoidosis-associated pulmonary hypertension: Clinical features and outcomes in Arab patients. *Ann Thorac Med.* Apr 2010;5(2):86-91.
5. Habersberger J, Manins V, Taylor AJ. Cardiac sarcoidosis. *Intern Med J.* Apr 2008;38(4):270-277.
6. Westney G, Mims A, Yuan MS, Rust G. Sarcoidosis Comorbidity and Expenditures in a Health Outcomes Management Company. *Am J Respir Crit Care Med.* 2009;179:A2262.
7. Myint AM, Kim YK, Verkerk R, Scharpe S, Steinbusch H, Leonard B. Kynurenine pathway in major depression: evidence of impaired neuroprotection. *J Affect Disord.* Feb 2007;98(1-2):143-151.
8. O'Connor JC, Lawson MA, Andre C, et al. Induction of IDO by bacille Calmette-Guerin is responsible for development of murine depressive-like behavior. *J Immunol.* Mar 1 2009;182(5):3202-3212.
9. Bralley J, Lord R. Treatment of chronic fatigue syndrome with specific amino acid supplementation. *J App Nutr.* 1994;46(3):74-78.
10. Bowery NG, Smart TG. GABA and glycine as neurotransmitters: a brief history. *Br J Pharmacol.* Jan 2006;147 Suppl 1:S109-119.
11. Iovieno N, Dalton ED, Fava M, Mischoulon D. Second-tier natural antidepressants: Review and critique. *J Affect Disord.* Jun 24.
12. Lakhan SE, Vieira KF. Nutritional therapies for mental disorders. *Nutr J.* 2008;7:2.
13. Bell KM, Potkin SG, Carreon D, Plon L. S-adenosylmethionine blood levels in major depression: changes with drug treatment. *Acta Neurol Scand Suppl.* 1994;154:15-18.
14. Benke D, Barberis A, Kopp S, et al. GABA A receptors as in vivo substrate for the anxiolytic action of valerenic acid, a major constituent of valerian root extracts. *Neuropharmacology.* Jan 2009;56(1):174-181.
15. Goracci A, Fagiolini A, Martinucci M, et al. Quality of life, anxiety and depression in sarcoidosis. *Gen Hosp Psychiatry.* Sep-Oct 2008;30(5):441-445.
16. Ebe Y, Ikushima S, Yamaguchi T, et al. Proliferative response of peripheral blood mononuclear cells and levels of antibody to recombinant protein from Propionibacterium acnes DNA expression library in Japanese patients with sarcoidosis. *Sarcoidosis Vasc Diffuse Lung Dis.* Oct 2000;17(3):256-265.
17. Gupta D, Agarwal R, Aggarwal AN, Jindal SK. Molecular evidence for the role of mycobacteria in sarcoidosis: a meta-analysis. *Eur Respir J.* Sep 2007;30(3):508-516.
18. Newman LS, Rose CS, Bresnitz EA, et al. A case control etiologic study of sarcoidosis: environmental and occupational risk factors. *Am J Respir Crit Care Med.* Dec 15 2004;170(12):1324-1330.
19. Schiepers OJ, Wichers MC, Maes M. Cytokines and major depression. *Prog Neuropsychopharmacol Biol Psychiatry.* Feb 2005;29(2):201-217.
20. Miura H, Ozaki N, Sawada M, Isobe K, Ohta T, Nagatsu T. A link between stress and depression: shifts in the balance between the kynurenine and serotonin pathways of tryptophan metabolism and the etiology and pathophysiology of depression. *Stress.* 2008;11(3):198-209.
21. Blaylock RL. A possible central mechanism in autism spectrum disorders, part 1. *Altern Ther Health Med.* Nov-Dec 2008;14(6):46-53.
22. Muller N, Schwarz MJ. The immune-mediated alteration of serotonin and glutamate: towards an integrated view of depression. *Mol Psychiatry.* Nov 2007;12(11):988-1000.
23. Kincses ZT, Toldi J, Vecsei L. Kynurenines, neurodegeneration and Alzheimer's disease. *J Cell Mol Med.* Jul 12.
24. Ille R, Spona J, Zickl M, et al. „Add-On"-therapy with an individualized preparation consisting of free amino acids for patients with a major depression. *Eur Arch Psychiatry Clin Neurosci.* Jun 2007;257(4):222-229.
25. Smith KA, Fairburn CG, Cowen PJ. Relapse of depression after rapid depletion of tryptophan. *Lancet.* Mar 29 1997;349(9056):915-919.

26. Bhattacharjee A, Bansal M. Collagen structure: the Madras triple helix and the current scenario. *IUBMB Life.* Mar 2005;57(3):161-172.

# 10 Respiratory Disorders

## Asthma

*More than 22 million Americans suffer with asthma (including 7 million children), accounting for almost 15 million physician visits per year.[1] The incidence of asthma in children more than doubled through the 1980s and 1990s and remains at historically high levels.[2] Asthma in adults also continues to increase, with 20% of obese individuals having been diagnosed with the condition.[3] Asthma is frequently associated with dermatitis and rhinitis, together termed the atopic triad. The annual cost of asthma in the United States in the year 2000 was estimated to be nearly $18 billion.[4] While medications are clearly an important tool in asthma management, there is evidence suggesting that excessive use of some may be associated with increased risk of death.[5] Asthma antecedents and triggers include antibiotics, infections, food, microbial and environmental antigens, smoking, alcohol use, and stress.[5-8] Minimizing these exposures may help reduce reliance on medication and thereby reduce risk of death. Moreover, evaluating and treating underlying nutrient imbalances may also help to reduce the incidence of asthma.*

### 54-Year-Old Female with Chronic Asthma

| | |
|---|---|
| **Symptoms and Conditions** | Chronic asthma |
| **Medications** | leukotriene inhibitors with albuterol |
| **Tests Used** | Plasma fatty acids and lipid peroxides |
| **Imbalances Identified** | Chronic omega fatty acid deficiency and elevated lipid peroxides |
| **Treatments** | Omega-3 and -6 fatty acids; vitamins A, C, E; zinc and selenium |
| **Outcome** | Resolution of asthma |
| **Discussion/ Significance** | Imbalances in the omega-3- and 6- derived eicosanoids have been associated with an increased incidence of asthma.[9] Laboratory evaluation of omega-3 and -6 fatty acids provides individualized treatment direction that may aid in relieving eicosanoid imbalances. In the case of this patient, treatment of specific fatty acid deficiencies resulted in a complete resolution of symptoms, cessation of medication, and normalization of oxidative stress. Fatty acid imbalances may be a strong etiologic factor in a subgroup of asthma sufferers. Further research into this safe, individualized approach to treating asthma is warranted. |

# CASE HISTORY

DP was 54 years old when she presented with chronic, poorly controlled asthma. She had experienced minimal success in achieving lasting control of her condition with the use of leukotriene inhibitors and albuterol. DP decided to seek integrative care for assistance in the management of her condition.

> Fatty acid imbalances may be a strong etiologic factor in a subgroup of asthma sufferers.

Note that this case includes comprehensive laboratory assessments, but discussion has been limited to fatty acids and lipid peroxides, because they were the main areas both of the imbalance and of the treatment focus.

## Initial Laboratory Results

**Laboratory tests ordered and rationale:**

1. **Plasma fatty acids**: Evaluation of fatty acid imbalances potentially associated with the pathophysiology of asthma.
2. **Lipid peroxides**: Evaluation of oxidative stress potentially associated with the pathophysiology of asthma.

***0040 Fatty Acids - Plasma*** — *Methodology: Capillary Gas Chromatography/Mass Spectrometry*

Ranges are for ages 13 and over

Percentile Ranking by Quintile: 1st | 2nd | 3rd | 4th | 5th (20% | 40% | 60% | 80%)

| | Results uM | | Quintile markers | 95% Reference Interval |
|---|---|---|---|---|
| ***Polyunsaturated Omega-3*** | | | | |
| 1 Alpha Linolenic (18:3n3) | 20 | | 20 | 13 - 80 |
| 2 Eicosapentaenoic (20:5n3) | 4 | L | 17 | 5 - 210 |
| 3 Docosapentaenoic (22:5n3) | 7 | L | 16 | 11 - 50 |
| 4 Docosahexaenoic (22:6n3) | 59 | | 59 | 31 - 213 |
| ***Polyunsaturated Omega-6*** | | | | |
| 5 Linoleic (18:2n6) | 454 | L | 930; 1,669 | 821 - 2,032 |
| 6 Gamma Linolenic (18:3n6) | 10 | | 7; 33 | 5 - 46 |
| 7 Eicosadienoic (20:2n6) | 4.5 | L | 6.4; 15.3 | 5.2 - 22.5 |
| 8 Dihomogamma Linolenic (20:3n6) | 13 | L | 34; 102 | 27 - 140 |
| 9 Arachidonic (20:4n6) | 325 | | 201; 451 | 158 - 521 |
| 10 Docosadienoic (22:2n6) | <0.23 | | 0.9 | <= 2.0 |
| 11 Docosatetraenoic (22:4n6) | 2.8 | L | 3.7; 13.8 | 2.6 - 18.1 |
| ***Polyunsaturated Omega-9*** | | | | |
| 12 Mead (20:3n9) | 8.5 | H | 5.3 | <= 8.3 |

**Figure 1. Plasma fatty acids.** Multiple omega-3 and -6 deficiencies with mead elevation.

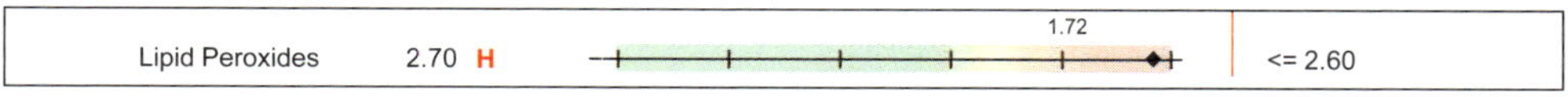


**Figure 2. Lipid peroxides.** Elevated lipid peroxidation demonstrated increased oxidative stress. (Units: nmol/mL)

# Initial Assessment

- Chronic asthma
- Multiple omega-3 and -6 fatty acid deficiencies
- Oxidative stress

# Initial Plan

- Omega-3-and -6 fatty acids including:
  - eicosapentaenoic acid (EPA) 1400 mg and docosapentaenoic acid (DHA) 925 mg, 1 tsp PO BID
  - gamma linolenic acid (GLA) 500 mg, 1 capsule PO BID
- Antioxidant support blend (per 2 caps): Vitamins A 10,000 IU, E 400 IU and C 500 mg; zinc 15 mg, and selenium 100 mg, 4 caps PO QD

**Treatment plan rationale:** Higher doses of EPA and DHA were introduced to relieve the marked deficiencies identified upon testing and to help reduce the amount of arachidonic acid (AA) relative to EPA. EPA will compete with AA for desaturase enzymes, thereby reducing the amount of AA that is produced.[10] Moreover, providing higher amounts of EPA will support anti-inflammatory resolvin and eicosanoid production. GLA was introduced to support production of dihomo-gamma-linolenic acid (DGLA), which is the fatty-acid precursor of the omega-6 anti-inflammatory eicosanoids. An antioxidant blend was introduced to quench the increased oxidative activity indicated by the elevated lipid peroxidation.

**In the United States, asthma in adults continues to increase, particularly among those with obesity, where 20% have been diagnosed with the condition at some point. In children, asthma continues at historically high levels.**

# One-Year Follow-up

DP stated that her asthma ceased to be a problem once she began taking the fatty acids and antioxidants. She also stated that she no longer required her medications.

## One-Year Follow-Up Laboratory Results

**0040 Fatty Acids - Plasma** *Methodology: Capillary Gas Chromatography/Mass Spectrometry*

Ranges are for ages 13 and over

Percentile Ranking by Quintile: 1st | 2nd | 3rd | 4th | 5th (20% | 40% | 60% | 80%)

| | Results uM | | Quintile markers | 95% Reference Interval |
|---|---|---|---|---|
| ***Polyunsaturated Omega-3*** | | | | |
| 1 Alpha Linolenic (18:3n3) | 17 | L | 20 | 13 - 80 |
| 2 Eicosapentaenoic (20:5n3) | 32 | | 17 | 5 - 210 |
| 3 Docosapentaenoic (22:5n3) | 35 | | 16 | 11 - 50 |
| 4 Docosahexaenoic (22:6n3) | 94 | | 59 | 31 - 213 |
| ***Polyunsaturated Omega-6*** | | | | |
| 5 Linoleic (18:2n6) | 595 | L | 930; 1,669 | 821 - 2,032 |
| 6 Gamma Linolenic (18:3n6) | 35 | H | 7; 33 | 5 - 46 |
| 7 Eicosadienoic (20:2n6) | 9.4 | | 6.4; 15.3 | 5.2 - 22.5 |
| 8 Dihomogamma Linolenic (20:3n6) | 100 | | 34; 102 | 27 - 140 |
| 9 Arachidonic (20:4n6) | 471 | H | 201; 451 | 158 - 521 |
| 10 Docosadienoic (22:2n6) | 0.9 | | 0.9 | <= 2.0 |
| 11 Docosatetraenoic (22:4n6) | 6.7 | | 3.7; 13.8 | 2.6 - 18.1 |
| ***Polyunsaturated Omega-9*** | | | | |
| 12 Mead (20:3n9) | 4.7 | | 5.3 | <= 8.3 |

**Figure 3. Follow-up plasma fatty acids.** Improvement shown in EPA and DHA; alpha linolenic and linoleic acids were still low; both gamma linolenic and arachidonic acids were higher than on initial testing.

| | | | |
|---|---|---|---|
| Lipid Peroxides | 1.00 | 1.72 | <= 2.60 |

**Figure 4. Follow-up lipid peroxides.** Significant reduction in oxidative stress from baseline. (Units: nmol/mL)

## One-Year Follow-up Plan

- Continue EPA and DHA supplementation
- Add 2 TBS freshly-ground flax seed for ALA support
- Continue general antioxidant support or switch to high-potency multivitamin and mineral supplement
- Discontinue GLA supplementation
- Decrease arachidonic acid-containing foods (shrimp, non-organic red meats, egg yolks) and other foods associated with inflammation (sugars and other simple carbohydrates)

**Treatment plan rationale:** Given the good clinical response, EPA and DHA were continued. Alpha linolenic acid (ALA) was found to be low normal, so ground flax seed was introduced as a good dietary source. GLA was discontinued because its level appeared to increase upon repeat testing. The fact that GLA can be metabolized to AA may be the reason that AA had increased upon repeated testing. AA levels may also rise as a result of ingestion of AA-containing foods and simple carbohydrates, which may lead to increased AA production via insulin.[11] ALA has been shown to be a potent inhibitor.

# DISCUSSION

Asthma is a type 1 hypersensitivity immune response, initiated by sensitized Th2 cells and driven by mast cells and B cell-produced immunoglobulin E, among other immunocompounds. Of the many toxic substances released during the immune cascade, the arachidonic acid-derived pro-inflammatory eicosanoid compounds (series 2 prostaglandins and series 4 leukotrienes) are key in producing many of the symptoms, including the wheezing, breathlessness, coughing and chest tightness associated with asthma.[12] (Figure 5)

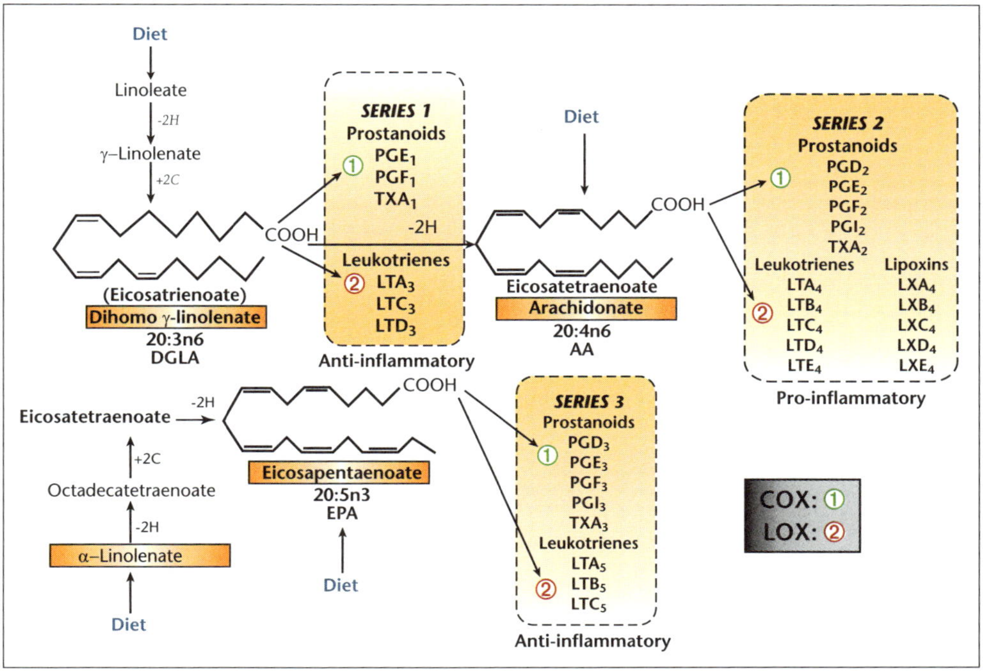


**Figure 5. Eicosanoid products of DGLA, AA, and EPA.** These eicosanoid products may be grouped as primarily anti-inflammatory or pro-inflammatory. Modulating dietary habits can alter the balance of the fatty acid substrates, supporting the production of pro- or anti-inflammatory eicosanoids. Strengthening anti-inflammatory eicosanoid production may help to reduce the incidence and severity of asthma attacks.

Causes of asthma include genetic predisposition, infection, GERD, and obesity; environmental antigens, pollutants, irritants, emotional factors and stress.[6] Food reactions, including allergy and sensitivity, also play a role in asthma.[7] The genetic and epigenetically-linked atopic triad includes asthma, hay fever, and dermatitis. Antibiotic exposure early in life also predisposes to asthma.[8]

Pronounced imbalances in eicosanoid metabolism have been found in asthma suffers and atopic individuals.[13] Treatment with omega-3 fatty acids has been shown to improve outcome in some asthma suffers and to increase the level of urinary anti-inflammatory eicosanoids.[13-17]

**The incidence of asthma continues to be alarming, and deaths from asthma are high. Laboratory identification of fatty acid imbalance and lipid peroxidation may help guide interventions.**

Initial assessment of DP's plasma fatty acids (Figure 1) demonstrated very low levels of anti-inflammatory omega-3 and -6 fatty acids, EPA and DGLA, which are precursors of the anti-inflammatory resolvins and eicosanoids. Imbalances in the pro- and anti-inflammatory eicosanoids have been found in asthma patients.[13] Indeed, childhood ingestion of fish or fish oil high in anti-inflammatory fatty acids has been associated with reduced incidence of asthma. The inverse of this finding points to ramifications of long-term anti-inflammatory fatty acid deficiency.[15] Moreover, GLA is used to increase levels of DGLA. It, too has shown great promise as a tool in asthma management.[17]

Figure 1 of DP's findings also demonstrated long-term fatty acid deficiency as indicated by mead acid elevation. [18] Mead is an omega-9 non-essential polyunsaturated fatty acid (PUFA). Mead production is suggested to be the body's attempt to produce adequate PUFA when there is an insufficiency of essential PUFA such as EPA or GLA. However, mead is not an eicosanoid precursor. Its main role appears to be in membrane fluidity.

Increased lipid peroxidation indicative of oxidative stress (Figure 2), has been implicated in the pathogenesis of asthma.[19, 20] The elevated finding demonstrated the need for antioxidant support.

Treatment for DP was designed to normalize the fatty acid deficiencies by using supplemental DHA, EPA, and GLA. A combination of antioxidants was also prescribed to minimize lipid peroxidation.

On follow-up, DP reported remarkable improvement in her condition. Her asthma was resolved and she stated that for many months, she had no longer required her medications. Figures 3 and 4 demonstrated improved anti-inflammatory fatty acid levels and reduced lipid peroxidation. Her mead acid level was also normal, demonstrating resolution of the long-term deficiency. Her AA and GLA, however, were still elevated. It was recommended that DP discontinue GLA supplementation and avoid excess amounts of AA-containing foods such as red meat and pro-inflammatory foods such as sugars and simple carbohydrates, all of which may contribute to AA elevation.[11, 21]

# CONCLUSION

This case may be unusual in that full resolution of asthma was achieved by treating fatty acid imbalances and improving antioxidant status. Eicosanoid imbalances, however, have a strong etiopathogenic role in asthma, and anti-inflammatory fatty acid precursors may be an important adjunctive therapy for most patients, especially given the risks associated with commonly used medications.

There is probably a continuum of degree of response to fatty acid supplementation, depending on the extent of imbalance. Identifying the cohort of asthma sufferers who demonstrate omega-3 fatty acid deficiencies and following their response to intervention through a well-designed research trial may have a similar outcome as this case.

The incidence of asthma continues to be alarming, and deaths from asthma are high.[22] Identification of imbalances in fatty acids, specifically eicosanoid precursors, as well as of increased lipid peroxidation may illuminate the pathophysiology of an individual's asthma presentation. Treatment based on the findings may improve outcome for asthma sufferers.

---

**Author: Kara Fitzgerald, ND**

## References


1. Asthma Prevalence, Health Care Use and Mortality: United States. 2003-05. Centers for Disease Control Web Site. http://www.cdc.gov/nchs/data/hestat/asthma03-05/asthma03-05.htm. Accessed March 1, 2010.
2. Akinbami L. The State of Childhood Asthma, United States, 1980–2005. Centers for Disease Control Web Site. http://www.cdc.gov/nchs/data/ad/ad381.pdf. Accessed March 1, 2010.
3. McHugh MK, Symanski E, Pompeii LA, Delclos GL. Prevalence of asthma among adult females and males in the United States: results from the National Health and Nutrition Examination Survey (NHANES), 2001-2004. *J Asthma.* Oct 2009;46(8):759-766.
4. The Cost of Asthma. Asthma and Allergy Foundation of America Web Site. http://www.aafa.org/display.cfm?id=6&sub=63. Accessed March 1, 2010.
5. Abramson MJ, Bailey MJ, Couper FJ, et al. Are asthma medications and management related to deaths from asthma? *Am J Respir Crit Care Med.* Jan 2001;163(1):12-18.
6. emedicine. Asthma. http://www.emedicinehealth.com/asthma/article_em.htm. Accessed 6/23/2010, 2010.
7. Gillman A, Douglass JA. What do asthmatics have to fear from food and additive allergy? *Clin Exp Allergy.* May 26 2010.
8. Marra F, Marra CA, Richardson K, et al. Antibiotic use in children is associated with increased risk of asthma. *Pediatrics.* Mar 2009;123(3):1003-1010.
9. Mickleborough TD, Rundell KW. Dietary polyunsaturated fatty acids in asthma- and exercise-induced bronchoconstriction. *Eur J Clin Nutr.* Dec 2005;59(12):1335-1346.
10. Raz A. Dietary fish oil inhibits delta-6-desaturase activity in vivo. *Journal of the American Oil Chemists' Society.* 1998;75(2):241-245.
11. Persaud SJ, Muller D, Belin VD, et al. The role of arachidonic acid and its metabolites in insulin secretion from human islets of langerhans. *Diabetes.* Jan 2007;56(1):197-203.
12. Barrios RJ, Kheradmand F, Batts L, Corry DB. Asthma: pathology and pathophysiology. *Arch Pathol Lab Med.* Apr 2006;130(4):447-451.
13. Broughton KS, Johnson CS, Pace BK, Liebman M, Kleppinger KM. Reduced asthma symptoms with n-3 fatty acid ingestion are related to 5-series leukotriene production. *Am J Clin Nutr.* Apr 1997;65(4):1011-1017.

14. Fetterman JW, Jr., Zdanowicz MM. Therapeutic potential of n-3 polyunsaturated fatty acids in disease. *Am J Health Syst Pharm.* Jul 1 2009;66(13):1169-1179.

15. Laerum BN, Wentzel-Larsen T, Gulsvik A, et al. Relationship of fish and cod oil intake with adult asthma. *Clin Exp Allergy.* Nov 2007;37(11):1616-1623.

16. Mickleborough TD, Tecklenburg SL, Montgomery GS, Lindley MR. Eicosapentaenoic acid is more effective than docosahexaenoic acid in inhibiting proinflammatory mediator production and transcription from LPS-induced human asthmatic alveolar macrophage cells. *Clin Nutr.* Feb 2009;28(1):71-77.

17. Lindemann J, David Pampe E, Peterkin JJ, Orozco-Cronin P, Belofsky G, Stull D. Clinical study of the effects on asthma-related QOL and asthma management of a medical food in adult asthma patients. *Curr Med Res Opin.* Dec 2009;25(12):2865-2875.

18. *Laboratory Evaluations for Integrative and Functional Medicine.* Atlanta: Metametrix Institute; 2008.

19. Sharma A, Bansal S, Nagpal RK. Lipid peroxidation in bronchial asthma. *Indian J Pediatr.* Sep 2003;70(9):715-717.

20. Wood LG, Gibson PG, Garg ML. Biomarkers of lipid peroxidation, airway inflammation and asthma. *Eur Respir J.* Jan 2003;21(1):177-186.

21. Li D, Ng A, Mann NJ, Sinclair AJ. Contribution of meat fat to dietary arachidonic acid. *Lipids.* Apr 1998;33(4):437-440.

22. McCoy L, Redelings M, Sorvillo F, Simon P. A multiple cause-of-death analysis of asthma mortality in the United States, 1990-2001. *J Asthma.* Nov 2005;42(9):757-763.

# 11 Toxic Exposures

## Lead Toxicity

*Despite a steady decline in blood lead levels (BLLs) in children and adults, exposure to lead is still relatively common in the United States.[1, 2] In children, although the main exposure source continues to be lead-containing paint, lead-contaminated foods and toys have been identified as well.[3] In adults, the chief exposure sources include storage battery manufacturing, construction and home improvement (painting, paperhanging and decorating). Other sources include contaminated foods, medicines and liquids.[4] Over 300,000 children below five years of age have elevated BLLs.[5] In the adult population, toxic BLLs are much less common and are primarily seen in industry.[4] BLLs well within the CDC action level of 10 µg/dL, however, have been associated with clinically relevant symptoms. In the young adult U.S. population, there was more than twice the incidence of major depression and almost five times the incidence of panic disorder in persons with BLLs at 2.11 µg/dL or higher as compared to those with levels in the first quintile (0.7 µg/dL or less).[6] In another study, BLL levels of 3.6 µg/dL were associated with a 55% increase in cardiovascular mortality as compared to those at or below 1.9 µg/dL.6. BLLs well within the CDC limit of 10 µg/dL may be clinically significant, which suggests that the toxic effects of lead may be impacting far more individuals than previously thought.*

### 16-Year-Old Female with Neurologic Effects of Lead Toxicity

| | |
|---|---|
| **Additional Symptoms and Conditions** | Episodic ataxia, severe fatigue, muscle twitching, and difficulty concentrating; unable to attend high school; post-Lyme disease syndrome |
| **Tests Used** | Urine, erythrocyte, and whole blood lead; water source of lead |
| **Imbalances Identified** | Lead toxicity |
| **Treatments** | IV EDTA Chelation and essential elements |
| **Outcome** | After two years of treatment for lead toxicity, her symptoms improved enough for her to resume high school. She was able to graduate with minimal delay and begin college. She completed her freshman year without incident. |
| **Discussion/ Significance** | Successful treatment of lead toxicity is challenging, therefore limiting exposure is vital. However, because even low levels of lead exposure may be problematic, a chelator-provoked urine or whole blood lead assessment may be a prudent addition to annual or semi-annual preventative medical screenings. |

# CASE HISTORY

JP was 16 years old in 2005 when she presented with recent onset episodic ataxia, severe fatigue, muscle twitching, and difficulty concentrating. On account of the severity of her symptoms, she required medical leave from high school. Since she had been diagnosed, three years prior, with Lyme disease, from which she never completely recovered, her problem was diagnosed as post-Lyme disease syndrome (PLD).

**JP was 16 years old in 2005 when she presented with recent onset episodic ataxia, severe fatigue, muscle twitching, and difficulty concentrating... Water testing revealed that the drinking fountain water had lead levels of 205 ppb; the upper limit for acceptable EPA lead level is 15 ppb.**

As part of a comprehensive evaluation, JP was tested for lead exposure using an IV EDTA-provoked urine test (Figure 1-B). JP's lead level was found to be more than 10 times the (non-chelated) upper limit range of 5 μg/24 hours. The result was considered to be significant, and a diagnosis of lead toxicity was made. JP was treated primarily with IV EDTA and essential elements. She had a screening for lead in 2002 (Figure 1-A) that demonstrated normal levels.

It was discovered that the lead exposure source was a single school water fountain from which the patient and her friends had been regularly drinking for three years. Water testing revealed that the drinking fountain water had lead levels of 205 ppb; the upper limit for acceptable EPA lead-level is 15 ppb (Figure 1-C). Further investigation revealed that the water fountain had been recalled by the manufacturer on account of a faulty refrigeration holding tank that was leaching lead into the water. The school was unaware of the recall. Although JP's friends described similar neurological symptoms, JP's response appeared to be more severe. It was speculated that her reaction may have been complicated by post-Lyme syndrome.

With ongoing IV EDTA treatment, JP's lead levels slowly dropped to normal over a two-year period (Figures 1-D, E, and F). She continued to experience symptoms of lead toxicity through early 2007. In the summer of 2007, symptoms subsided enough to allow her to return to high school in the autumn. She was able to graduate high school in 2008. In June of 2009, her physician was happy to report that JP had completed her freshman year of college.

NOTES

# Significant Laboratory Results 2002–2007

**Laboratory tests ordered and rationale:**

1. **EDTA-provoked urine lead**: A reliable measure of the toxic fraction of the total body lead burden[7]
2. **Erythrocyte lead**: RBCs readily take up lead from blood,[8] and may therefore reflect toxicity.
3. **Whole blood lead**: Assessment of recent lead exposure, most common specimen used[9]
4. **Water tested for lead**: Establishment of lead exposure source

| | Result | | 95% Reference Interval |
|---|---|---|---|
| ***A. 2002 RBC Lead Levels (pre-exposure)*** | | | |
| Lead | 0.04 | | <= 0.10 |
| ***B. 2005 24-hour Urine Lead Levels (with EDTA Provoction)*** | | | |
| Lead | 42 µg/24 hour | H | < 5 µg/24 hour |
| ***C. 2005 Water Lead Levels*** | | | |
| Lead | 205 ppb | H | < 15 ppb |
| ***D. RBC Lead 2006*** | | | |
| Lead | 0.117 | H | <= 0.030 |
| ***E. Whole Blood Lead 2006*** | | | |
| Lead | 12 | H | < 10 µg/dl |
| ***F. Whole Blood Lead 2007*** | | | |
| Lead | 1.9 µg/dl | | < 10 µg/dl |

**Figure 1. Test results.** Lead measurements in different specimens over time

Lead damage includes the hemopoietic, musculoskeletal, cardiac, nervous and genitourinary systems. Rapid diagnosis and treatment are hindered by the variable clinical presentation, make the diagnosis of lead toxicity difficult.

# DISCUSSION

Human exposure to toxic metals has been excessive since industrialization, and it continues to be common despite efforts to limit the exposure.[1,2] Lead damage includes the hemopoietic, musculoskeletal, cardiac, nervous and genitourinary systems.[10] Rapid diagnosis and treatment are hindered by the variable clinical presentation, making the diagnosis of lead toxicity difficult.[11]

In this case, three years of regular lead exposure had occurred before the patient was diagnosed with lead toxicity and the source identified. The patient's exposure to the lead-contaminated water started in the very year of her Lyme disease diagnosis. It is possible that the lead exposure exacerbated the symptoms of Lyme disease or that the symptoms of lead toxicity were mistaken for Lyme disease (or the later diagnosis of post-Lyme disease syndrome), all of which can show impaired neurological function and therefore present similarly.[12-14] Fortunately, the lead toxicity and exposure source were eventually identified, with the result that appropriate treatment could be initiated. Figure 1 showed lead measurements in different specimen over time. A normal BLL was achieved in 2007 and correlated with symptom improvement.

While this case is demonstrative of frank lead toxicity, BLLs less than 4 µg/dL have been associated with cardiovascular disease, depression and panic disorder. Subclinical BLL has also been associated with increased all-cause mortality (3.6 µg/dL).[6] In children, levels at or below 2.2 µg/dL were associated with increased incidence of ADHD.[15] Lowered IQ has also been strongly demonstrated in multiple studies in children with lower BLLs.[16]

Because BLLs below the CDC cutoff of 10 µg/dL are clinically significant in both children and adults,[17-19] recommendations to lower the current CDC cutoff of 10 µg/dL have been proposed. However, it has been argued that there may be no safe threshold for lead exposure.[175, 6, 1115, 16] As the toxic effects of ever lower amounts of lead have been recognized over time, action levels for exposure have likewise been reduced over time (Figure 2).

**In children, levels at or below 2.2 µg/dL were associated with increased incidence of ADHD. Lowered IQ has also been demonstrated in multiple studies in children with lower BLLs.**

The primary sources of occupational lead exposure are found in battery manufacturing, construction and home improvement industries.[4] Non-occupational exposures include water, food, dust, paints, leaded gasoline, soil and kitchen utensils.[3, 10] Certain herbal and calcium (bone, dolomite) supplements have been associated with high lead levels.[20] As illustrated in this case, most occurrences of lead poisoning are due to oral ingestion and absorption through the gut.

Since successful treatment of lead toxicity is challenging, limiting exposure to lead is of prime importance. If exposure does occur, however, early identification and treatment will improve outcomes. Annual or semi-annual testing for lead toxicity using (provoked) urine to identify total body burden, or whole blood to identify recent exposure may be prudent.[7,9] For treatment, research demonstrates the efficacy of IV CaNa(2) ethylenediaminetetraacetic acid (EDTA) in reducing soft tissue lead levels.[21] Since chelation will remove essential elements, regular laboratory assessment of, and treatment with, essential elements should be conducted. Adjunctive nutrient support for the lead-exposed patient is also important. Supplementation with calcium has been shown to reduce lead levels in pregnant women,[22] and antioxidants have been shown to lower lead levels and to be protective against lead-induced oxidative damage.[23] In children, nutritional therapy, especially that involving the essential elements iron, zinc and calcium, may be warranted.

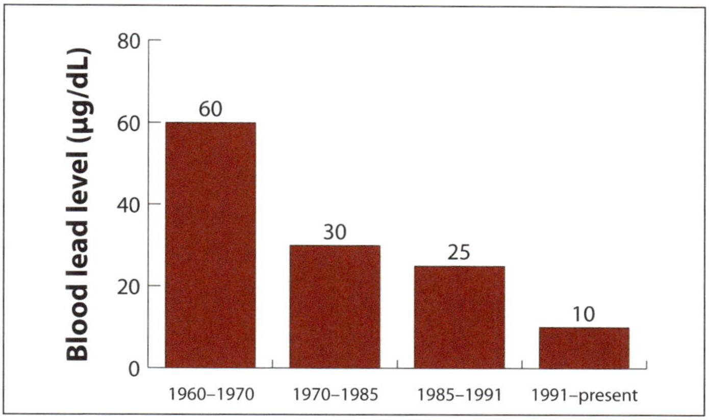


**Figure 2. CDC blood lead levels that require action have lowered over time.** Most recent data (not shown here) recommend action in children at levels below 10 µg/dL.[18, 25]

# CONCLUSION

In this case, the patient experienced years-long debilitation resulting from lead toxicity. Fortunately, the source of lead exposure was identified and removed, and on-going chelation and nutrient therapy allowed the patient to resume her life with presumably normal function. It is possible, however, that the diagnosis of lead toxicity was delayed in this case because the symptoms may have been similar to Lyme disease (or post-Lyme disease syndrome), conditions with which the patient was concurrently diagnosed.

Because lead can interfere with metabolic function in most organ systems, symptoms associated with lead toxicity are often insidious and may mimic other conditions, making diagnosis of lead toxicity elusive. Furthermore, numerous conditions have been associated with lead exposure at levels well within normal limits, including cardiovascular disease, major depression, panic disorder and ADHD. Because of these findings, it has been recommended that the CDC lead action level of 10 µg/dL be lowered, although research suggests that there may be no safe threshold for lead exposure.

Although avoidance of lead exposure is optimal, it may be unrealistic. Therefore, early diagnosis and treatment of lead toxicity is imperative. Laboratory testing for lead using provoked urine or whole blood assay should be included as a part of any annual or semi-annual preventive medicine protocol.

---

**Authors: Kara Fitzgerald, ND; Christie Egeston, MS**
**Case Clinician: Kathy Keipura, MD**

## References


1. Lord RS, Bralley JA, eds. *Laboratory Evaluations for Integrative and Functional Medicine.* 2nd ed. Duluth, GA: Metametrix Institute; 2008.
2. Howard Hu MD, M.P.H., Sc.D. *HUMAN HEALTH AND HEAVY METALS EXPOSURE*: MIT press; 2002.
3. CDC. Lead Prevention Tips. http://www.cdc.gov/nceh/lead/tips.htm. Accessed May 12, 2010.
4. CDC. Adult Blood Lead Epidemiology and Surveillance – United States, 2003. *MMWR.* 2006;55(32):876-879.
5. Warniment C, Tsang K, Galazka SS. Lead poisoning in children. *Am Fam Physician.* Mar 15;81(6):751-757.
6. Bouchard MF, Bellinger DC, Weuve J, et al. Blood lead levels and major depressive disorder, panic disorder, and generalized anxiety disorder in US young adults. *Arch Gen Psychiatry.* Dec 2009;66(12):1313-1319.
7. ATSDR. Toxicological Profile for Lead http://www.atsdr.cdc.gov/toxprofiles/tp13.pdf, pg. 230.
8. ATSDR. Toxicological Profile for Lead. http://www.atsdr.cdc.gov/toxprofiles/tp13-c3.pdf, p. 204.
9. ATSDR. Toxicological Profile for Lead. http://www.atsdr.cdc.gov/toxprofiles/tp13-c3.pdf, p. 1.
10. Papanikolaou NC, Hatzidaki EG, Belivanis S, Tzanakakis GN, Tsatsakis AM. Lead toxicity update. A brief review. *Med Sci Monit.* Oct 2005;11(10):RA329-336.
11. Coon T, Miller M, Shirazi F, Sullivan J. Lead toxicity in a 14-year-old female with retained bullet fragments. *Pediatrics.* Jan 2006;117(1):227-230.
12. Pfister HW, Rupprecht TA. Clinical aspects of neuroborreliosis and post-Lyme disease syndrome in adult patients. *Int J Med Microbiol.* May 2006;296 Suppl 40:11-16.
13. Lockitch G. Perspectives on lead toxicity. *Clin Biochem.* Oct 1993;26(5):371-381.
14. Goyer RA. Lead toxicity: from overt to subclinical to subtle health effects. *Environ Health Perspect.* Jun 1990;86:177-181.
15. Nigg JT, Nikolas M, Mark Knottnerus G, Cavanagh K, Friderici K. Confirmation and extension of association of blood lead with attention-deficit/hyperactivity disorder (ADHD) and ADHD symptom domains at population-typical exposure levels. *J Child Psychol Psychiatry.* Jan 2010;51(1):58-65.
16. Needleman HL, Gatsonis CA. Low-level lead exposure and the IQ of children. A meta-analysis of modern studies. *JAMA.* Feb 2 1990;263(5):673-678.
17. Canfield RL, Henderson CR, Jr., Cory-Slechta DA, Cox C, Jusko TA, Lanphear BP. Intellectual impairment in children with blood lead concentrations below 10 microg per deciliter. *N Engl J Med.* Apr 17 2003;348(16):1517-1526.
18. CDC. Interpreting and Managing Blood Lead Levels <10 µg/dL in Children and Reducing Childhood Exposures to Lead. http://www.cdc.gov/mmwr/preview/mmwrhtml/rr5608a1.htm.
19. Rossi E. Low level environmental lead exposure - a continuing challenge. *Clin Biochem Rev.* May 2008;29(2):63-70.
20. Ross EA, Szabo NJ, Tebbett IR. Lead content of calcium supplements. *Jama.* Sep 20 2000;284(11):1425-1429.
21. Seaton CL, Lasman J, Smith DR. The effects of CaNa(2)EDTA on brain lead mobilization in rodents determined using a stable lead isotope tracer. *Toxicol Appl Pharmacol.* 1999;159(3):153-160.
22. Ettinger AS, Lamadrid-Figueroa H, Tellez-Rojo MM, et al. Effect of calcium supplementation on blood lead levels in pregnancy: a randomized placebo-controlled trial. *Environ Health Perspect.* Jan 2009;117(1):26-31.
23. Patrick L. Lead toxicity part II: the role of free radical damage and the use of antioxidants in the pathology and treatment of lead toxicity. *Altern Med Rev.* Jun 2006;11(2):114-127.
24. Goyer RA. Lead toxicity: current concerns. *Environ Health Perspect.* Apr 1993;100:177-187.
25. ATSDR. Toxicological Profile for Lead. http://www.atsdr.cdc.gov/toxprofiles/tp13.pdf.

# Environmental Organic Toxins

*There are nearly 80,000 chemicals on the market in the United States, with 1,000 new chemicals introduced annually.[1] Most of these chemicals are largely unregulated, and the toxic effects of many have either not been studied or have been understudied. While occupational exposure to known toxicants continues to be a major problem world-wide,[2] many such compounds are also encountered in normal daily life. These exposures are particularly concerning, given that a study found more than 200 chemicals, including bis-phenol A,[3] in newborn cord blood and that the half-life of certain aliphatic toxins may exceed 15 years.[4] Common classes of environmental toxins found in human specimens include volatile solvents, polychlorinated biphenyls, phthalates, pesticides and dioxins.[5, 6] These compounds may be encountered in foods, plastics, body lotions and other common household items. Synergistic toxicity among multiple chemicals is suspected, although research is still forthcoming.[7]Disease conditions associated with environmental toxins involve all organ systems, with endocrine and central nervous systems being particularly vulnerable.[5] Cancers, diabetes, neurodevelopmental and neurodegenerative, psychiatric, reproductive, allergic, respiratory, musculoskeletal and autoimmune disorders have all been associated with environmental toxin exposure.[5, 8-12] In view of the aforementioned body-burden of chemicals—many of them known toxicants—avoidance of exposure is the primary recommended intervention, if difficult to achieve. Evidenced-based post-exposure treatment options are few, despite an urgent need for them.*

## 43-Year-Old Male with Volatile Solvent-Induced Neurotoxicity

| | |
|---|---|
| **Additional Symptoms and Conditions** | Bipolar disorder, memory loss, insomnia, hypothyroidism |
| **Medications** | Lithium, clonazapam, diphenhydramine, levothyroxine |
| **Tests Used** | Blood volatile solvents, oxidative stress markers, organic acids, amino acids, intradermal food allergy testing |
| **Imbalances Identified** | Elevated volatile solvents, oxidative stress, $B_6$ insufficiency, amino acid insufficiency, multiple food allergies |
| **Treatments** | Volatile solvent avoidance, intravenous nutrients including minerals, amino acids and vitamins, melatonin and sauna therapy |
| **Outcome** | Memory deficits resolved, bipolar hypomania lessened, insomnia improved, lithium dosage reduced; clonazapam, diphenhydramine, levothyroxine stopped |
| **Discussion/ Significance** | Environmental organic toxins are ubiquitous and thought to be an etiopathogenic factor in many diseases. Although exposure to these toxins is unavoidable, widely accepted evidenced-based treatment options are scant. In this case, the patient's chronic exposure to volatile solvents in the workplace resulted in significantly impaired memory and was involved in the precipitation of adult-onset bipolar disorder. Along with avoidance of toxin exposure, IV nutrient therapy, sauna and a nutrient-rich hypoallergenic organic diet led to an improvement in, or resolution of, all symptoms. |

# CASE HISTORY

RS was 43 years old when he presented with a history of progressive memory impairment and diagnosis of a three-year-long bipolar disorder. The bipolar presentation consisted primarily of hypomania with severe insomnia; his affect was otherwise generally flat, his speech was not fluent, and he was more dull than depressed. He could be irritable and easily roused to anger, although he was not violent. RS presented as awake, alert and oriented to person, place and time, but his memory deficits rendered him incapable of reliable recall. Thus, RS was dependant on his wife for memory support, including for his own medical history. RS's wife thought that there had been a slow, but steady decline in his mental function over many years. The bipolar diagnosis seemed to be an extension of the mental decline, rather than a cause of it. Previously, he was a generally happy, hardworking individual with a positive outlook on life. RS had undergone extensive medical evaluations over the years, including laboratory and imaging by numerous specialists. All findings were unremarkable, although a diagnosis of mercury toxicity had been made at one point. Intravenous chelation therapy using dimercaptosuccinic acid (DMSA) and 2,3-dimercapto-1-propanesulfonic acid (DMPS) was completed, but not apparently helpful.

> Disease conditions associated with environmental toxins involve all organ systems, with endocrine and central nervous systems being particularly vulnerable.

RS was prescribed lithium and clonazepam for the bipolar disorder which were of limited benefit. He took diphenhydramine for insomnia, which was also of only limited benefit. He took numerous supplements including fish oil, vitamins C, E, B complex and $B_{12}$, garlic, and essential minerals.

RS had been unable to perform many of his work duties for the six months prior to his initial clinic visit. He was an executive and co-owner in his family's fabric printing business for over 10 years, but had been experiencing hallucination and mania at work, significantly diminishing his capacity to function. His wife noted that historically his symptoms improved when he was away from the business for a period of time, although in the recent past these improvements were less apparent. She explained that at work, he was chronically exposed to many chemicals, including solvents, pigments and dyes. There was no family history of neurodegenerative or psychiatric conditions, including memory loss, dementia and bipolar disorder.

RS ate a standard American diet. He did not consume alcohol, use tobacco, or engage in recreational drug use. Apart from the noted memory deficits, RS's physical exam was unremarkable, including his neurological evaluation. RS's past medical history included chronic sinusitis, hypothyroidism (treated with levothyroxine) and onychomycosis. He reported no known drug, food or environmental allergies.

# Initial Laboratory Results

**Laboratory tests ordered and rationale:**

1. **Volatile solvents**: RS's history was compelling for chronic occupational solvent exposure, which is documented to cause neuropsychiatric conditions including memory loss and dementia.[2]
2. **Multiprofile panel**: A comprehensive direct and functional assessment of nutrient status was conducted using organic acids, amino acids, and oxidative stress markers. The panel evaluates nutrient deficits, oxidative and inflammatory stressors that may contribute to the etipathogenesis of the presenting condition. Only the significant findings are discussed.
3. **Intradermal food allergy testing (completed in-office, results not shown)**: Immunological reactions to foods have been associated with chronic sinusitis and psychiatric complaints including depression and anxiety.[13,14] IFAT is contraindicated in individuals at risk for anaphylaxis. RS demonstrated a positive response to: milk, egg, wheat, corn, tomato and potato.

| | Results (ppb) | | Percentile Ranking by Quintile (1st, 2nd, 3rd, 4th, 5th; 20%, 40%, 60%, 80%) | 95th Percentile (ppb) |
|---|---|---|---|---|
| Hexane | >700 | H | 500.0 | <= 700.0 |
| 2-Methylpentane | 123.0 | H | 68.0 | <= 84.0 |
| 3-Methylpentane | 260.0 | H | 103.0 | <= 128.0 |

**Figure 1. Volatile solvents.** Evaluation revealed extremely elevated levels

| | | | | |
|---|---|---|---|---|
| Lipid Peroxides | 2.70 | H | 1.72 | <= 2.60 |
| 8-Hydroxy-2-deoxyguanosine ** | 14.0 | H | 5.3 | <= 7.6 |

** Units for 8-Hydroxy-2-deoxyguanosine are ng/mg creatinine

**Figure 2. Oxidative stress markers.** High oxidative stress was present in cellular membrane as evidenced by the elevated lipid peroxides and in DNA, as indicated by the DNA damage marker 8-Hydroxy-2-deoxyguanosine (8OH-2'dG). (Lipid peroxide units: nmol/mL)

| | | | | |
|---|---|---|---|---|
| Xanthurenate | 1.40 | H | 0.47 | <= 0.74 |

**Figure 3. Urinary organic acids.** Elevated xanthurenate was suggestive of vitamin $B_6$ deficiency. (Units: µg/mg creatinine)

| Ranges: Ages 13 and over | Results umol/L | | Quintile Ranking (1st / 2nd / 3rd / 4th / 5th) | | 95% Reference Interval |
|---|---|---|---|---|---|
| **Essential Amino Acids** | | | | | |
| *Limiting Amino Acids* | | | | | |
| 1. Lysine | 121 | | 117 | 203 | 99 - 234 |
| 2. Methionine | 17 | | 16 | 26 | 14 - 30 |
| 3. Tryptophan | 41 | | 35 | 59 | 30 - 67 |
| *Branched Chain Amino Acids* | | | | | |
| 4. Isoleucine | 29 | L | 40 | 72 | 33 - 89 |
| 5. Leucine | 62 | L | 80 | 137 | 68 - 161 |
| 6. Valine | 118 | L | 143 | 240 | 123 - 282 |
| *Other Essential Amino Acids* | | | | | |
| 7. Phenylalanine | 45 | | 43 | 64 | 39 - 74 |
| 8. Histidine | 53 | | 48 | 72 | 41 - 82 |
| 9. Threonine | 58 | L | 76 | 151 | 63 - 181 |
| *Conditionally Essential Amino Acids* | | | | | |
| 10. Arginine | 33 | L | 48 | 96 | 37 - 114 |
| 11. Taurine | 34 | | 31 | 73 | 26 - 100 |
| 12. Glycine | 131 | L | 162 | 348 | 136 - 430 |
| 13. Serine | 52 | L | 66 | 115 | 57 - 133 |
| **Functional Categories** | | | | | |
| *Vascular Function* | | | | | |
| 14. Arginine | 33 | L | 48 | 96 | 37 - 114 |
| 15. Taurine | 34 | | 31 | 73 | 26 - 100 |
| *Neurotransmitters and Precursors* | | | | | |
| 16. Phenylalanine | 45 | | 43 | 64 | 39 - 74 |
| 17. Tyrosine | 23 | L | 38 | 70 | 29 - 80 |
| 18. Tryptophan | 41 | | 35 | 59 | 30 - 67 |
| 19. Glutamic Acid | 20 | L | 29 | 95 | 23 - 136 |
| 20. Taurine | 34 | | 31 | 73 | 26 - 100 |
| *Sulfur Amino Acids (Glutathione - related)* | | | | | |
| 21. Methionine | 17 | | 16 | 26 | 14 - 30 |
| 22. Taurine | 34 | | 31 | 73 | 26 - 100 |

**Figure 4. Plasma amino acids.** Multiple essential and non-essential amino acids levels were low. (Units: µmol/L)

## Initial Assessment

- Volatile solvent-induced neurotoxicity (presenting as memory impairment)
- Bipolar disorder
- Multiple food allergies
- Nutrient insufficiencies
- Oxidative stress
- Hypothyroidism
- Chronic sinusitis
- Onychomycosis

## Initial Plan

- Avoid highly polluted areas, including work environment
- Install home air filtration system and water filter
- Comprehensive plan for work environment to be implemented prior to returning: reduce reliance on toxic chemicals, evaluate alternative options, install factory-wide exhaust and air filtration systems.
- Organic hypoallergenic rotation diet based on intradermal testing (avoid milk, egg, wheat, corn, tomato and potato)
- Filtered water intake: ½ body weight in ounces per day
- Preservative-free intravenous nutrient protocol (administered 2 × per week) for 12 sessions
  - IV ingredients: glutathione, 600 mg; taurine, 2 gm; ascorbic acid 12.5 gm; B complex vitamins 50 mg each of $B_1$, $B_2$, $B_3$, $B_5$ and $B_6$; magnesium sulfate, 5 gm; and 2 cc of a trace minerals solution containing 8 µg Cr, 0.2 mg Mn, 40 µg Se, 0.8 mg Cu, and 2 mg Zn with sodium bicarbonate to neutralize the low pH of ascorbic acid
- Continue at-home supplement protocol
- Sauna therapy, 2 sessions per week (A non-toxic, glue-free, aged-wood sauna was used)

**Treatment plan rationale:** The extremely high levels of volatile solvents (VS) in RS's blood and his years-long neurodegeneration suggested that he—and likely others at his business—were being chronically poisoned. It was therefore imperative that he continue to avoid the work environment during early treatment, and that a safer workspace be established, which involved the installation of high-quality air filtration and ventilation systems and a reduction in the use of toxic chemicals. Furthermore, a comprehensive plan involving air and water filtration and a hypoallergenic, organic diet to minimize toxic exposure was initiated at home. Both anxiety and depression have been associated with food reactions, and thus it is possible that his positive findings on intradermal testing were exacerbating his toxicity symtoms.[13, 14]

The recognized interventions for acute VS toxicity are toxin avoidance and supportive therapies based on presentation of symptoms that frequently consist of nephrological, pulmonological, cardiovascular and gastrointestinal problems.[2] Permanent neurological damage in the chronically exposed individual is not uncommon.[2] However, integrative clinicians working with the VS-exposed patient find that high-dose, long term IV nutrient therapy and regular sauna—both of which are designed to support phase I and II liver detoxification—are useful treatments that may reverse symptomology.[15-17] That being the case, both therapies were started with this patient, individualized according to his nutrient needs as identified on laboratory analysis.

## One-Month Follow-up

With some recall difficulty, RS discussed how he had responded to treatment over the month previous, which suggested improvement in his memory, as he had not been able to provide such a history at his initial office visit. His wife also thought that RS's mood was more stable. Although RS was sleeping better, he reported that insomnia was still an issue. There was no change to the treatment plan.

## Four-Month Follow-up

RS reported that he felt physically and emotionally stronger. His affect was no longer flat, and his speech was once again fluent. A trial visit to his company resulted, however, in a return of symptoms. Insomnia continued to be a periodic challenge. He had not experienced sinusitis since the start of treatment. A six-week course of IV nutrient therapy was reinstated; otherwise, there was no change to the treatment plan.

A follow-up volatile solvents test was ordered.

NOTES

# Eight-Month Follow-up

RS was well enough to resume working. He felt happy, and his memory was restored. He did not feel excessively angry or aggressive. He was able to tolerate the work environment (which had been cleaned up considerably) without a recurrence of symptoms. His lithium was reduced and his clonazapam was stopped, as he no longer required it. (Lithium is known to induce hypothyroidism. It was hoped that reduction in his dosage might improve his thyroid function.[18]) Insomnia continued to be an occasional issue. Overall, he showed remarkable improvement. He and his family were very pleased and grateful for his recovery. Melatonin 3 mg/QHS was added to his treatment plan, no other changes were made.

**Along with avoidance of toxin exposure, IV nutrient therapy, sauna and a nutrient-rich hypoallergenic organic diet led to an improvement in, or resolution of, all symptoms.**

## Eight-Month Follow-up Laboratory Results

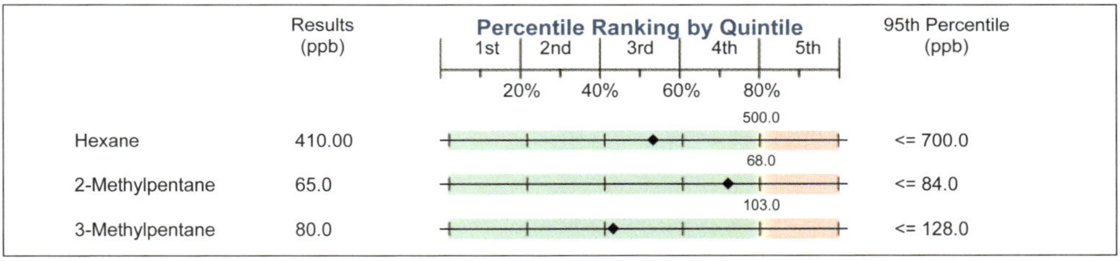


**Figure 5. Follow-up volatile solvents.** Significant improvement from baseline levels was found.

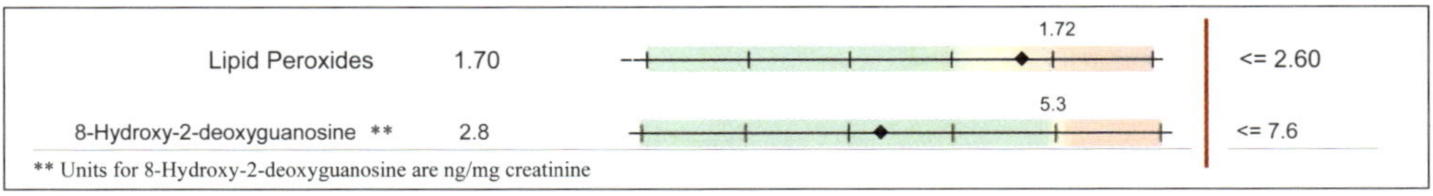


**Figure 6. Follow-up oxidative stress markers.** Significant improvement in both markers was found. (Lipid peroxide units: nmol/mL)

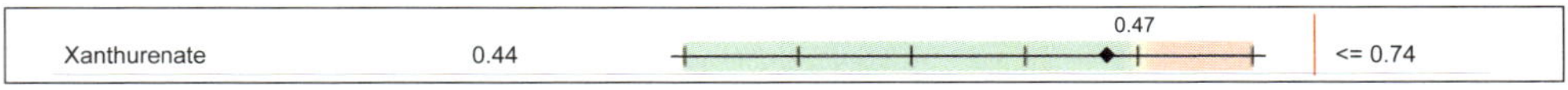


**Figure 7. Follow-up urinary organic acids.** Xanthurenate level was within normal limits, demonstrating improved functional vitamin $B_6$ status. (Units: µg/mg creatinine)

| Ranges: Ages 13 and over | Results umol/L | Quintile Ranking (1st, 2nd, 3rd, 4th, 5th) | 95% Reference Interval |
|---|---|---|---|
| ***Essential Amino Acids*** | | | |
| ***Limiting Amino Acids*** | | | |
| 1. Lysine | 201 | 117 – 203 | 99 - 234 |
| 2. Methionine | 21 | 16 – 26 | 14 - 30 |
| 3. Tryptophan | 58 | 35 – 59 | 30 - 67 |
| ***Branched Chain Amino Acids*** | | | |
| 4. Isoleucine | 47 | 40 – 72 | 33 - 89 |
| 5. Leucine | 115 | 80 – 137 | 68 - 161 |
| 6. Valine | 222 | 143 – 240 | 123 - 282 |
| ***Other Essential Amino Acids*** | | | |
| 7. Phenylalanine | 60 | 43 – 64 | 39 - 74 |
| 8. Histidine | 61 | 48 – 72 | 41 - 82 |
| 9. Threonine | 111 | 76 – 151 | 63 - 181 |
| ***Conditionally Essential Amino Acids*** | | | |
| 10. Arginine | 75 | 48 – 96 | 37 - 114 |
| 11. Taurine | 70 | 31 – 73 | 26 - 100 |
| 12. Glycine | 201 | 162 – 348 | 136 - 430 |
| 13. Serine | 85 | 66 – 115 | 57 - 133 |
| ***Functional Categories*** | | | |
| ***Vascular Function*** | | | |
| 14. Arginine | 75 | 48 – 96 | 37 - 114 |
| 15. Taurine | 70 | 31 – 73 | 26 - 100 |
| ***Neurotransmitters and Precursors*** | | | |
| 16. Phenylalanine | 60 | 43 – 64 | 39 - 74 |
| 17. Tyrosine | 59 | 38 – 70 | 29 - 80 |
| 18. Tryptophan | 58 | 35 – 59 | 30 - 67 |
| 19. Glutamic Acid | 51 | 29 – 95 | 23 - 136 |
| 20. Taurine | 70 | 31 – 73 | 26 - 100 |
| ***Sulfur Amino Acids (Glutathione - related)*** | | | |
| 21. Methionine | 21 | 16 – 26 | 14 - 30 |
| 22. Taurine | 70 | 31 – 73 | 26 - 100 |

**Figure 8. Follow-up plasma amino acids.** Levels demonstrated significant improvement from baseline. (Units: µmol/L)

## 24-Month Follow-up

RS continued to thrive. He no longer required clonazapam or diphenhydramine. His lithium dose was minimal and well-tolerated.

### 24-Month Follow-up Laboratory Results

| | Results (ppb) | Percentile Ranking by Quintile (1st, 2nd, 3rd, 4th, 5th; 20%, 40%, 60%, 80%) | 95th Percentile (ppb) |
|---|---|---|---|
| Hexane | 200.00 | 500.0 | <= 700.0 |
| 2-Methylpentane | 33.0 | 68.0 | <= 84.0 |
| 3-Methylpentane | 20.0 | 103.0 | <= 128.0 |

**Figure 9. Volatile Solvents.** After two years of treatment, volatile solvents were at low levels.

# DISCUSSION

Organic solvents are ubiquitous worldwide; sources include paints, paint thinners, pharmaceuticals, degreasing agents, adhesives, printing inks, pesticides, cosmetics and cleaners. Solvent exposure is common. Without appropriate precautions, including limiting exposure, protective clothing and sufficient ventilation, toxic exposure levels may be achieved. Additionally, solvent co-exposures, nutrient deficiencies, or genetic weaknesses in liver detoxification pathways may potentiate toxic effects.[19]

Hexane specifically is found in petroleum compounds, including paint, glues, adhesives, gasoline, automobile exhaust and jet fuel and jet exhaust. N-hexane is also used to extract oil from grain and protein from soy. Interestingly, it has been suggested that its use in the latter capacity may be the current greatest contributor to hexane emissions.[20]

In this case, the patient's baseline blood level of the solvent n-hexane and its isomers 2-methylpentane and 3-methylpentane (hereafter collectively referred to as hexane) were markedly elevated—well above the laboratory's 95$^{th}$ reference interval—suggesting occupational exposure (Figure 1). However, it was determined that the patient was not exposed to high levels of hexane outside the work environment, and he had not been in the work environment for six months prior to the baseline assessment. The half-life of hexane is variable depending on tissue type. In blood, it is understood to be about 92 minutes, but is greater than 10 days in adipose tissue. Partition coefficient data, which may be used to assess uptake and distribution of organotoxins in mammals, demonstrates that hexane preferentially bioaccumulates in fat.[21,22] Thus, it may be that while the patient was not under current exposure, hexane was mobilized from adipose tissue during lipolysis, thereby allowing for a higher blood level to be maintained, even during non-exposure. This has been demonstrated to occur with other lipophilic organotoxins during weight loss.[23] The fact that his blood hexane levels dropped to below detection over the course of his treatment

(Figures 1, 5 and 9) lend support to the hypothesis. However, the data on human adipose bioaccumulation and liberation of hexane are scant.

Another consideration is that the patient was under current exposure, but because of the great variety of toxicant sources, many of which are difficult to detect, it is common that the exact origins of elevated toxicants remains unknown. One must therefore proceed on the laboratory evidence of exposure and the results of the many studies showing potential biochemical or cellular effects that may manifest as diseases in humans, regardless of knowledge of source.

Memory impairment and neuropsychiatric changes were the chief effects thought to be attributed to hexane toxicity in this case. Neurotoxicity due to solvent exposure has been well studied; symptoms are even predictable by certain psychological tests

Hexane toxicity symptoms typically initiate in the periphery, with neurological damage being the most common and well-documented effect in humans. Neurotoxicity resulting from hexane inhalation of as little as 58 ppm daily over a period of years has been found in humans. Research has found hexane toxicity associated with damage to most organ systems, including the neurological, reproductive, renal, gastroenterological, endocrine and immunological, in animals, along with increased incidence of cancers and developmental issues.[19] A recent case involving the use of n-hexane as a cleaning agent in a company developing touch screen applications resulted in the death of an employee. It was later reported that severe n-hexane poisoning at the company was found in the case of 61 other employees.[24, 25]

Memory impairment and neuropsychiatric changes were the chief effects thought to be attributed to hexane toxicity in this case. Neurotoxicity due to solvent exposure has been well studied; symptoms are even predictable by certain psychological tests.[26] Psychological effects from exposure to fabric screen-printing chemicals have been documented—a particularly significant finding, given the patient's ownership of a fabric printing business.[27] Studies have suggested that chronic, high-level solvent exposure might be associated with a syndrome of personality change, memory impairment, and neurological deficits that is termed solvent neurotoxicity.[2] A categorization of these neurobehavioral changes has been created that identifies severity of exposure and progression of damage.[28] The mechanism of such changes has been attributed to alteration in neuronal membrane and modification of CNS oxidative metabolism.[29] GABA and glutamatergic neuronal alterations have been specifically implicated in CNS solvent toxicity. Hexane-induced peripheral nervous-system damage has been associated with demyelination.[29]

It is not surprising that high levels of oxidative stress in the forms of lipid peroxidation (indicating excess damage to lipid membranes) and 8-hydroxy 2' deoxyguanosine (8-OHdG)—a marker of oxidation damage to the DNA[30]—were identified in this individual (Figure 2). Solvent-induced free-radical activity has been a well-documented molecular mechanism of toxicity.[31] N-hexane-mediated damage is thought to occur through the production of free radicals, including hydroxyl radicals.[19] Many studies have shown an increase, compared with controls or according to solvent exposure levels, of 8-OHdG in solvent-exposed subjects.[32-34] Increased lipid peroxidation was found in workers engaged in a profession involving exposure to solvents for more than five years.[35]

Individuals with nutrient insufficiencies and/or genetic limitations involved in liver detoxification and biotransformation pathways may be particularly vulnerable to the toxic effects of hexane.[19] In this case, functional evidence suggesting $B_6$ deficiency, as indicated by elevated xanthurenic acid, was identified (Figure 3).[36] Low plasma amino-acid levels were also found (Figure 4). Amino acids are key substrates in phase II liver detoxification and in antioxidation; $B_6$ is required for transaminase reactions involved in the production of amino acids including glutathione, taurine and glycine—key detoxification and antioxidant compounds. Thus, low levels of these may have impacted the patient's ability to eliminate the solvents, potentiating their toxic effects.

As discussed above in the treatment rationale, interventions were designed to eliminate toxin exposure at home and at work, and to assist in removal of the body burden. A whole food, hypoallergenic, organic diet, IV nutrient therapy based on laboratory findings and sauna therapy were the main interventions employed. This approach has been demonstrated to be useful in treating chemically-exposed individuals.[15,16] Follow-up visits showed clear clinical improvements, demonstrating the efficacy of the approach used. At the 8- and 24-month follow-up visits, hexane levels were obtained that showed a continued reduction from baseline to acceptable levels (Figures 5 and 9). Oxidant stress markers, as well as xanthurenate and plasma amino acid levels, were also obtained at the 8-month follow-up visit (Figures 6, 7 and 8). All findings showed significant improvement, corroborating clinical improvements.

**It is not surprising that high levels of oxidative stress in the forms of lipid peroxidation and 8-hydroxy 2′deoxyguanosine (8-OHdG) —a marker of oxidation damage to the DNA—were identified in this individual. Solvent-induced free-radical activity has been a well-documented molecular mechanism of toxicity.**

# CONCLUSION

Environmental organic toxins are ubiquitous and, in the U.S., their compounds are found in high numbers in most individuals. The effects of many of these compounds on health are not yet well-characterized, on account of limited toxicology study, although etiopathogenic links to many diseases are strongly suspected.

Occupational solvent exposure-related toxicity is better understood, but continues with relatively little regulatory intervention. Fortunately, the recognition of the widespread reliance on industrial volatile solvents and of their toxicity to humans and the environment has led to the development of Green Chemistry—a specific field of chemistry devoted to the development of less-toxic alternatives.[37]

It took comprehensive laboratory evaluation and persistent management of this case to bring about a successful outcome. Today, the patient is grateful and feels like a healthy, much younger man. He uses sauna regularly and is once again running the family business, but he no longer uses or is exposed to toxic compounds. He continues to reduce his lithium dose under careful supervision, and is planning to taper off the medication. He does not require any other medications.

A worldwide public health crisis associated with environmental toxin exposure appears imminent. Limiting the introduction and use of toxic or untested chemical compounds, and making available effective assessments and treatments is essential to the health and wellbeing of the planet and its inhabitants.

---

**Authors: Kara Fitzgerald, ND; Terry Pollock, MS**
**Case Clinician: Adrienne Sprouse, MD**

## References

1. Senate Committee on Environmental Quality. http://www.aroundthecapitol.com/billtrack/analysis.html?aid=36558. Accessed 11/08/2010, 2010.
2. Dick FD. Solvent neurotoxicity. *Occup Environ Med.* Mar 2006;63(3):221-226, 179.
3. EWG. Body Burden - The Pollution in Newborns. http://www.ewg.org/reports/bodyburden2/execsumm.php. Accessed 11/12/2010, 2010.
4. Ritter R, Scheringer M, Macleod M, Moeckel C, Jones KC, Hungerbuhler K. Intrinsic Human Elimination Half-Lives of Polychlorinated Biphenyls Derived from the Temporal Evolution of Cross-Sectional Biomonitoring Data from the UK Population. *Environ Health Perspect.* Oct 7 2010.
5. Crinnion WJ. Environmental medicine, part one: the human burden of environmental toxins and their common health effects. *Altern Med Rev.* Feb 2000;5(1):52-63.
6. Boas M, Frederiksen H, Feldt-Rasmussen U, et al. Childhood exposure to phthalates: associations with thyroid function, insulin-like growth factor I, and growth. *Environ Health Perspect.* Oct 2010;118(10):1458-1464.
7. NIH. Reducing Environmental Cancer Risk: What We Can Do Now. http://deainfo.nci.nih.gov/advisory/pcp/annualReports/pcp08-09rpt/PCP_Report_08-09_508.pdf. Accessed 11/11/2010, 2010.
8. Stein Y, Finkelstein Y, Levy-Nativ O, Bonne O, Aschner M, Richter ED. Exposure and susceptibility: schizophrenia in a young man following prolonged high exposures to organic solvents. *Neurotoxicology.* Sep 2010;31(5):603-607.
9. Fontham ET, Thun MJ, Ward E, et al. American Cancer Society perspectives on environmental factors and cancer. *CA Cancer J Clin.* Nov-Dec 2009;59(6):343-351.
10. Crinnion WJ. Environmental medicine, part 4: pesticides - biologically persistent and ubiquitous toxins. *Altern Med Rev.* Oct 2000;5(5):432-447.
11. Hyman MA. Environmental toxins, obesity, and diabetes: an emerging risk factor. *Altern Ther Health Med.* Mar-Apr;16(2):56-58.
12. ACAM. Heel Workshop - Toxic Exposure Related Chronic Musculoskeletal Conditions. http://www.acamnet.org/site/c.ltJWJ4MPIwE/b.6076139/k.8D02/HEEL_Workshop.htm. Accessed 11/12/2010, 2010.
13. Atkinson W, Sheldon TA, Shaath N, Whorwell PJ. Food elimination based on IgG antibodies in irritable bowel syndrome: a randomised controlled trial. *Gut.* Oct 2004;53(10):1459-1464.
14. Chad Z. Allergies in children. *Paediatr Child Health.* Oct 2001;6(8):555-566.
15. Rea W. Reduction of Chemical Sensitivity by Means of Heat Depuration, Physical Therapy and Nutritional Supplementation in a Controlled Environment. *Journal of Nutritional and Environmental Medicine.* 1996;6(2):141-148.
16. Krop J. Chemical Sensitivity After Intoxication at Work with Solvents: Response to Sauna Therapy. *Journal of Alternative and Complementary Medicine.* 1998;4(1):77-86.
17. Cecchini M, LoPresti V. Drug residues store in the body following cessation of use: impacts on neuroendocrine balance and behavior--use of the Hubbard sauna regimen to remove toxins and restore health. *Med Hypotheses.* 2007;68(4):868-879.
18. Johnston AM, Eagles JM. Lithium-associated clinical hypothyroidism. Prevalence and risk factors. *Br J Psychiatry.* Oct 1999;175:336-339.
19. CDC. n-Hexane. *Tox Profiles* [http://www.atsdr.cdc.gov/toxprofiles/tp113-c5.pdf. Accessed 11/11/2010, 2010.

20. Behind the Bean - The Heroes and Charlatans of the Natural and Organic Soy Foods Industry. http://www.cornucopia.org/soysurvey/OrganicSoyReport/behindthebean_color_final.pdf. Accessed 11/11/2010, 2010.

21. EPA. Toxicological Review of n-Hexane. http://www.epa.gov/IRIS/toxreviews/0486tr.pdf. Accessed 12/10/2010, 2010.

22. Gargas ML, Burgess RJ, Voisard DE, Cason GH, Andersen ME. Partition coefficients of low-molecular-weight volatile chemicals in various liquids and tissues. *Toxicol Appl Pharmacol.* Mar 15 1989;98(1):87-99.

23. Imbeault P, Chevrier J, Dewailly E, et al. Increase in plasma pollutant levels in response to weight loss in humans is related to in vitro subcutaneous adipocyte basal lipolysis. *Int J Obes Relat Metab Disord.* Nov 2001;25(11):1585-1591.

24. Kutlu G, Gomceli YB, Sonmez T, Inan LE. Peripheral neuropathy and visual evoked potential changes in workers exposed to n-hexane. *J Clin Neurosci.* Oct 2009;16(10):1296-1299.

25. ABC. Workers poisoned while making iPhones. http://www.abc.net.au/news/stories/2010/10/26/3048024.htm. Accessed 11/11/2010, 2010.

26. Bockelmann I, Pfister EA, Peters B, Duchstein S. Psychological effects of occupational exposure to organic solvent mixtures on printers. *Disabil Rehabil.* Jul 8 2004;26(13):798-807.

27. White RF, Proctor SP, Echeverria D, Schweikert J, Feldman RG. Neurobehavioral effects of acute and chronic mixed-solvent exposure in the screen printing industry. *Am J Ind Med.* Aug 1995;28(2):221-231.

28. Human aspects of solvent neurobehavioral effects. *Neurotoxicology.* Winter 1986;7(4):43-56.

29. INCHEM. n-Hexane. *International Programme on Chemical Safety* [http://www.inchem.org/documents/ehc/ehc/ehc122.htm. Accessed 11/11/2010, 2010.

30. Valavanidis A, Vlachogianni T, Fiotakis C. 8-hydroxy-2' -deoxyguanosine (8-OHdG): A critical biomarker of oxidative stress and carcinogenesis. *J Environ Sci Health C Environ Carcinog Ecotoxicol Rev.* Apr 2009;27(2):120-139.

31. Dundarz MR, Turkbay T, Akay C, et al. Antioxidant enzymes and lipid peroxidation in adolescents with inhalant abuse. *Turk J Pediatr.* Jan-Mar 2003;45(1):43-45.

32. Sajous L, Botta A, Sari-Minodier I. [Urinary 8-hydroxy-2'-deoxyguanosine: a biomarker of environmental oxidative stress?]. *Ann Biol Clin (Paris).* Jan-Feb 2008;66(1):19-29.

33. Pilger A, Rudiger HW. 8-Hydroxy-2'-deoxyguanosine as a marker of oxidative DNA damage related to occupational and environmental exposures. *Int Arch Occup Environ Health.* Oct 2006;80(1):1-15.

34. Abder-Rahman HA, Nusair S. 8-Hydroxy-2'-deoxyguanosine (8-OHdG) as a short-term predictor of regional and occupational health problems. *J Uoeh.* Sep 1 2007;29(3):247-258.

35. Loseva MI, Shpagina LA, Sharapov VI, Sazonova OV, Grek OR. [Fatty acids in erythrocyte membranes and the status of lipid peroxidation in painters]. *Gig Tr Prof Zabol.* 1991(2):19-21.

36. Miller JW, Ribaya-Mercado JD, Russell RM, et al. Effect of vitamin B-6 deficiency on fasting plasma homocysteine concentrations. *Am J Clin Nutr.* Jun 1992;55(6):1154-1160.

37. Anastas PT, Williamson TC, eds. *Green Chemistry: Designing Chemistry for the Environment.* Washington, DC: American Chemical Society; 1996; No. 626.

# Appendix A

## Introduction to the Functional Medicine Matrix

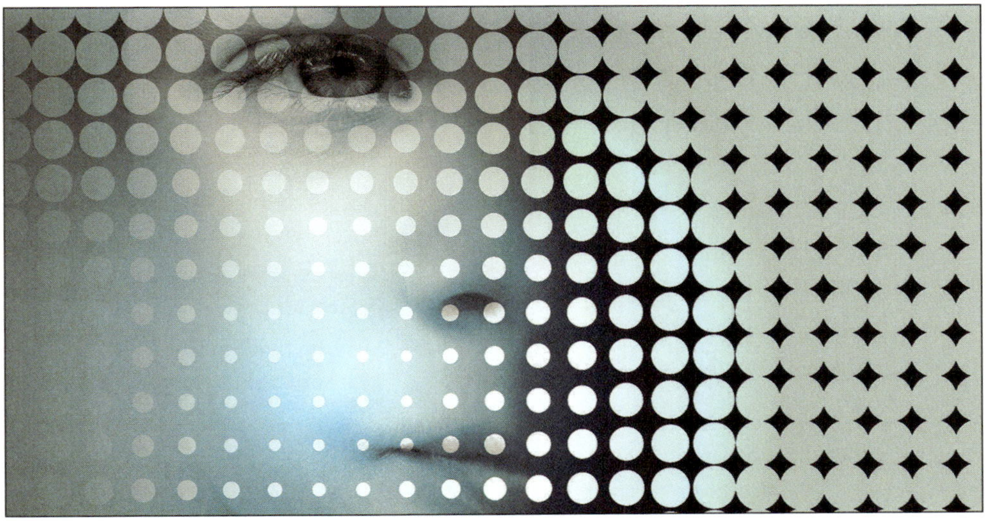

The goal of the functional medicine approach to patient care is to understand fully when, why and how the person became ill and then use that knowledge to restore health. Every health condition begins with dysfunction in one or more of the body's fundamental physiological systems (assimilation, defense and repair, energy, biotransformation/elimination, communications, and structure). Analyzing all the elements of the patient's story (including genetic, lifestyle, and environmental influences, as well as antecedents, triggers, and mediators), presenting signs and symptoms, and laboratory findings is done through a matrix focused on functionality in these basic organizing systems.

This process requires analytic thinking and a willingness on the part of the clinician to reflect deeply on underlying biochemistry and physiology. The foundational scientific principles of how the human organism functions—and how its systems communicate and interact—are essential to the process of linking ideas about multifactorial causation with the perceptible effects we call disease or dysfunction.

To assist clinicians in this process, The Institute for Functional Medicine has identified and organized a set of *core clinical imbalances* that are linked to the basic physiological processes. These serve to marry the mechanisms of disease with the manifestations and diagnoses of disease. Many common underlying pathways of disease are reflected in these clinical imbalances. The list below is not definitive, but some of the most common examples are provided.

Once imbalances have been identified, and the source clarified, interventions can directly address the underlying cause(s) of dysfunction. The Case-at-a-Glance files in this Appendix have been organized according to the functional medicine matrix in order to provide concrete examples of how to structure information and design therapy more effectively.

- Assimilation Imbalances
  - Digestion
  - Absorption
  - Microbiota/GI
  - Respiration
- Defense and Repair Imbalances
  - Immune system
  - Inflammatory processes
  - Infection and microbiota
- Energy Imbalances
  - Energy regulation
  - Mitochondrial function
- Biotransformation and Elimination Imbalances
  - Toxicity
  - Detoxification
- Communication Imbalances
  - Endocrine
  - Neurotransmitter
  - Immune messengers
  - Cognition
- Structural Integrity Imbalances
  - From the subcellular membranes to the musculoskeletal system
- Mental, Emotional, Spiritual
  - Cognitive function, perceptual patterns
  - Emotional regulation, grief, anger, sadness, etc
  - Meaning and purpose, relationship with something greater

For more information, please see www.functionalmedicine.org.

# Case at a Glance: Migraine and Depression

## History of Present Illness

BB presented at age 40 with a 20-year history of common migraine, depression, anxiety and fatigue. She experienced four to six migraines each week for which she took eletriptan hydrobromide and ibuprofen. They were worse at her menses, and triggered by jogging. She also experienced significant bloating and cramps with her menses. She used an etonogestrel/ethinyl estradiol vaginal ring for birth control, but reported that it did not alter her headache pattern. She also had mild environmental allergies. BB ate a standard American diet (SAD). Her physical exam was unremarkable. A standard battery of laboratory testing previously ordered included a complete blood count, comprehensive metabolic panel, and thyroid and iron studies; all results were within normal limits.

See Table A1 on following page.

**Table A1. Case at a Glance: Migraine and Depression Organized According to the Functional Medicine Matrix**

(Refer to full case presentation for details, including treatment rationale, case discussion, and references.)

| Clinical Assessment | Laboratory Results | Initial Recommended Treatment |
|---|---|---|
| | Defense and Repair (e.g., Immune, Inflammation, Infection/Microbiota) | |
| • Common migraine<br>• Food sensitivities<br>• Intestinal hyperpermeability<br>• Depression<br>• Anxiety<br>• Fatigue<br>• Hx of environmental allergies | • Multiple IgG4 food sensitivities<br>• Multiple low plasma amino acids | • Elimination/Rotation Diet: Eliminate all foods with IgG4 levels of +4 and +5 for one month. Foods with +1 to +3 reactions should be consumed no more often than twice per week. Reintroduction phase: after one month of avoidance, rotate IgG4 +4 and +5 foods into diet no more than twice per week.<br>• *Lactobacillus* and *Bifidobacterium* species 20 billion CFU: 1 capsule QD<br>• Glutamine: 5000 mg 1 tsp PO BID<br>• EPA/DHA: 1 capsule PO BID |
| | Communication (e.g., Endocrine, Neurotransmitters, Immune Messengers) | |
| • Common migraine<br>• Dysmenorrhea<br>• Depression<br>• Anxiety<br>• Fatigue | • Multiple low plasma amino acids<br>• Low 5-HIAA<br>• Low-normal urine HVA, VMA | • Custom amino acids (10 g per 1 tsp): Start with 0.25 tsp PO QAM and increase dose by 0.25 tsp until reaching 1.5 tsp QAM<br>• EPA/DHA: 1 capsule PO BID<br>• Women's specific multivitamin and mineral supplement taken as directed |
| | Fundamental Lifestyle Factors: Nutrient Imbalances | |
| • Migraine<br>• Dysmenorrhea<br>• Multiple amino acid insufficiencies | • Multiple low plasma amino acids | • Women's specific multivitamin and mineral supplement taken as directed |
| | Assimilation (e.g., Digestion, Absorption, Microbiota/GI, Respiration) | |
| • Intestinal hyperpermeability<br>• Maldigestion/ malabsorption | • Multiple IgG4 food sensitivities<br>• Multiple low plasma amino acids<br>• Multiple low plasma amino acids | • Elimination/Rotation Diet, probiotics, glutamine (described above)<br>• Custom amino acid powder (described above) |

# Three-Month Follow-up

BB reported feeling more energetic and happy. She found her mood to be much more even, without the big swings between anxiety and depression she experienced in the past. The frequency of migraine attacks was reduced to once per month, accompanying her menses. When she did experience one, it was reduced in intensity and didn't always require medication. She also reported some improvement in bloating and cramps during menses. Previously, she experienced migraine attacks "all the time" and took medication at least weekly.

She did continue to get occasional exertion-induced migraines during exercise, which required eletriptan. She admitted that the rotation diet (especially avoidance of eggs and dairy) was difficult, but it was a significant factor in minimizing migraine attacks, even those associated with her menstrual cycle and exercise. She believed that, if she could fully comply with the diet, she would reduce the incidence of migraines even further.

# Case at a Glance: ADHD

## History of Present Illness

LC presented at age 12 with attention deficit hyperactivity disorder (ADHD), dysgraphia, environmental allergies, asthma, insomnia, eczema, canker sores, migraine headaches, muscle cramps, stomach pain, nausea and diarrhea. LC was first diagnosed with ADHD at age 5. He repeated kindergarten because of attention and behavioral difficulties. He began methylphenidate (Ritalin®) in first grade and continued to take it through fourth grade, although his behavior did not change significantly. The drug was discontinued in fourth grade due to growth retardation. Off the medication, he gained weight and increased his intake of junk food and deli meats. He continued to have trouble focusing in school and was still disruptive. He had never received a positive teacher report. He had severe dysgraphia, but excelled in math. His medications included: cetirizine (Zyrtec®), albuterol, levalbuterol inhaler (Xopenex®), flunisolide (Nasarel or AeroBid®), cimetidine (Tagamet®), acetaminophen, and ibuprofen. He liked pasta, sweets, and ice cream despite the fact that he felt better avoiding dairy.

See Table A2 on following page.

## Six-Month Follow-up

LC's mother reported that he was free from his chronic symptoms for the first time in his life. His dysgraphia improved dramatically (see "Figure 6" on page 79 in full case presentation). He no longer required his medications, including antihistamines (cetirizine and cimetidine), bronchodilators, steroid inhaler, acetaminophen, and ibuprofen. His mood and behavior stabilized, and his ability to focus improved greatly. His hyperactivity symptoms, including disruptiveness, irritability, and anxiety, were gone. His hives, asthma, runny nose and postnasal drip, anal itching, stomachaches, nausea, diarrhea, headaches, muscle cramps, and sensitivity to loud noises were all completely resolved. He slept soundly at night. He was doing well in school, academically and socially (see mother's comments in full case presentation). LC tolerated supplements and dietary changes well, because he felt so much better when he followed the plan.

**Table A2. Case at a Glance: ADHD Organized According to the Functional Medicine Matrix**

(Refer to full case presentation for details, including treatment rationale, case discussion, and references.)

| Clinical Assessment | Laboratory Results | Initial Recommended Treatment |
|---|---|---|
| | Fundamental Lifestyle Factors: Nutrient Imbalances | |
| • Nutrient deficiencies<br>• Fatty acid imbalance<br>• Anxiety<br>• Muscle spasms<br>• Audio sensitivity<br>• Hyperkeratosis pilaris | • Low essential minerals<br>• Low vitamins A, E, beta carotene<br>• Elevated AA/EPA ratio<br>• Low $B_6$ (organic acid markers)<br>• Elevated saturated and trans fatty acids | • Zinc citrate<br>• Magnesium glycinate<br>• Multivitamin/mineral<br>• EPA/DHA<br>• Pyridoxal 5′ phosphate<br>• Dietary changes as noted below |
| | Defense and Repair (e.g., Immune, Inflammation, Infection/Microbiota) | |
| • Hypovitaminosis D<br>• Food sensitivities<br>• Intestinal hyperpermeability<br>• ADHD<br>• Asthma, allergies, headache, hives, sinusitis<br>• Atopic dermatitis<br>• Aphthous stomatitis | • Low serum vitamin D<br>• Multiple + IgG food sensitivities<br>• Elevated IgG antigliadin antibodies | • Vitamin $D_3$<br>• Dietary changes: Modified elimination diet based on test results. No dairy, peanuts, gluten, sugar, or trans fatty acids. Reduce saturated fat intake. Whole foods, minimally processed, organic diet. (Nutritionist comments available in full case presentation.) |
| | Assimilation (e.g., Digestion, Absorption, Microbiota/GI, Respiration) | |
| • Yeast overgrowth<br>• GERD, IBS, Pruritus ani<br>• Nausea | • Elevated lymphocyte/ neutrophil ratio<br>• +IgG food sensitivities, IgG antigliadin antibodies | • Fluconazole<br>• Broad spectrum probiotics |
| | Biotransformation & Elimination (e.g., Toxicity, Detoxification) | |
| • Mild lead toxicity<br>• ADHD<br>• Food additives | • Elevated 6-hour urine lead after 250 mg DMPS (2,3-dimercapto-1-propane-sulphonic acid) provocation | • After 2 months on treatment protocol: Start DMSA (refer to full case presentation for details)<br>• Dietary changes as noted above |
| | Communication (e.g., Endocrine, Neurotransmitters, Immune Messengers) | |
| • ADHD, Dysgraphia<br>• Insomnia | • Low-normal plasma tryptophan<br>• Low-normal urine HVA, 5-HIAA | • 5-HTP 50–100 mg QHS as needed for sleep |

# Case at a Glance: Psoriatic Arthritis

## History of Present Illness

MP was 56 years old when he presented to the clinic with psoriatic arthritis. Over the previous year, his symptoms had progressively worsened, with increased pain, decreased range of motion, and swelling in his feet, ankles, hands and knees. He walked with a limp and had difficulty climbing stairs. His left shoulder was also frequently painful. He was taking etodolac (Lodine®), methotrexate, and adalimumab (Humira®), which did not adequately control his symptoms. He maintained a highly demanding career as a university professor and researcher. He drank alcohol and caffeinated beverages regularly. He meditated 15 minutes each morning. He had a positive family history for rheumatoid arthritis, sero-negative inflammatory arthritis, schizophrenia and inflammatory bowel disease.

See Table A3 on following page.

## Five-Month Follow-up

MP was markedly improved, stating that he hadn't felt so good in years. He reported an 80% reduction in overall pain, with improved mobility and decreased swelling. He was able to walk upstairs and his limp was gone. Morning pain and stiffness were gone. He had not used adalimumab (Humira) for two months and reduced methotrexate from 15 to 5 mg per week. He was following the dietary recommendations and taking the supplements. He eliminated caffeine and reduced alcohol intake considerably.

Reflux and migraines were gone. His mood improved, and he was less irritable. He lost weight. He was no longer constipated. He was still under a great deal of stress, working 80 hours a week, but meditation continued to be helpful.

NOTES

**Table A3. Abbreviated Assessments, Laboratory Findings and Treatments Organized According to the Functional Medicine Matrix**

(Refer to full case presentation for details, including treatment rationale, case discussion, and references.)

| Clinical Assessment | Laboratory Results | Initial Recommended Treatment |
|---|---|---|
| | Defense and Repair (e.g., Immune, Inflammation, Infection/Microbiota) | |
| • Gluten sensitivity<br>• Intestinal hyperpermeability<br>• Multiple IgG food sensitivities<br>• Hypovitaminosis D<br>• Psoriatic arthritis, nails, skin<br>• Blepharitis, aphthous stomatitis<br>• FMH: autoimmunity | • + celiac gene (*HLA DQ2*)<br>• +IgG to 27 foods<br>• Low vitamin D and magnesium<br>• Elevated arachidonic acid and lipid peroxides | • Anti-inflammatory medicinal food<br>• EPA/DHA<br>• Vitamin $D_3$<br>• Dietary changes: Gluten and dairy free. Avoid yeast and eggs. Eat whole, low glycemic foods, good fats & protein. D/C alcohol, caffeine, sugar. |
| | Communication (e.g., Endocrine, Neurotransmitters, Immune Messengers) | |
| • Metabolic syndrome<br>• Suspected fatty liver<br>• Subclinical hypothyroidism<br>• Migraine headaches<br>• FMH: HD, DM, HTN, psychiatric disorders | • Elevated triglycerides, FBS, insulin, cholesterol<br>• Low-normal HDL<br>• Elevated ALT<br>• High normal TSH | • Methyl donors ($B_{12}$, folic acid, and $B_6$)<br>• Amino acids (taurine, glycine, N-acetyl-cysteine, methionine)<br>• High-dose multivitamin and mineral without iron<br>• Dietary changes as noted above |
| | Assimilation (e.g., Digestion, Absorption, Microbiota/GI, Respiration) | |
| • GERD<br>• Chronic constipation<br>• GI yeast overgrowth<br>• Family history IBD | • DNA stool analysis:<br>• +3 Candida sp. | • 450 billion CFU probiotic<br>• Fluconazole 100 mg: 1 tab QD × 30 days |
| | Biotransformation & Elimination (e.g., Toxicity, Detoxification) | |
| • Mercury toxicity (multiple amalgams) | • Negative whole blood toxic metals<br>• Urine toxic metals | • Methyl donors ($B_{12}$, folic acid, and $B_6$)<br>• Amino acids as noted above<br>• High-dose multivitamin and mineral without iron |
| | Mental/Emotional/Spiritual | |
| • High-stress work life<br>• Depression<br>• Family history of psychiatric illness | • Low serum vitamin D<br>• Elevated arachidonic acid<br>• High-normal TSH<br>• Low-normal free T3 and free T4 | • Continue daily meditation practice<br>• Vitamin $D_3$ 5000 IU<br>• EPA/DHA<br>• Dietary changes as noted above<br>• Methyl donors ($B_{12}$, folic acid, and $B_6$)<br>• Amino acids as noted above<br>• High-dose multivitamin and mineral without iron |

# Case at a Glance: Volatile Solvent-Induced Neurotoxicity

## History of Present Illness

RS was 43 years old when he presented with a history of progressive memory impairment and diagnosis of a three-year-long bipolar disorder. The bipolar presentation consisted of hypomania with severe insomnia. He took lithium and clonazepam for the bipolar disorder and diphenhydramine for insomnia. All were reported to be of limited benefit. RS was dependent on his wife for memory support, including for his own medical history. RS's wife thought there had been a steady decline in his mental function over many years. The bipolar diagnosis seemed to be an extension of the mental decline, rather than a cause of it. Previously, he was a generally happy, hardworking individual. RS had been unable to work for six months. He had been an executive in his family's fabric printing business for over 10 years, but had been experiencing hallucination and mania at work. His wife noted that historically his symptoms improved when he was away from the business for a period of time, although in the recent past these improvements were less apparent. He was chronically exposed to many chemicals, including solvents, pigments, and dyes. There was no family history of neurodegenerative or psychiatric conditions, including memory loss, dementia, or bipolar disorder. RS ate a standard American diet. He did not consume alcohol, use tobacco, or engage in recreational drug use. He took fish oil, vitamins C, E, B complex, $B_{12}$, garlic, and essential minerals. His medical history included chronic sinusitis, hypothyroidism (treated with levothyroxine), and onychomycosis. He reported no known drug, food, or environmental allergies. Extensive previous medical evaluations were unremarkable. Apart from the noted memory deficits, RS's physical exam was unremarkable.

See Table A4 on following page.

## Eight-Month Follow-up

RS was well enough to resume working. He felt happy, and his memory was restored. He did not feel excessively angry or aggressive. He was able to tolerate the work environment (which had been cleaned up considerably) without a recurrence of symptoms. His lithium was reduced and his clonazepam was stopped, as he no longer required it. (Lithium is known to induce hypothyroidism. It was hoped that reduction in his dosage might improve his thyroid function.[18]) Insomnia continued to be an occasional issue. Overall, he showed remarkable improvement. He and his family were very pleased and grateful for his recovery. Melatonin 3 mg/QHS was added to his treatment plan; no other changes were made.

**Laboratory follow-up revealed nontoxic levels of volatile solvents.**

## Table A4. Case at a Glance: Volatile Solvent-Induced Neurotoxicity Organized According to the Functional Medicine Matrix

(Refer to full case presentation for details, including treatment rationale, case discussion, and references.)

| Clinical Assessment | Laboratory Results | Initial Recommended Treatment |
|---|---|---|
| | **Biotransformation & Elimination** (e.g., Toxicity, Detoxification) | |
| • Volatile solvent-induced neurotoxicity<br>• Bipolar disorder<br>• Oxidative stress | • Significantly elevated volatile solvents: hexane, 2-methylpentane, and 3-methylpentane<br>• Elevated oxidative stress markers 8OH-2'dG and lipid peroxides | • Avoidance of highly polluted areas, including work environment<br>• Installation of home air filtration system and water filter<br>• Comprehensive plan for work environment to be implemented prior to returning: reduce reliance on toxic chemicals, evaluate alternative options, install factory-wide exhaust and air filtration systems.<br>• Sauna therapy, 2 sessions per week (A non-toxic, glue-free, aged-wood sauna was used.)<br>• Filtered water intake: ½ body weight in ounces per day<br>• Preservative-free intravenous nutrient protocol (administered 2 X per week) for 12 sessions: IV Ingredients: glutathione, 600 mg; taurine, 2 gm; ascorbic acid 12.5 gm; B complex vitamins, 50 mg each of $B_1$, $B_2$, $B_3$, $B_5$, and $B_6$; magnesium sulfate, 5 gm; and 2 cc of a trace minerals solution containing 8 µg Cr, 0.2 mg Mn, 40 µg Se, 0.8 mg Cu, and 2 mg Zn with sodium bicarbonate to neutralize the low pH of ascorbic acid. |
| | **Defense and Repair** (e.g., Immune, Inflammation, Infection/Microbiota) | |
| • Multiple food allergies<br>• Chronic sinusitis<br>• Onychomycosis | • Intradermal food allergy testing (IFAT) positive for multiple foods | • Organic hypoallergenic rotation diet based on intradermal testing (avoid milk, egg, wheat, corn, tomato and potato)<br>• Filtered water intake: as above |
| | **Energy** (e.g., Energy Regulation, Mitochondrial Function) | |
| • Oxidative stress | • Elevated 8OH-2'dG<br>• Elevated lipid peroxides | • Preservative-free intravenous nutrient protocol (see above); continue at-home supplement protocol |
| | **Communication** (e.g., Endocrine, Neurotransmitters, Immune Messengers) | |
| • Hypothyroidism<br>• Bipolar disorder<br>• Insomnia | • Previously diagnosed | • Levothyroxine<br>• Lithium, clonazepam<br>• Diphenhydramine (changed to melatonin at 8 month F/U) |
| | **Fundamental Lifestyle Factors: Nutrient Imbalances** | |
| • Nutrient deficiencies | • Low $B_6$ (organic acid marker)<br>• Low plasma amino acids | • Preservative-free intravenous nutrient protocol (see above); continue at-home supplement protocol |

# Appendix B

## Table B1. Select Laboratory Imbalances and Clinical Conditions

| Clinical Conditions | Underlying Imbalances: IgG, IgE, IgA Food-Specific Antibodies* | GI Microbial Imbalance** | GI Inflammation Patterns*** | Organic Acid Imbalances | Oxidative stress | Fatty Acid Imbalances | Amino Acid Imbalances | Genetic | Metallo- or Organotoxicity | Nutrient Imbalances: Vitamins | Nutrient Imbalances: Essential Elements | Other Significant Laboratory Tests |
|---|---|---|---|---|---|---|---|---|---|---|---|---|
| Adrenal Fatigue | | | | | | | | | | | | X- salivary cortisol, TSH, insulin |
| Amyotrophic Lateral Sclerosis | | | | | | X | | | | | | |
| Atopic Dermatitis | X | | X | | | | | | | | | X- serum IgA deficiency |
| Attention Deficit Hyperactivity Disorder | X | X | X | X- NT | | X | | | X- lead | X | X | X-CBC |
| Chronic Asthma | | | | | X | X | | | | | | |
| Depression and Sarcoidosis | | | | X- NT, QUIN | | | X | | | | | |
| Hemochromatosis | | | | | | | | X | X- multiple toxic metals | | X- Fe overload | |
| Idiopathic Gastrointestinal Pain | X | X | X | | X | | | | | | | |
| Migraine Headaches and Depression | X | | | X- NT | | | X | | | | | |
| Mitochondrial Disease | | X | | X- MITO | | | | X | | | | |
| Neurologic Effects of Lead Toxicity | | | | | | | | | X- lead | | | |
| Paroxysmal Supraventricular Tachycardia | | | | | | | X | | | | X | |
| Pervasive Developmental Disorder | X | X | X | X- MITO, BV, S | X | X | | X | X | X | X | X- urine polypeptides |
| Psoriatic Arthritis | X | X | X | | | X | X | X | | X | X | X- metabolic, thyroid |
| Resistant Hypertension | | | | X- QUIN | X | | | | | X | X | X- ADMA; hsCRP |
| Rheumatoid Arthritis and Osteoporosis | X | X | X | X- MITO, QUIN, S, NT | X | X | X | | | X | X | X- autoimmune, thyroid, bone resporption, hsCRP |
| Statin-Induced Myopathy | | | | X- MITO | | | | | | X | | |
| Type 2 Diabetes Mellitus | | | | X- MITO, BV | X | X | | | | X | X | X- metabolic, lipids, thyroid |
| Ulcerative Colitis | X | X | X | | | | | | | | | |
| Volatile Solvent Neurotoxicity | X-IFAT | | | x- BV | X | | X | | X- volatile solvents | | | |

*See following page for Table B1 legend and additional details...*

Varied clinical conditions can present with shared underlying etiopathogenic factors, as this table illustrates. Conversely, close inspection of the laboratory data and clinical history suggests that similar clinical conditions may present with different underlying imbalances, such as the two autoimmune and depression cases. Note that a blank category in the table does not rule out a positive finding. Check the case study to confirm which tests were used. This table may be useful as a tool for testing considerations for a given condition.

| Abbreviations used in Table B1 | |
|---|---|
| MITO | Mitochondrial markers |
| BV | B vitamin markers |
| NT | Neurotransmitter markers |
| QUIN | Quinolinate |
| 5-HIAA | 5-hydroxyindoleacetate |
| Fe | Iron |
| IFAT | Intradermal food allergy testing |
| ADMA | Asymmetric dimethylarginine |
| hsCRP | High sensitivity C-reactive protein |
| TSH | Thyroid stimulating hormone |
| S | Sulfur |
| CBC | Complete blood count |

* Including anti-gliadin antibodies
** Fungal, bacterial or parasitic
*** Including intestinal hyperpermeability, IgA abnormalities, lactoferrin elevation

# Appendix C

## Web-based Medical and Scientific Resources

### Integrative and Functional Medicine Organizations

- American Academy of Anti-Aging Medicine (A4M) • www.worldhealth.net
- Autism Research Institute (Defeat Autism Now – DAN!) • www.autism.com
- Metametrix Institute • www.metametrixinstitute.org
  - Educational resources on laboratory science, including blogs, books and seminars
  - Additional books published by Metametrix Institute:
    - *Metametrix Handbook: Clinical Reference Manual.* Lord RS, Bralley JA, Fitzgerald K, eds. 2nd ed. Duluth, GA: Metametrix Institute; 2010.
    - *Laboratory Evaluations for Integrative and Functional Medicine.* Lord RS, Bralley JA, eds. 2nd ed. Duluth, GA: Metametrix Institute; 2008.
- Metametrix Clinical Laboratory • www.metametrix.com
  - The Learning Center contains educational resources including articles, books, presentations and case studies related to laboratory science.
- National Center for Complementary and Alternative Medicine • nccam.nih.gov
- The American Academy of Environmental Medicine • www.aaemonline.org
- The American Association of Naturopathic Physicians • www.naturopathic.org
- The American College for the Advancement of Medicine • www.acam.org
- The Institute for Functional Medicine • www.functionalmedicine.org
- The Institute of Women's Health & Integrative Medicine • www.instituteofwomenshealth.com

### Science Resources

- PubMed – National Library of Medicine • www.ncbi.nlm.nih.gov/pubmed
- The Centers for Disease Control and Prevention • www.cdc.gov
- Dr. Bruce Ames • www.bruceames.org

## Medical Resources

- Epocrates Online • www.epocrates.com/products/online/
- MD consult • www.mdconsult.com
- Medscape • www.emedicine.medscape.com
- Merck Manual • www.merckmanuals.com
- Natural Standard • www.naturalstandard.com
  - Subscription: Evidenced-based information on complementary and alternative medicine
- WebMD • www.webmd.com

## Nutrition Resources

- American Clinical Board of Nutrition • www.acbn.org
- Celiac.com • www.celiac.com
- Linus Pauling Institute • lpi.oregonstate.edu
- NIH Office of Dietary Supplements • ods.od.nih.gov
- USDA Nutrient Database • www.nal.usda.gov/fnic/foodcomp/search/

## Toxicity Resources

- Environmental Working Group • www.ewg.org
- EPA Mercury Fish Advisory • www.epa.gov/hg/advisories.htm
- Everyday Exposures • www.everydayexposures.com/

## Botanical Medicine Resources

- American Botanical Council Herbal Information • abc.herbalgram.org
- Dr. Duke's Phytochemical and Ethnobotanical Databases • www.ars-grin.gov/duke/
- Medherb • www.medherb.com

## Nutritional Biochemistry and Metabolic Pathways

- ExPASy Proteomics Server • www.expasy.ch/enzyme/
- Unipathway • www.grenoble.prabi.fr/obiwarehouse/unipathway
- The Medical Biochemistry Page • themedicalbiochemistrypage.org/
- Citric Acid Cycle Pathway • www.metametrix.com/learning-center/metabolic-pathways/2009/citric-acid-cycle

# Appendix D

## Select Supplement Companies

### Allergy Research Group

2300 N. Loop Road
Alameda, CA 94502

Tel: 510.263.2000
Fax: 510.263.2100
Email: info@allergyresearchgroup.com
Web site: www.allergyresearchgroup.com

### Apex Energetics

16592 Hale Ave.
Irvine, CA 92606

Tel: 949.251.0152
Fax: 949.251.0153
Email: info@apexenergetics.com
Website: www.apexenergetics.com

### Biocodex

1250 Bayhill Drive, Suite 315
San Bruno, CA 94066

Tel: 650.243.5320
Fax: 650.589.1196
Website: www.biocodexusa.com

### Biotics Research Corporation

6801 Biotics Research Dr
Rosenberg, TX 77471

Toll-Free: 800.231.5777
Tel: 281.344.0909
Fax: 281.344.0725
Website: www.bioticsresearch.com

### Cardiovascular Research/ Ecological Formulas

1061 Shary Circle
Concord, CA 94518-2407

Tel: 925.827.2636
Toll-Free: 800.888.4585
Website: www.ecologicalformulas.net

### Custom Probiotics

2947 Honolulu Ave. Unit B
Glendale, CA 91214

Tel: 818.248.3529
Toll-Free: 800.219.8405
Fax: 818.248.6343
Email: info@customprobiotics.com
Website: www.customprobiotics.net

### Designs for Health

Designs for Health Corporate Offices
2 North Road
East Windsor, CT 06088

800-FOR-HEALTH (800.367.4325)
Email: info@designsforhealth.com
Website: www.designsforhealth.com

*Continued on following pages...*

## Douglas Laboratories

600 Boyce Road
Pittsburgh, PA 15205

Tel: 412.494.0122
Toll-Free: 800.245.4440
Website: www.douglaslabs.com

## Herb Pharm

P.O. Box 116
Williams, OR 97544

Tel: 800.348.4372
Fax: 800.545.7392
Email: info@herb-pharm.com
Website: www.herb-pharm.com

## Integrative Therapeutics, Inc.

825 Challenger Drive
Green Bay, WI 54311

Tel: 800.931.1709
Fax: 800.380.8189
Email: info@integrativeinc.com
Web site: www.integrativeinc.com

## J R Carlson

15 College Drive
Arlington Heights, IL 60004-1985

Tel: 827.255.1600
Toll-Free: 888.234.5656
Fax: 847.255.1605
Website: www.carlsonlabs.com

## Kirkman Laboratories

6400 SW Rosewood Street
Lake Oswego, OR 97035

Tel: 503.694.1600
Toll-Free: 800.245.8282
Fax: 503.682.0838
Email: sales@kirkmanlabs.com
Website: www.kirkmanlabs.com

## Klaire Laboratories

(Division of ProThera – see following page)

## Life Extension

1100 W. Commercial Blvd
Fort Lauderdale, FL 33309

Tel: 800.678.8989
Website: www.lifeextension.com

## Metabolic Maintenance

Metabolic Maintenance Products
68994 N. Pine St
PO Box 940
Sisters OR 97759

800.772.7873 or 541.549.7800
FAX: 541.549.3299
Email: info@metabolicmaintenance.com
Website: www.metabolicmaintenance.com

## Metagenics

100 Avenida La Pata
San Clemente, CA 92673

Tel: 949.366.0818
Toll-Free: 800.692.9400

9770 44th Ave N.W. Suite 100
Gig Harbor, WA 98332

Toll-Free: 800.843.9660
Website: www.metagenics.com

## Nordic Naturals

94 Hangar Way
Watsonville, CA 95076

Tel: 831.724.6200 x1
Toll-Free: 800.662.2544 x1
Fax: 831.724.5263
Email: prosales@nordicnaturals.com
Website: www.nordicnaturals.com

## Ortho Molecular Products

1991 Duncan Place
Woodstock, IL 60098

Tel: 815.337.0089
Fax: 800.476.4664
Website: www.orthomolecularproducts.com

## Phytopharmica

825 Challenger Drive
Green Bay, WI 54311

Tel: 800.553.2370
Fax: 920.469.4444
Website: www.phytostore.com

## ProThera

10439 Double R Blvd
Reno, NV 89521

Toll-Free: 888.488.2488
Tel: 775.850.8800
Fax: 775.850.8810
Website: www.protherainc.com

## Pure Encapsulations

490 Boston Post Road
Sudbury, MA 01776

Toll-Free: 800.753.2277
Fax: 888.783.2277
Website: www.purecaps.com

## Thorne

25820 Hwy 2 West
Sandpoint, ID 83864

Tel: 800.228.1966
Fax: 800.747.1950
Email: info@thorne.com
Website:www.thorne.com

## Vital Nutrients

45 Kenneth Dooley Dr.
Middletown CT 06457

Tel: 888.328.9992
Fax: 860.638.3651
Website:www.vitalnutrients.net

## Vitanica

P.O. BOX 1299
Tualatin, OR 97062

Tel: 503.692.5085
Toll-Free: 800.572.4712
Fax: 503.692.5685
Email: inquiries@vitanica.com
Website: www.vitanica.com

## VSL

9841 Washingtonian Blvd., Ste. 500
Gaithersburg, MD 20878-7352

Tel: 301.948.1041
Fax: 301.948.1862
Website: www.vsl3.com

## Wise Woman Herbals

P.O. Box 279
Creswell, OR 97426

Tel: 800.532.5219
Fax: 800.476.6518
Email: info@wisewomanherbals.com
Web site: www.wisewomanherbals.com

## Xymogen

725 S. Kirkman Road
Orlando, FL 32811

Tel: 800.647.6100
Website: www.xymogen.com

# Select Compounding Pharmacies

## College Compounding Pharmacy

3505 Austin Bluffs Parkway
Colorado Springs, CO 80918

Tel: 800.888.9358 or 719.262.0022
Fax: 800.556.5893 or 719.262.0035
Patient Email:
inforequest@collegepharmacy.com
Practitioner Email:
info@collegepharmacy.com
Website: www.collegepharmacy.com

## Wellness Compounding Pharmacy

3401 Independence Drive
Suite 231
Birmingham, AL 35209

Toll Free: 800.227.2627
Fax: 205.871.2568 or 800.369.0302
Email: info@wellnesshealth.com
Website: www.wellnesshealth.com

# Select Distribution Companies

## Emerson Ecologics

7 Commerce Drive
Bedford, NH 03110

Tel: 800.654.4432
Fax: 800.718.7238
Email: cs@emersonecologics.com
Web site: www.emersonecologics.com

## Natural Standard

One Davis Square
Somerville, MA 02144

Tel: 617.591.3300
Fax: 617.591.3399
Email: questions@naturalstandard.com
Website: http://naturalstandard.com

# Quality Assurance Analysis of Nutritional Products

## ConsumerLab.com

333 Mamaroneck Avenue
White Plains, NY 10605

Tel: 914.722.9149
Toll Free: 888.502.5100
Email: info@consumerlab.com
Website: www.consumerlab.com